Prediction and Change
of Health Behavior

Applying the Reasoned Action Approach

Prediction and Change of Health Behavior

Applying the Reasoned Action Approach

EDITED BY

Icek Ajzen
University of Massachusetts, Amherst

Dolores Albarracín
University of Florida

Robert Hornik
University of Pennsylvania

LEA LAWRENCE ERLBAUM ASSOCIATES, PUBLISHERS
2007   Mahwah, New Jersey   London

Senior Acquisitions Editor: Debra Riegert
Editorial Assistant: Rebecca Larsen
Cover Design: Tomai Maridou
Full-Service Compositor: MidAtlantic Books and Journals, Inc.

Lawrence Erlbaum Associates, Inc., Publishers
10 Industrial Avenue
Mahwah, New Jersey 07430
www.erlbaum.com

**CIP information for this volume can be obtained by contacting the
Library of Congress.**

ISBN 978–0–8058–5926–3 — 0–8058–5926–8 (case)
ISBN 978–0–8058–6282–9 — 0–8058–6282–X (paper)
ISBN 978–1–4106–1677–7 — 1–4106–1677–0 (e-book)

Books published by Lawrence Erlbaum Associates are printed on
acid-free paper, and their bindings are chosen for strength and durability.

Printed in the United States of America

10 9 8 7 6 5 4 3 2 1

This book is dedicated to Martin Fishbein, our teacher, colleague, and friend

> —who taught his students to think
> —his colleagues to think straight
> —social psychologists to think like him
> —his detractors to think again
> —administrators to think big
> —his wife Debby to think for him
> —his friends to think the world of him, and
> —commercial sex workers to think "condoms"

Contents

Preface

This book is based on a symposium held in honor of Martin Fishbein's 70th birthday in March 2006 at the Annenberg School for Communication, University of Pennsylvania. The book's chapters are organized around two broad themes that reflect Marty's major research interests: *Attitudes and Behavior* and *Health Promotion*. Marty first started to work on a theory of attitudes while pursuing his dissertation research at UCLA. This theory, later to be called the expectancy-value model, has become the dominant conceptual framework for thinking about attitude formation and change. After receiving his PhD in 1961, he accepted a position in Social Psychology and Communication at the University of Illinois in Urbana-Champaign. It was at Illinois that Marty pursued, in collaboration with Icek Ajzen, his landmark work on the nature of attitudes and their relation to behavior, culminating in what became known as the theory of reasoned action. It is fair to say that this theory has had a profound impact not only on basic attitude research but also on the application of social psychology to the solution of social problems. Indeed, from the outset, Marty was not content with knowledge for its own sake; he wanted to use his work to understand behavior in real-world settings. In the 1970s, these efforts were focused primarily on voting choice and consumer behavior, but in the 1980s, his interests shifted to the health domain. In 1988–89 he served as a consultant for NIMH on AIDS research and in 1992 he took an extended leave from the University of Illinois to go to the Centers for Disease Control in Atlanta where he joined in the effort to deal with behavioral aspects of the AIDS epidemic. Marty did not return to Illinois but instead, in 1997, accepted the Harry C. Coles Distinguished Professorship at the Annenberg School for Communication where he has continued his basic research on attitudes and his applied work as Director of the Health Communication Area of the Annenberg Public Policy Center.

The collection of papers and commentaries in this book illustrates the breadth and depth of the reasoned action approach pioneered by Martin Fishbein. The first part is devoted largely to theoretical issues surrounding the reasoned action approach while the second part deals with applications of this approach in the health domain. In the opening chapter, Ajzen and Albarracín provide an overview of the reasoned action approach with emphasis on the theories of reasoned action and planned behavior, followed by a discussion of intervention research in the framework of this approach. Subsequent chapters in the first part address a number of conceptual issues related to the reasoned action approach: The problem of measurement correspondence, the logic of the double negative in behavioral beliefs and outcome evaluations, and the contributions of attitudes and subjective norms to the prediction of intentions (Trafimow); the role of emotions in a reasoned action approach (Cappella); how to deal with the prediction of classes of behaviors as opposed to single actions (Hornik); and the role of implicit versus explicit attitudes in the prediction of behavior (Jaccard and Blanton). The final two papers in this section are commentaries by Triandis and by Ottati and Krumdick.

The book's second part opens with a chapter that examines the moderating effect of perceived behavioral control on the intention-behavior relation (Yzer), followed by several chapters dealing with issues related to the application of a reasoned action approach to behavioral interventions: a general discussion of considerations related to the selection of a behavioral criterion (Middlestadt); an application of reasoned action theory to understanding risky sexual behavior in rural Zimbabwe (Kasprzyk and Montaño); and insights derived from the theory for predicting HIV transmission risks among people infected with HIV (Wolitski and Zhang). These chapters are discussed in commentaries by Sherr and by Gorn.

The final section features a chapter by Rietmeijer on using a reasoned action approach to AIDS prevention by means of serosorting; a chapter by Pick who reports on her experiences trying to apply this approach in a marginalized population of Latin American women; and a chapter by Jemmott and Jemmott describing research in which reasoned action theory was used to design and evaluate AIDS risk reduction interventions. Commentaries on these chapters are provided by Kalichman and by Holtgrave. In the book's final chapter, Martin Fishbein reflects on the different contributions and his own work within the reasoned action approach.

Any student of human social behavior will find a wealth of information in this volume. Those unfamiliar with the reasoned action approach are provided with a general introduction and discussion of outstanding issues. But this book is perhaps of greatest interest to graduate students and practitioners interested in understanding and modifying human behavior by relying on a reasoned action approach. With its many illustrations of applications in the health domain, it will be especially valuable to public health practitioners, nurses, and other health professionals as well as social and clinical psychologists interested in health psychology.

We would like to acknowledge the generous support of the symposium provided by the Annenberg School for Communication and by the Annenberg Public Policy Center. These contributions helped bring together a group of researchers—some of Marty's former students and post-docs and well as present collaborators and colleagues—dedicated to advancing the reasoned action approach in their own work. We hope that the collection of chapters in this book serves to illustrate the achievements and promise of the reasoned action approach.

Icek Ajzen
Dolores Albarracín
Robert Hornik

Contributors

Icek Ajzen, Department of Psychology, University of Massachusetts, Amherst.

Dolores Albarracín, Department of Psychology, University of Florida.

Hart Blanton, Department of Psychology, Texas A&M University.

Joseph N. Cappella, Annenberg School for Communication, University of Pennsylvania.

Martin Fishbein, Annenberg School for Communication, University of Pennsylvania.

Gerald Gorn, Department of Marketing, Hong Kong University of Science & Technology, China.

David Holtgrave, Department of Health, Behavior & Society, Johns Hopkins University.

Emily Hopkins, Denver Health, Department of Preventive Medicine and Biometrics, Denver, CO.

Robert Hornik, Annenberg School for Communication, University of Pennsylvania.

James Jaccard, Department of Psychology, Florida International University.

John B. Jemmott, Annenberg School for Communication, University of Pennsylvania.

Loretta Sweet Jemmott, School of Nursing, University of Pennsylvania.

Seth C. Kalichman, Department of Psychology, University of Connecticut.

Danka Kasprzyk, Battelle Seattle Research Center, Seattle, WA 98109.

Nathaniel D. Krumdick, Department of Psychology, Loyola University.

Susan E. Middlestadt, Department of Applied Health Science, Indiana University.

Daniel Montaño, Battelle Seattle Research Center, Seattle, WA 98109.

Victor Ottati, Department of Psychology, Loyola University.

Susan Pick, IMIFAP, Col. Insurgentes Mixcoac, Mexico City, Mexico.

Cornelis A. Rietmeijer, Denver Health, Department of Preventive Medicine and Biometrics, Denver, CO.

Lorraine Sherr, Department of Primary Care and Population Science, University College, London, United Kingdom.

David Trafimow, Department of Psychology, New Mexico State University.

Harry Triandis, Department of Psychology, University of Illinois.

Richard Wolitski, Centers for Disease Control, Division of HIV/AIDS Prevention, Atlanta, GA.

Marco Yzer, School of Journalism and Mass Communication, University of Minnesota.

Jun Zhang, Centers for Disease Control, Division of HIV/AIDS Prevention, Atlanta, GA.

Prediction and Change of Health Behavior

Applying the Reasoned Action Approach

PART 1

Attitudes and Behavior

CHAPTER 1

Predicting and Changing Behavior: A Reasoned Action Approach

Icek Ajzen

University of Massachusetts

Dolores Albarracín

University of Florida

If you were told of a miraculous potion that could prevent all manner of illness—from cancer to cardiovascular disease, AIDS to malaria, diabetes to Alzheimer's—you would be justifiably skeptical. And if, after reviewing the evidence, you found that the medicine had no more curative effects than a placebo, you would reject the claim and return to a more realistic search for the diverse causes and cures of these illnesses. Psychological research, by comparison, seems at times to obey a different set of rules. Our attempts to predict and explain human behavior tend to rely on broad dispositional constructs: locus of control, sensation seeking, trust in doctors, self-consciousness, liberalism–conservatism, dominance, hedonism, prejudice, self-esteem, authoritarianism, altruism, achievement motivation, and so on ad infinitum. The oft documented failure of such constructs to predict behavior has done little to undermine confidence in their utility.

Self-esteem is a good case in point. Low self-esteem is often considered a major cause of problem behavior. In 1994, Robyn Dawes (1994) wrote a scathing critique of a report (Mecca, Smelser, & Vasconcellos, 1989) by a task force on self-esteem and social responsibility established by the California State Assembly. In their report, the task force reviewed the voluminous literature on self-esteem and found virtually no evidence for any effects of self-esteem on child maltreatment, academic achievement, unwanted teenage pregnancy, crime and violence, chronic welfare dependency, or alcoholism and drug use. Nevertheless, the contributors clung to their preconceived ideas regarding the importance of self-esteem and suggested that interventions to increase self-esteem be encouraged. A more recent review of the literature (Baumeister, Campbell, Krueger, & Vohs, 2003) again documented the lack of evidence for a relation between self-esteem and problem behavior among adolescents: "Most studies on self-esteem and smoking have failed to find any significant relationship, even with very large samples and the correspondingly high statistical power... Large, longitudinal investigations have tended to yield no relationship between self-esteem and either drinking in general or heavy, problem drinking in particular... Self-esteem does not appear to prevent early sexual activity or teen pregnancy" (p. 35). We do not wish to claim, of course, that self-esteem is a useless construct. All else equal, we might well prefer that people feel good about themselves, but it is important to recognize that this construct does little to advance our understanding of the determinants of human social behavior.

Other instances of injudicious reliance on dispositional constructs abound. For example, not much more encouraging than the findings regarding self-esteem are the results of research on racial prejudice and discriminatory behavior. In two recent meta-analyses (Schütz & Six, 1996; Talaska, Fiske, & Chaiken, 2004) of the relevant literature, the average correlations between measures of prejudice and discrimination were .29 (based on 46 data sets) and .26 (based on 136 data sets), respectively. Correlations of comparable magnitude were reported in recent research that, instead of measuring attitudes explicitly, obtained implicit measures by means of the Implicit Association Test (Greenwald, McGhee, & Schwartz, 1998) or evaluative priming (Fazio, Jackson, Dunton, & Williams, 1995). Like explicit measures of prejudice, implicit measures tend to have relatively low correlations even with nonverbal behaviors that are not consciously monitored (for reviews, see Ajzen & Fishbein, 2005; Fazio & Olson, 2003). Nevertheless, there is no readily apparent diminution in work on this construct. Again, we do not wish to give the impression that racial, ethnic, and gender prejudices are unimportant, but we have to realize that prejudice does not account for a great deal of variance in any particular behavior.

THE REASONED ACTION APPROACH

Evidence of this kind led Fishbein (1967a; Fishbein & Ajzen, 1972, 1975) more than 30 years ago to question reliance on global dispositions. Instead of studying the role of self-esteem, prejudice, internal-external locus of control, or some other global disposition, he suggested that we direct our attention to the particular behavior of interest and try to identify its determinants. Much prior theory and research had focused on one or another global disposition that might serve as an overarching causal agent and then tried to rely on this disposition to account for many different types of behavior in the disposition's domain of application. By contrast, Fishbein and Ajzen proposed that we identify a particular behavior and then look for antecedents that can help to predict and explain the behavior of interest, and thus potentially provide a basis for interventions designed to modify it.

Of course, this quest would be quite unrealistic if we had to assume that each behavior is determined by a unique set of antecedents. The reasoned action model that emerged in response to the challenge, now known as the theory of planned behavior, actually identified a small set of causal factors that should permit explanation and prediction of most human social behaviors. Briefly, according to the theory, a central determinant of behavior is the individual's *intention* to perform the behavior in question. As they formulate their intentions, people are assumed to take into account three conceptually independent types of considerations. The first are readily accessible or salient beliefs about the likely consequences of a contemplated course of action, beliefs which, in their aggregate, result in a favorable or unfavorable *attitude toward the behavior*. A second type of consideration has to do with the perceived normative expectations of relevant referent groups or individuals. Such salient normative beliefs lead to the formation of a *subjective norm*—the perceived social pressure to perform or not to perform the behavior. Finally, people are assumed to take into account factors that may further or hinder their ability to perform the behavior, and these salient control beliefs lead to the formation of *perceived behavioral control*, which refers to the perceived capability of performing the behavior. As a general rule, the more favorable the attitude and subjective norm with respect to a behavior, and the greater the perceived behavioral control, the stronger should be an individual's intention to perform the behavior under consideration. Finally, given a sufficient degree of *actual* control over the behavior, people are expected to carry out their intentions when the opportunity arises. Intention is thus assumed to be the immediate antecedent of behavior. However, because many behaviors pose difficulties of execution that may limit volitional control, it is useful to consider perceived behavioral control in addition to intention. To the extent that perceived behavioral control is veridical, it can serve as a proxy for actual control and contribute to the prediction of the behavior in question. A schematic representation of the theory is shown in Figure 1–1.

Expectancy-Value Model

The three major determinants in the theory of planned behavior—attitudes toward the behavior, subjective norms, and perceptions of behavioral control—are traced to corresponding sets of behavior-related beliefs. The relation between beliefs and overall evaluative attitude is embodied in the most popular model of attitude formation and structure, the expectancy-value model (see Feather, 1959, 1982). One of the first and most complete statements of the model can be found in Fishbein's (1963; 1967b) summation theory of attitude. In this theory, people's evaluations of, or attitudes toward, an object are determined by their salient or readily accessible beliefs about the object, where a belief is defined as the subjective probability that the object has a certain attribute (Fishbein & Ajzen, 1975). The terms *object* and *attribute* are used in the generic sense and they refer to any discriminable aspect of an individual's world. When applied to attitudes toward a behavior, the object of interest is a particular action and the attributes are the action's anticipated outcomes. For example, a person may believe that physical exercise (the attitude object) reduces the risk of heart disease (the attribute).

Each belief thus associates a behavior with a certain outcome. According to the expectancy-value model, a person's overall attitude toward performing a behavior is determined by the subjective values or evaluations of the outcomes

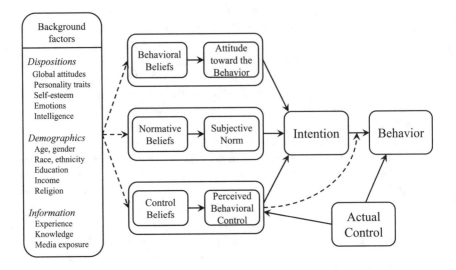

FIGURE 1–1.   The theory of planned behavior.

associated with the behavior and by the strength of these associations. Specifically, the evaluation of each outcome contributes to the attitude in direct proportion to the person's subjective probability that the behavior will lead to the outcome in question. The basic structure of the model is shown in the equation below, where A_B is the attitude toward the behavior, b_i is the strength of the belief that the behavior will lead to outcome i, e_i is the evaluation of outcome i, and the sum is over all salient outcomes (see Fishbein & Ajzen, 1975).

$$A_B \propto \sum b_i e_i \qquad\qquad 1$$

A similar logic applies to the relation between normative beliefs and subjective norm, and the relation between control beliefs and perceived behavioral control. Normative beliefs refer to the perceived behavioral expectations of important referent individuals or groups such as the person's family, friends, coworkers, and health professionals. These normative beliefs—in combination with the motivation to comply with the different referents—determine the prevailing subjective norm regarding the behavior. Finally, control beliefs have to do with the perceived presence of factors that can facilitate or impede performance of a behavior. It is assumed that the perceived power of each control factor to impede or facilitate performing the behavior contributes to perceived control in direct proportion to the person's subjective probability that the control factor is present.

Basically, then, the theory assumes that human social behavior follows reasonably from the information or beliefs people possess about the behavior under consideration. These beliefs originate in a variety of sources: personal experiences, formal education, radio, newspapers, TV, the Internet and other media, interactions with family and friends, and so forth. No matter how beliefs were acquired, they are assumed to produce attitudes, subjective norms, and perceptions of control with regard to the behavior, and thus guide the formation of behavioral intentions and actual performance of the behavior.

To summarize briefly, Fishbein and Ajzen's response to the failure of global dispositions, and in particular of global attitudes, to predict behavior was twofold. First, they suggested that we shift focus from global dispositions, such as attitudes toward broad objects, groups, institutions, or policies to behavior-specific dispositions, such as intentions to perform the behavior, attitudes toward the behavior, subjective norms regarding the behavior, and perceptions of control over performing the behavior. This shift constituted a revolution in the theorizing of social scientists who for decades had relied almost exclusively on global dispositions in their attempts to explain social behavior. In fact, Fishbein and Ajzen's insight has yet to reach many investigators as is evidenced by the continuing reliance on global dispositions in diverse areas of research. Second, Fishbein and Ajzen proposed that we apply the well-established expectancy-value model of general attitudes to the study of attitudes toward a behavior and that we extend its logic to the other antecedents of intentions as well. This approach is reminiscent of behavioral decision theory and its dominant theoretical framework, the subjective expected utility model (see Edwards, 1954). Both models focus on specific behavioral options and assume that an option's perceived attributes determine a person's decision. However, the expectancy-value model makes fewer psychometric assumptions, is more descriptive of the decision-making process, and is consistent with work on the psychological limitations of human judgments and decisions (see Ajzen, 1996). We return to this last point in the following discussion of misconceptions about the reasoned action approach.

Background Factors

Though focusing on determinants closely linked to a behavior of interest, the theory of planned behavior does not deny the importance of global dispositions, demographic factors, or other kinds of variables often considered in social psychology and related disciplines. In fact, the reasoned action approach recognizes the potential importance of such factors but, as can be seen in Figure 1–1, they are considered background variables that can influence behavior indirectly by affecting behavioral, normative, and control beliefs. However, whether a particular background factor does indeed have an impact on beliefs is an empirical question. Furthermore, given the large number of potentially relevant background factors, it is difficult to know which should be considered without a content-specific theory to guide selection in the behavioral domain of interest. Content theories of this kind are not part of the reasoned action model but can complement it by identifying relevant background factors and thereby extending our understanding of a behavior's determinants (see Petraitis, Flay, & Miller, 1995). With the aid of the theory of planned behavior we can not only examine whether a given background factor is related to the behavior of interest but also explain such an effect by tracing it to differences in behavior-relevant beliefs, attitudes, subjective norms, perceptions of behavioral control, and intentions.

The proposition that behavior follows from information or beliefs about the behavior is not unique to the reasoned action model developed by Fishbein and Ajzen (see Fishbein et al., 2001). Among other theories consistent with this proposition are the health belief model (Rosenstock, Strecher, & Becker, 1994; Strecher, Champion, & Rosenstock, 1997), social cognitive theory (Bandura, 1986, 1997), the theory of subjective culture and interpersonal relations (Triandis, 1972, 1977), the information-motivation-behavioral skills model (Fisher & Fisher, 1992), and the theory of trying (Bagozzi & Warshaw, 1990). For example, Bandura's well-known social cognitive theory relies on outcome expectancies or behavioral beliefs and, more importantly, on the construct of self-efficacy to explain behavior. It deals with the same kinds of variables as the theory of planned behavior, but subdivides them into a greater number (see, e.g., Bandura, 1998). Thus, instead of a single intention, it distinguishes between proximal and distal goals; instead of beliefs about behavioral consequences and social norms, it refers to physical, social, and self-evaluative outcome expectations; and instead of a single factor referring to perceived behavioral control, it draws a distinction between beliefs about self-efficacy on one hand and beliefs about personal and situational versus system impediments on the other. Similarly, in his theory of subjective culture and interpersonal relations Triandis considers intentions, facilitating factors, perceived consequences of performing a behavior, and perceived social influences to be important determinants of behavior, but he also includes habit and emotion as additional factors.

Misconceptions

Though widely accepted and applied, some aspects of the theory of planned behavior—and of the reasoned action approach in general—are frequently misconstrued.

Reasoned versus rational action. Foremost among misconceptions is the supposition that in a reasoned action approach people are assumed to behave rationally, basing their decision on a dispassionate weighing of all relevant information. In actuality, all the theory assumes is that behavioral intentions follow reasonably from beliefs about performing the behavior. People may hold few or many beliefs. Some beliefs persist over time, some are forgotten, and new beliefs are formed. However, there is no assumption in reasoned action models that these beliefs are veridical. On the contrary, the theory recognizes that beliefs, although often quite accurate, can be biased by a variety of cognitive and motivational processes, that they may derive from invalid or selective information, be self-serving, or otherwise fail to correspond to reality. However, once a set of beliefs is formed it provides the cognitive foundation from which attitudes, perceived social norms, and perceptions of control—and ultimately intentions—are assumed to follow in a reasonable and consistent fashion.

Deliberative versus automatic processes.   The theory of planned behavior is also often misinterpreted as implying that people form a conscious intention prior to carrying out each and every behavior. In reality, the theory assumes that, after repeated opportunities for performance of a given behavior, deliberation is no longer required because the intention to perform (or not perform) the behavior is activated spontaneously in a behavior-relevant situation (see Ajzen & Fishbein, 2000). In other words, the behavior has become so routine that it is initiated with minimal conscious effort or attention. Many behaviors in everyday life are of this kind: We brush our teeth, leave the house for work, put on a seat belt, walk up stairs, and so forth without prior conscious deliberation. There is no need to assume that such behaviors are activated automatically or unconsciously, without prior intentions—only that the intentions are activated spontaneously without much conscious effort.

A related issue has sometimes been raised with respect to the formal structure of the expectancy-value model of attitudes. The equation used to compute an attitude estimate on the basis of accessible beliefs may seem to imply that people go through a complex mental calculus, involving multiplication of belief strength by outcome evaluation and summation of the resulting product terms. In actuality, although the investigator does perform these computations, people are *not* assumed to do so. It is merely proposed that attitude formation can be *modeled* in this fashion. The psychological processes involved in arriving at an attitude are assumed to take account of belief strength as well as outcome evaluation, roughly in the form described by the formal model: The more strongly a belief is held, and the more positive or negative the outcome evaluation, the greater is the belief's expected contribution to the overall attitude. The same is true of the models describing the relations between normative beliefs and subjective norms, and the relations between control beliefs and perceived behavioral control.

Indeed, the processes described in the expectancy-value model are assumed to occur automatically and often below conscious awareness. Fishbein's (1963; 1967b) original summation model described attitude formation as the automatic conditioning of evaluative reactions to the attitude object. Similarly, although couched in more cognitive, information-processing terminology, the expectancy-value model of attitudes in the theory of planned behavior does *not* assume deliberate and conscious attitude construction. Instead, our attitudes toward a behavior are assumed to be formed automatically and inevitably as we acquire new information about the behavior's outcomes, and as the subjective values of these outcomes become linked to the behavior. These attitudes are immediately available when we are confronted with the behavior. The same logic applies to the formation and automatic activation of subjective norms and of perceived behavioral control.

Empirical Support

A large number of studies have applied the theory of planned behavior to examine the psychological antecedents of actions in various domains, and more recently, attempts have also been made to use the theory as a framework for behavioral interventions. In this chapter, we focus on health-related behaviors, but our conclusions hold equally well for behavior in other domains. It is beyond the scope of this chapter to review the large body of research that has applied the theory of planned behavior in the health domain (for summaries, see Albarracín, Johnson, Fishbein, & Muellerleile, 2001; Godin & Kok, 1996; Hausenblas, Carron, & Mack, 1997). Suffice it to note that, generally speaking, the theory has been well supported. Thus, with regard to the prediction of behavior, many studies have substantiated the predictive validity of behavioral intentions. A few sample applications in the health domain are shown in Table 1–1. It can be seen that intentions can be highly predictive of various health-related behaviors. Indeed, meta-analyses of studies dealing with specific health behaviors, such as condom use and exercise, have revealed a strong link between intentions and behavior, with mean correlations ranging from .44 to .56 (Albarracín et al., 2001; Godin & Kok, 1996; Hausenblas et al., 1997; Sheeran & Orbell, 1998). Also, it has been found that the addition of perceived behavioral control can improve prediction of behavior considerably, especially when performance of the behavior is difficult. For example, in a general sample of smokers, a measure of perceived behavioral control accounted for an additional 12% of the variance in smoking behavior over and above intentions; and among postnatal women, the increase in explained behavioral variance due to perceived behavioral control was 34% (Godin, Valois, Lepage, & Desharnais, 1992).

Regarding the antecedents of intentions, Table 1–2 summarizes the results of a few recent studies that attempted to predict behavioral intentions in the health domain. It can be seen that the theory of planned behavior accounted for appreciable variance in people's intentions to perform a diverse set of behaviors: physical exercise, using illicit drugs, eating a low-fat diet, consuming dietary products, and performing breast self-examinations. And here, too, meta-analyses of the empirical literature have provided strong evidence to show that intentions to perform health-related behaviors can be predicted with considerable accuracy from measures of attitudes toward the behavior, subjective norms, and perceived behavioral control or self-efficacy, with mean correlations ranging from .63 to .71 (Albarracín et al., 2001; Godin & Kok, 1996; Hagger, Chatzisarantis, & Biddle, 2002; Sheeran & Taylor, 1999).

Overall, then, the theory of planned behavior has done quite well across a variety of behavioral domains. Still, one may wonder about the relatively large amount of variance that often remains unaccounted for. Some of the unexplained variance may be due to random measurement error. This suggestion is supported by structural equation modeling which usually results in a good fit between model and data and a high proportion of explained variance once measurement unreliability is taken into account (see, e.g., Bamberg & Schmidt, 1994; Blue, Wilbur, & Marston-Scott, 2001; Davis, Ajzen, Saunders, & Williams, 2002; Levin, 1999). In some studies, low predictive validity is due to lack of variance in the behavioral criterion, or inappropriate operationalization of the predictor or criterion measures. Even with these limitations, meta-analyses provide strong support for the reasoned action approach, particularly when one considers that prior to the

TABLE 1–1
Correlations Between Health-Related Intentions and Behaviors

Behavior	Intention-behavior correlation
Using birth control pills (see Ajzen & Fishbein, 1980, ch. 11)	.85
Breast vs. bottle feeding (Manstead, Proffitt, & Smart, 1983)	.82
Using ecstasy drugs (Orbell, Blair, Sherlock, & Conner, 2001)	.75
Having an abortion (Smetana & Adler, 1980)	.96
Donating blood (Giles & Cairns, 1995)	.75
Using homeopathic medicine (Furnham & Lovett, 2001)	.75

Note: All correlations are significant (p < .01).

TABLE 1–2
Prediction of Intentions from Attitude Toward the Behavior (AB), Subjective Norm (SN),
and Perceived Behavioral Control (PBC)

Intention	Correlation coefficients			Regression coefficients			
	A_B	SN	PBC	A_B	SN	PBC	R
Physical exercise (Courneya, 1995)	.51	.47	.48	.22	.17	.18	.62
Using cannabis (Conner & McMillan, 1999)	.70	.55	.69	.42	.11	.43	.81
Eating a low-fat diet (Armitage & Conner, 1999)	.68	.43	.59	.36	.16	.33	.78
Consuming dairy products (Kim, Reicks, & Sjoberg, 2003)	.42	.33	.48	.38	.11*	.30	.65
Breast self-examination (Norman & Hoyle, 2004)	.56	.52	.80	.26	.03*	.70	.85

*Not significant; all other coefficients p < .05.

introduction of the theories of reasoned action and planned behavior, most studies accounted for no more than 10% of the variance in behavior (see Wicker, 1969).

The Cognitive Foundation of Intentions and Behavior

Substantive information about the considerations that guide decisions to perform a given behavior is obtained by examining the behavioral, normative, and control beliefs that provide the basis for attitudes, subjective norms, and perceptions of behavioral control. A recent review of research on physical exercise (Downs & Hausenblas, 2005) provides summary information for this particular domain and can serve as an illustration. The authors surveyed 47 investigations that had conducted elicitation studies to identify salient behavioral, normative, and control beliefs about exercising. Salient behavioral beliefs associated exercising with such advantages as improved physical and psychological health, control of body weight, improved daily functioning, increased energy, stress relief, and relaxation. Salient negative outcomes of exercising had to do with pain and injury, fatigue, and time expenditure. The most frequently mentioned salient normative referents were family members, friends, and health-care professionals. Finally, the most frequently listed control factors that could interfere with exercising were health-related problems (injury, pain), inconvenience, lack of energy, lack of time, and lack of social support. Salient facilitating factors included convenience, pleasure derived from exercise, and social support.

This analysis of exercise beliefs also showed that, in the context of expectancy-value formulations, behavioral beliefs accounted for over 54% of the variance in direct measures of attitude toward exercising, normative beliefs for almost 56% of the variance in direct measures of subjective norms, and control beliefs for about 34% of the variance in direct measures of perceived behavioral control. Examination of differences in behavioral, normative, and control beliefs between individuals who exercise and those who do not can provide useful information about the kinds of considerations that are the most influential determinants of this behavior and that may be targeted most effectively in behavioral interventions.

BEHAVIORAL INTERVENTIONS AND PERSUASIVE COMMUNICATIONS

According to the reasoned action approach, changes in behavior can be brought about by changing people's intentions to perform the behavior in question. A recent meta-analysis (Webb & Sheeran, 2006) provides strong support for this expectation. This meta-analysis examined 47 studies in which an intervention program was found to significantly strengthen intentions to perform a behavior of interest. The analysis showed conclusively that these changes also led to subsequent changes in behavior. An important question, therefore, has to do with strategies that can be used to effectively change the antecedents of behavioral intentions and thus modify behavior. The remainder of this chapter discusses research that has examined possible strategies in the health domain.

Changing the Psychological Antecedents of Intentions

The reasoned action approach has guided many interventions designed to prevent disease and promote health. In these interventions, attempts are made to induce favorable attitudes, norms, and/or perceived control with respect to a health-related behavior. For example, in the domain of condom use to prevent HIV/AIDS, Albarracín McNatt, Klein (2003) and Albarracín, Gillette, (2005) identified several intervention strategies relevant for a reasoned action approach. One strategy entails attempts to modify attitudes by means of *attitudinal arguments*. These programs usually consist of assertions that condom use has personally beneficial consequences for one's physical health or psychological comfort. Another strategy comprises arguments to increase favorable norms with respect to condom use (*normative arguments*). These arguments are often designed to convince an audience that its social network supports condom use. In addition, interventions can also contain behavioral scripts about strategies that yield successful performance of the behavior. These scripts can be transmitted verbally, within persuasive arguments, or as part of a behavioral skills training based on Kelly et al.'s (1991) approach. For example, a persuasive message may describe how successful condom use depends on preparatory actions such as carrying condoms around all the time or discussing condom use with potential partners (*behavioral skills arguments*). Similarly, a widely accepted strategy is to ask participants to role-play condom application or negotiation (*behavioral skills training*). Presumably, the behavioral practice and the instructional feedback facilitate acquisition of necessary behavioral skills. As a result of teaching behavioral skills, interventions of this type presumably increase perceived behavioral control.

Albarracín and her colleagues (2005) conducted a comprehensive meta-analysis of the outcomes of HIV-prevention interventions to increase condom use published between 1986 and 2004. As part of this project, over 350 interventions and around 100 control groups were selected, comprising a large number of countries and U.S. states. For each of these groups or conditions, the researchers calculated amount of change in behavior (e.g., increases in condom use frequency) and change in various psychological variables. Of interest to this chapter, they calculated change in *actual condom use*, *attitudes* with regard to condom use (whether one thinks that condom use is good and desirable), *norms* about the use of condoms (beliefs that others support one's use of condoms), *perceptions of control* over the behavior (perceiving that one can do it if one wants to), and *intentions* to use condoms.

Changing behavior by changing attitudes and perceived behavioral control. Albarracín et al. (2005) distinguished between what they termed *active* and *passive* interventions. Overall, interventions with strategies that required *activities* by the recipients (behavioral skills training, HIV counseling and testing, or client-tailored counseling, termed *active interventions*) were more effective than interventions that relied exclusively on presented material without the recipients engaging in specific activities (termed *passive interventions*). Within passive interventions, the most effective strategies were attitudinal arguments discussing the beneficial outcomes of using condoms and behavioral-skills arguments explaining how to best implement condom use. The distribution of condoms to participants was also effective when the intervention was passive. Within active interventions (those including behavioral skills training, HIV counseling and testing, and/or client-tailored counseling), effective strategies included presenting attitudinal and control/behavioral skills arguments (two passive strategies often included in active interventions) and training people in the management of their moods and situations in which drugs and alcohol are involved (one of the strategies that characterized active interventions).

Of course, the finding that an intervention with attitudinal and behavioral-control contents is effective at changing behavior does not necessarily validate the reasoned action approach. Like any treatment, behavioral interventions may work for any number of reasons. For example, an intervention to improve condom use attitudes may increase condom use because it is accompanied by the provision of condoms or arguments to increase HIV threat. Thus, one must verify that the behavioral change produced by the attitudinal or control arguments was mediated by changes in attitudes and perceived behavioral control (while controlling for other strategies).

Figure 1–2 summarizes the findings from path analyses fit to test mediational models for the effects of attitudinal arguments and self-management training (Albarracín et al., 2005). Sobel (1982) tests were calculated and are presented along with the path coefficients; a significant test indicates significant mediation. The figure shows that the effects of attitudinal and behavioral-skills arguments on behavior were positive and significant across passive and active interventions. However, the positive effects of attitudinal arguments on behavior change were mediated by changes in attitudes. Similarly, the analyses in the bottom half of the

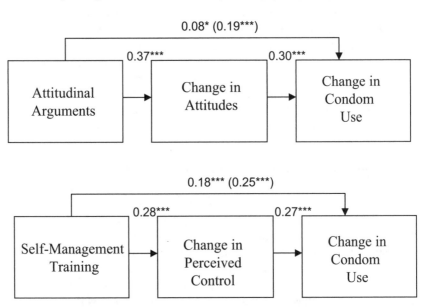

FIGURE 1–2. Path analyses to determine the mediating effects of change in specific psychological variables on changes in condom use. Panel A: Effects of attitudinal arguments. Panel B: Effects of self-management training. Both models also included all the strategies that were coded in the meta-analysis. However, the other paths are not presented for simplicity. Path coefficients are standardized. The direct path when the mediator was not included appears between parentheses. Sobel tests were significant unless indicated as ns. Adapted from Albarracín et al. (2005).

figure indicate that the positive influence of behavioral-skills arguments on condom use change was mediated by control perceptions. The analyses are simplified for display purposes; they controlled for other possible influences such as condom provision and threat-inducing arguments.

Changing behaviors by changing norms. The outcomes of HIV-prevention interventions also illustrate how changing norms can produce changes in behaviors. Durantini et al. (2006) used the same meta-analytic procedures as Albarracín et al. (2005) to investigate the impact of source characteristics and demographic similarity between the source and the recipient on actual behavioral changes after the interventions. Some researchers have argued that persuasive communications (and therefore behavioral interventions) should use experts as sources (Hovland, Janis, & Kelley, 1953). However, there is also extensive work and policy favoring the use of laypersons selected from the target community (Freire, 1972; Putnam, 1911; in the domain of HIV prevention, see Kelly et al., 1997). Although there are some deeply held beliefs about these issues, there have been no direct comparisons. Researchers have compared control groups with peer-led interventions, or control groups with expert led interventions. The key comparison between expert and peer sources, however, was absent prior to this meta-analysis of source effects.

By dividing interventions into ones presented by experts (e.g., public health educators, physicians, nurses, research staff) and ones presented by lay community members (e.g., community leaders, artists, religious ministers), the meta-analysis by Durantini and her colleagues (2006) could establish what type of source is more effective. Findings indicated that, overall, expert sources were more effective than lay community members. Moreover, as shown in the top part of Figure 1–3, these effects were mediated by norms (in addition to other factors) in various samples that differed in race (Black and White) as well as gender. This meta-analysis also showed that communicators similar to the audience produced greater changes in behavior than dissimilar communicators, and that the effect of source similarity was again mediated by changes in subjective norms. We return to this issue in the following section.

The Role of Background Factors in Interventions

In the reasoned action approach, background factors such as gender, ethnicity, and past behavior can influence intentions and behavior in two ways. First, the relative influence of attitudes, norms, and perceived control on intentions and behavior may vary as a function of a given background factor. Second, background factors can influence intentions and behavior by their effects on the proximal determinants, that is, beliefs, attitudes, subjective norms, and perceived behavioral control.

Background factors as moderators. Whether an intervention that targets norms, or attitudes, or perceived control will be influential appears to depend on the target population. The results from Durantini et al.'s (2006) review revealed that even when experts were generally effective, they were most effective for

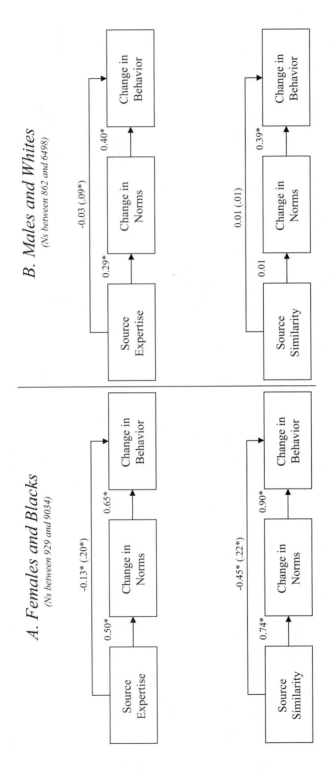

FIGURE 1–3. Path analyses for the effects of expertise and demographic similarity. Models were fit using pair-wise deletion procedures to maintain the number of groups included in the main analyses reported in this paper. The first number next to each path is a standardized path coefficient. The parenthetical numbers correspond to the univariate correlations between expertise and each potential mediator. Sobel tests were significant whenever the source variable had a direct effect on behavior change. Adapted from Albarracín et al. (2005).

populations that typically have restricted power in society. That is, the beneficial impact of having an expert source was stronger for ethnic minorities and women than for ethnic majorities and men (see top part of Figure 1–3).

Notwithstanding the finding that experts are more effective than peers in unempowered populations, it also seems to be beneficial if the expert shares some of the characteristics of the audience. Thus, women and ethnic minorities were found to be sensitive to sources who share whatever characteristic makes that audience different from the mainstream (see bottom part of Figure 1–3). First women changed more in response to other women, and members of ethnic minorities changed more in response to other members of their ethnic group. Also, most populations whose behavior places them at risk for HIV (injection drug users, multiple partner heterosexuals, low condom users) benefited from having both an expert and somebody from their own group as intervention facilitators. In all of these cases, changes in norms mediated changes in behavior. For instance, the effect of demographic similarity among women and people of African backgrounds was mediated by norms (see bottom left diagram in Figure 1–3).

Whether normative arguments are effective is also contingent on the nature of the audience. For teens, receiving an HIV-prevention message that contains normative arguments was found to be better than not receiving these arguments. However, for adults, receiving these arguments was worse than not receiving them at all (see Albarracín et al., 2005).

Mediated effects of background factors.   The reasoned action approach assumes that attitudes and norms are formed spontaneously when specific beliefs develop. For instance, people may form a favorable attitude toward a behavior if they previously formed beliefs that the behavior has desirable outcomes. However, as noted earlier in this chapter, the fact that beliefs are implicated does not imply that the process is rational. To the contrary, beliefs have many sources. For example, Albarracín and Wyer (2000) led college students to believe that outside of awareness they had either supported or opposed the institution of comprehensive examinations at their university. Because the feedback was experimentally manipulated, the researchers were able to examine the causal influence of participants' perceived past behavior on both their later behavior decisions and the cognitive processes that mediated these decisions. This influence was studied under a variety of experimental conditions designed to influence the participant's ability to process information. It was found that at least in some of these conditions the influence of the past behavior induction was belief-mediated. Likewise, interventions that induce actual trial of a new behavior may have similar belief-mediated effects on later behavior (for limiting conditions, see Albarracín, Cohen, & Kumkale, 2003; Albarracín & McNatt, 2005).

CONCLUSION

The reasoned action approach, as embodied in the theory of planned behavior, has proven useful both as a conceptual framework for understanding the determinants of specific behaviors, notably in the health domain, and as a basis for designing effective behavioral interventions. A considerable amount of variance in behavior can be explained by considering intentions to engage in a behavior of interest as well as perceptions of control over the behavior. Intentions, in turn, are found to be well predicted from attitudes toward the behavior, subjective norms, and perceptions of behavioral control. Finally, salient beliefs about the behavior's outcomes, about the normative expectations of salient referents, and about facilitating and inhibiting factors can be examined to obtain a more detailed understanding of the cognitive foundation that underlies behavioral decisions. Consistent with this conceptual framework, behavior can be influenced by changing its theoretical antecedents. Thus, as expected, interventions directed at behavioral beliefs are found to influence attitudes, and by changing attitudes influence intentions and actions. Similar conclusions apply to interventions designed to change subjective norms or perceptions of behavioral control. Finally, also consistent with the theory, background factors such as personality, race, gender, and past actions have been found to influence behavior indirectly, by their effects on salient beliefs about the behavior.

REFERENCES

Ajzen, I. (1996). The social psychology of decision making. In E. T. Higgins & A. W. Kruglanski (Eds.), *Social psychology: Handbook of basic principles* (pp. 297–325). New York: Guilford Press.

Ajzen, I., & Fishbein, M. (1980). *Understanding attitudes and predicting social behavior.* Englewood Cliffs, NJ: Prentice Hall.

Ajzen, I., & Fishbein, M. (2000). Attitudes and the attitude-behavior relation: Reasoned and automatic processes. In W. Stroebe & M. Hewstone (Eds.), *European review of social psychology* (Vol. 11, pp. 1–33). Chichester, England: Wiley.

Ajzen, I., & Fishbein, M. (2005). The influence of attitudes on behavior. In D. Albarracín, B. T. Johnson & M. P. Zanna (Eds.), *Handbook of attitudes and attitude change: Basic principles* (pp. 173–221). Mahwah, NJ: Lawrence Erlbaum Associates.

Albarracín, D., Cohen, J. B., & Kumkale, G. T. (2003). When persuasive communications collide with behavior: Effects of post-message actions on beliefs and intentions. *Personality and Social Psychology Bulletin, 29,* 834–845.

Albarracín, D., Gillette, J., Earl, A., Glasman, L.R., Durantini, M.R., & Ho., M.H. (2005). A test of major assumptions about behavior change: A comprehensive look at HIV prevention interventions since the beginning of the epidemic. *Psychological Bulletin, 131,* 856–897.

Albarracín, D., Johnson, B. T., Fishbein, M., & Muellerleile, P. A. (2001). Theories of reasoned action and planned behavior as models of condom use: A meta-analysis. *Psychological Bulletin, 127,* 142–161.

Albarracín, D., & McNatt, P. S. (2005). Maintenance and decay of past behavior influences: Anchoring attitudes on beliefs following inconsistent actions. *Personality and Social Psychology Bulletin, 31,* 719–733.

Albarracín, D., McNatt, P. S., Klein, C., Ho, R., Mitchell, A., & Kumkale, G. T. (2003). Persuasive communications to change actions: An analysis of behavioral and cognitive impact in HIV prevention. *Health Psychology, 22,* 166–17.

Albarracín, D., & Wyer, R. S., Jr. (2000). The cognitive impact of past behavior: Influences on beliefs, attitudes, and future behavioral decisions. *Journal of Personality and Social Psychology, 79,* 5–22.

Armitage, C. J., & Conner, M. (1999). Distinguishing perceptions of control from self-efficacy: Predicting consumption of a low-fat diet using the theory of planned behavior. *Journal of Applied Social Psychology, 29*, 72–90.

Bagozzi, R. P., & Warshaw, P. R. (1990). Trying to consume. *Journal of Consumer Research, 17*, 127–140.

Bamberg, S., & Schmidt, P. (1994). Automobile or Bicycle? Empirical test of a Utility-Theory Approach. *Koelner Zeitschrift Fuer Soziologie und Sozialpsychologie, 46*, 80–102.

Bandura, A. (1986). *Social foundations of thought and action: A social cognitive theory.* Englewood Cliffs, NJ: Prentice Hall.

Bandura, A. (1997). *Self-efficacy: The exercise of control.* New York: Freeman.

Bandura, A. (1998). Health promotion from the perspective of social cognitive theory. *Psychology and Health, 13*, 623–649.

Baumeister, R. F., Campbell, J. D., Krueger, J. I., & Vohs, K. D. (2003). Does high self-esteem cause better performance, interpersonal success, happiness, or healthier lifestyles? *Psychological Science in the Public Interest, 4*, 1–44.

Blue, C. L., Wilbur, J., & Marston-Scott, M. V. (2001). Exercise among blue-collar workers: Application of the theory of planned behavior. *Research in Nursing and Health, 24*, 481–493.

Conner, M., & McMillan, B. (1999). Interaction effects in the theory of planned behavior: Studying cannabis use. *British Journal of Social Psychology, 38*, 195–222.

Courneya, K. S. (1995). Understanding readiness for regular physical activity in older individuals: An application of the theory of planned behavior. *Health Psychology, 14*, 80–87. (There is no citation.)

Davis, L. E., Ajzen, I., Saunders, J., & Williams, T. (2002). The decision of African American students to complete high school: An application of the theory of planned behavior. *Journal of Educational Psychology, 94*, 810–819.

Dawes, R. M. (1994). *House of cards: Psychology and psychotherapy built on myth.* New York: The Free Press.

Downs, D. S., & Hausenblas, H. A. (2005). Elicitation studies and the theory of planned behavior: A systematic review of exercise beliefs. *Psychology of Sport and Exercise, 6*, 1–31.

Durantini, M. R., Albarracín, D., Earl, A., & Mitchell, A.L. (2006). Conceptualizing the influence of social agents of change: A meta-analysis of HIV prevention interventions for different groups. *Psychological Bulletin, 132*, 212–248.

Edwards, W. (1954). The theory of decision making. *Psychological Bulletin, 51*, 380–417.

Fazio, R. H., Jackson, J. R., Dunton, B. C., & Williams, C. J. (1995). Variability in automatic activation as an unobtrusive measure of racial attitudes: A bona fide pipeline? *Journal of Personality and Social Psychology, 69*, 1013–1027.

Fazio, R. H., & Olson, M. A. (2003). Implicit measures in social cognition research: Their meaning and uses. *Annual Review of Psychology, 54*, 297–327.

Feather, N. T. (1959). Subjective probability and decision under uncertainty. *Psychological Review, 66*, 150–164.

Feather, N. T. (Ed.). (1982). *Expectations and actions: Expectancy—value models in psychology.* Hillsdale, NJ: Lawrence Erlbaum Associates.

Fishbein, M. (1963). An investigation of the relationships between beliefs about an object and the attitude toward that object. *Human Relations, 16*, 233–240.

Fishbein, M. (1967a). Attitude and the prediction of behavior. In M. Fishbein (Ed.), *Readings in attitude theory and measurement* (pp. 477–492). New York: Wiley.

Fishbein, M. (1967b). A consideration of beliefs and their role in attitude measurement. In M. Fishbein (Ed.), *Readings in attitude theory and measurement* (pp. 257–266). New York: Wiley.

Fishbein, M., & Ajzen, I. (1972). Attitudes and opinions. *Annual Review of Psychology,* 487–544.

Fishbein, M., & Ajzen, I. (1975). *Belief, attitude, intention, and behavior: An introduction to theory and research.* Reading, MA: Addison-Wesley.

Fishbein, M., Triandis, H. C., Kanfer, F. H., Becker, M., Middlestadt, S. E., & Eichler, A. (2001). Factors influencing behavior and behavior change. In A. Baum & T. A. Revenson (Eds.), *Handbook of health psychology.* Mahwah, NJ: Lawrence Erlbaum Associates.

Fisher, J. D., & Fisher, W. A. (1992). Changing AIDS-risk behavior. *Psychological Bulletin, 111*, 455–474.

Freire, P. (1972). *Pedagogy of the oppressed.* Harmondsworth, UK: Penguin.

Furnham, A., & Lovett, J. (2001). Predicting the use of complementary medicine: A test of the theories of reasoned action and planned behavior. *Journal of Applied Social Psychology, 31*, 2588–2620.

Giles, M., & Cairns, E. (1995). Blood donation and Ajzen's theory of planned behaviour: An examination of perceived behavioural control. *British Journal of Social Psychology, 34*, 173–188.

Godin, G., & Kok, G. (1996). The theory of planned behavior: A review of its applications to health-related behaviors. *American Journal of Health Promotion, 11*, 87–98.

Godin, G., Valois, P., Lepage, L., & Desharnais, R. (1992). Predictors of smoking behaviour: An application of Ajzen's theory of planned behaviour. *British Journal of Addiction, 87*, 1335–1343.

Greenwald, A. G., McGhee, D. E., & Schwartz, J. L. K. (1998). Measuring individual differences in implicit cognition: The implicit association test. *Journal of Personality and Social Psychology, 74*, 1464–1480.

Hagger, M. S., Chatzisarantis, N. L. D., & Biddle, S. J. H. (2002). A meta-analytic review of the theories of reasoned action and planned behavior in physical activity: Predictive validity and the contribution of additional variables. *Journal of Sport and Exercise Psychology, 24*, 3–32.

Hausenblas, H. A., Carron, A. V., & Mack, D. E. (1997). Application of the theories of reasoned action and planned behavior to exercise behavior: A meta-analysis. *Journal of Sport and Exercise Psychology, 19*, 36–51.

Hovland, C. I., Janis, I. L., & Kelley, H. H. (1953). *Communication and persuasion: Psychological studies of opinion change.* New Haven, CT: Yale University Press.

Kelly, J. A., Murphy, D. A., Sikkema, K. J., McAuliffe, T. L., Roffman, R. A., Solomon, L. J., Winett, R. A., Kalichman, S. C., & the Community HIV Prevention Research Collaborative (1997). Randomised, controlled, community-level HIV-prevention intervention for sexual-risk behavior among homosexual men in US cities. *The Lancet, 350*, 1500–1505.

Kelly, J. A., St. Lawrence, J. S., Diaz, Y. E., Stevenson, L. Y., Hauth, A. C., Brasfield, T. L., Kalichman, S. C., Smith, J. E., & Andrew, M. E. (1991). HIV risk behavior reduction following intervention with key opinion leaders of population: An experimental analysis. *American Journal of Public Health, 81*, 168–171.

Kim, K., Reicks, M., & Sjoberg, S. (2003). Applying the theory of planned behavior to predict dairy product consumption by older adults. *Journal of Nutrition Education and Behavior, 35*, 294–301. (There is no citation)

Levin, P. F. (1999). Test of the Fishbein and Ajzen models as predictors of health care worker's glove use. *Research in Nursing & Health, 22*, 295–307.

Manstead, A. S. R., Proffitt, C., & Smart, J. (1983). Predicting and understanding mothers' infant-feeding intentions and behavior: Testing the theory of reasoned action. *Journal of Personality and Social Psychology, 44*, 657–671.

Mecca, A. M., Smelser, N. J., & Vasconcellos, J. (Eds.). (1989). *The social importance of self-esteem.* Berkeley, CA: University of California Press.

Norman, P., & Hoyle, S. (2004). The theory of planned behavior and breast self-examination: Distinguishing between perceived control and self-efficacy. *Journal of Applied Social Psychology, 34*, 694–708.

Orbell, S., Blair, C., Sherlock, K., & Conner, M. (2001). The theory of planned behavior and ecstasy use: Roles for habit and perceived control over taking versus obtaining substances. *Journal of Applied Social Psychology, 31*, 31–47.

Petraitis, J., Flay, B. R., & Miller, T. Q. (1995). Reviewing theories of adolescent substance use: Organizing pieces in the puzzle. *Psychological Bulletin, 117*, 67–86.

Putnam, R.D. (1911). *Making democracy work.* Princeton, NJ: Princeton University Press.

Rosenstock, I. M., Strecher, V. J., & Becker, M. H. (1994). The health belief model and HIV risk behavior change. In R. J. DiClemente & J. L. Peterson (Eds.), *Preventing AIDS: Theories and methods of behavioral interventions. AIDS prevention and mental health* (pp. 5–24). New York, NY: Plenum Press.

Schütz, H., & Six, B. (1996). How strong is the relationship between prejudice and discrimination? A meta-analytic answer. *International Journal of Intercultural Relations, 20*, 441–462.

Sheeran, P., & Orbell, S. (1998). Do intentions predict condom use? Meta-analysis and examination of six moderator variables. *British Journal of Social Psychology, 37*, 231–250.

Sheeran, P., & Taylor, S. (1999). Predicting intentions to use condoms: A meta-analysis and comparison of the theories of reasoned action and planned behavior. *Journal of Applied Social Psychology, 29*, 1624–1675.

Smetana, J. G., & Adler, N. E. (1980). Fishbein's Value x Expectancy model: An examination of some assumptions. *Personality and Social Psychology Bulletin, 6*, 89–96. (There is no cite)

Sobel, M. E. (1982). Asymptotic confidence intervals for indirect effects in structural equation models. In S. Leinhardt (Ed.), *Sociological methodology 1982* (pp. 290–312). Washington, DC: American Sociological Association.

Strecher, V. J., Champion, V. L., & Rosenstock, I. M. (1997). The health belief model and health behavior. In D. S. Gochman (Ed.), *Handbook of health behavior research 1: Personal and social determinants* (pp. 71–91). New York: Plenum Press.

Talaska, C. A., Fiske, S. T., & Chaiken, S. (2004). *Predicting discrimination: A meta-analysis of the racial attitude-behavior literature.* Unpublished manuscript.

Triandis, H. C. (1972). *The analysis of subjective culture.* New York: Wiley.

Triandis, H. C. (1977). *Interpersonal behavior.* Monterey, CA: Brooks/Cole.

Webb, T. L., & Sheeran, P. (2006). Does Changing Behavioral Intentions Engender Behavior Change? A Meta-Analysis of the Experimental Evidence. *Psychological Bulletin, 132*, 249–268.

Wicker, A. W. (1969). Attitudes versus actions: The relationship of verbal and overt behavioral responses to attitude objects. *Journal of Social Issues, 25*, 41–78.

CHAPTER 2

Distinctions Pertaining to Fishbein and Ajzen's Theory of Reasoned Action

David Trafimow

New Mexico State University

Attitude has had a long sojourn as the most important concept in social psychology. Throughout much of the history of social psychology it seemed obvious that if an attitude is a "predisposition for behavior" and one wishes to predict behavior, a good understanding of attitude is desirable. So when research accumulated in the 1930s–1960s indicating that attitude is really a rather poor predictor of behavior (e.g., see Wicker, 1969 for a review), many expressed concern, and some even questioned the utility of the attitude construct (e.g., Calder & Ross, 1973; Campbell, 1963; DeFleur & Westie, 1958; 1963; Deutscher, 1966; 1969; Ehrlich, 1969; Kelman, 1974; Rokeach, 1967; Tittle & Hill, 1967). The failure of attitudes to predict behaviors also stimulated researchers to propose hosts of "other" variables that greatly increased the degree of conceptual entropy in the field. The main person responsible for changing this state of affairs was Martin Fishbein who, in combination with Icek Ajzen, suggested some proposals that eventually became known as the *theory of reasoned action* (e.g., Ajzen & Fishbein, 1980; Fishbein, 1963; 1967; 1980; Fishbein & Ajzen, 1975; Fishbein & Hunter, 1964; Fishbein & Raven, 1962). As even critics of the theory have acknowledged (e.g., Liska, 1984), this theory was largely responsible for rescuing the attitude construct and for having "imposed some conceptual order on the mushrooming 'other' variables research of the 1960s and early 1970s, and has strongly influenced the direction of attitude-behavior research over the last decade. Indeed, a substantial portion of the research has been designed to test, extend, and apply this model to a host of research areas" (p. 62). Several decades later, it seems worthwhile to gaze back and see what has changed. In fact, a great deal has been discovered since Fishbein's original research but as Manstead and van der Pligt (1998) pointed out in their introduction to a special issue of Journal of Applied Social Psychology on the theory of reasoned action and its extensions, attitude "seems once again to be the single most indispensable construct in social psychology. Certainly, the sheer amount of published research in the 1990s and new books on attitudes and attitude-related issues point to something of a renaissance of research interest in this field" (p. 1313). Given the resurgence of interest in this domain, this seems like an appropriate time to review some of the more important distinctions that have come out of research pertaining to the theory of reasoned action.

THE "RECEIVED" THEORY OF REASONED ACTION

The theory of reasoned action was largely concerned with why researchers had often obtained low attitude-behavior correlations and it addressed the issue in two ways. In the first place, it suggests that if a researcher wishes to predict behavior from attitude, it is better to use an attitude about a behavior rather than an attitude about an object. For example, if one wishes to predict whether employers will hire Hispanics, a substantially greater correlation between attitude and hiring behavior will be obtained if attitude towards "hiring Hispanics" is measured than if attitude towards "Hispanics" is measured. Secondly, Fishbein proposed that a behavior really contains four elements—action, target, time, and context—and the attitude and behavior measures must *correspond* with regard to each element if high correlations are to be expected. Researchers in the 1970s soon found out that simply by obeying this *principle of correspondence*, they could obtain attitude-behavior correlations that were substantially greater than the ($r = .3$) barrier that existed at the time (e.g., Wicker, 1969; see Mischel, 1968 for a more general statement about personality traits as predictors of behaviors).

Fishbein and Ajzen did not stop here. Based on the premise that behavior is the result of a "reasoned" process, they placed the principle of correspondence in the context of a larger theoretical structure. Put briefly, Fishbein and Ajzen assumed that people have beliefs about the performance of behaviors and they use these beliefs to decide whether or not to perform them. The assumption is not that people necessarily make "right" decisions—only that these decisions derive from beliefs that may or may not be accurate reflections of reality. The reasoning process can be described as follows. To start, people can have two kinds of beliefs about a behavior; these are behavioral and normative beliefs. Behavioral beliefs are beliefs about the likelihood of various consequences of the behavior and normative beliefs are beliefs about the likelihood that various important others think one should or should not perform the behavior. People also have evaluations of these beliefs. Particular behavioral beliefs can be evaluated with respect to whether the consequences, if they occurred, would be good or bad. Particular normative beliefs can be evaluated with respect to how important it is to comply with various important others. People construct an attitude on the basis of the sum of the products of behavioral beliefs and evaluations of those beliefs and they construct a subjective norm on the basis of the sum of the products of normative beliefs and how much they want to comply with each normative referent. These processes can be summarized by the following equations:

$$A = \Sigma b_i e_i \qquad\qquad 1$$

where A is attitude towards the behavior, b_i is strength of belief i about a consequence of the behavior, and e_i is evaluation of belief i.

$$SN = \Sigma n_i m_i \qquad\qquad 2$$

where ΣN is subjective norm towards the behavior, n_i is strength of normative belief i, and m_i is motivation to comply with a specific normative referent referred to by i.

Given that a person has constructed an attitude (A) and a subjective norm (SN) towards the behavior by the processes described above, he or she then weights the relative importance of the attitude and the subjective norm in determining whether or not to perform the behavior. This decision is termed a *behavioral intention (BI)*. Different people might use different attitudinal or normative weights to determine a behavioral intention towards a behavior or the same person might use different attitudinal or normative weights to form behavioral intentions for different behaviors. This weighting process is described by Equation 3.

$$BI = w_1 A + w_2 SN \qquad\qquad 3$$

where BI is the strength of the intention to perform or not perform a particular behavior, w_1 is the weight for attitude (A), and w_2 is the weight for subjective norm (SN).

Finally, behavioral intention determines behavior. This is not to say that people always do what they intend; people may change their intention before performing a behavior or find that the behavior is not under their voluntary control. In summary, the theory can be described as follows:

1. People use $\Sigma b_i e_i$ to form an attitude and $\Sigma n_i m_i$ to form a subjective norm.
2. People weight their attitude and subjective norm to form a behavioral intention.
3. People do what they intend to do unless they change their intention or the behavior is not under their control.

Using the theory outlined above to provide a basic structure, the remainder of this article will focus on distinctions that are either implied by the theory or are brought up by more recent additions to the theory.

DISTINCTIONS PERTAINING TO THE ATTITUDE CONCEPT

As the most historically emphasized variable in the theory of reasoned action, attitude has been examined particularly closely. This section focuses on distinctions that derive from how attitude is conceptualized by theory of reasoned action researchers.

The Implication of the Attitude-Intention Relation for Distinguishing Levels of Behaviors

Much evidence suggests that attitude is a strong predictor of behavioral intention. For example, Ajzen and Fishbein (1970) used attitudes towards cooperating or defecting in prisoner's dilemma games to predict intentions to do so and obtained correlations of .75 and .74 in the two games. Davidson and Jaccard (1975) used attitudes towards "having a child in the next two years" to predict intentions to do so and obtained a correlation of .80. Trafimow (1996) predicted intention to "get drunk" from attitudes to do so and obtained a correlation of .83. Trafimow and Miller (1996) predicted intentions of Virginia Tech football players to perform mental practice from attitudes towards doing so and obtained a correlation of .83. Ajzen and Fishbein (1977) reviewed many more examples of large correlations between attitude and behavioral intention.

Despite the many cases of impressive attitude-intention relations, there are also many cases where attitudes and intentions are not highly correlated. Does this mean that attitudes are not such great predictors of intentions after all, or does it mean something else? It may mean something else. Specifically, despite the emphasis Fishbein and Ajzen put on having measures that correspond, the vast majority of studies have employed attitude and intention measures that do not correspond with each other (e.g., see Courneya, 1994 for a recent review). In those cases where the degree of correspondence was systematically varied, findings have consistently demonstrated that noncorrespondent measures greatly decrease attitude-intention/behavior correlations (see Ajzen & Fishbein, 1977 for a review). Consider an elegant study by Davidson and Jaccard (1975) who attempted to predict intention to "have a child in the next two years" from the following measures: (1) attitude towards "having a child in the next two years," (2) "having children," or (3) "children." The first attitude measure is highly correspondent with the intention measure; the second attitude measure is correspondent with regard to action ("have"), target ("child/children"), and context (unspecified in both the attitude and intention measure), but not time ("in the next two years" versus unspecified); and the third attitude measure is correspondent with regard to target ("child/children") and context (unspecified in both measures), but not action ("have" versus unspecified) or time ("in the next two years" versus unspecified). Consistent with Fishbein's emphasis on the importance of correspondence, the first attitude measure was highly correlated with the intention measure ($r = .80$); but the second attitude measure, which only differed from the intention measure with respect to time, was weakly correlated with intention ($r = .23$), and the third attitude measure resulted in no correlation at all with intention ($r = -.038$). Others have performed similar demonstrations with behaviors pertaining to marijuana use (Albrecht & Carpenter, 1976), drinking (Schlegel, Crawford, & Sanborn, 1977), cutting class (Rokeach & Kliejunas, 1972), participation in psychological research (Wicker & Pomazal, 1971), and nuclear war (McClenney & Neiss, 1989). Kim and Hunter (1993) performed a meta-analysis where they rated the degree to which attitude and intention measures corresponded and obtained an impressively high average correlation ($r = .87$) when highly correspondent measures were used and various sources of error (e.g., attenuation due to unreliable measures) were statistically corrected. Thus, there is a great deal of evidence that attitude is an excellent predictor of intention when the attitude and intention measures correspond with each other.

The strong empirical evidence for the importance of correspondence of measurement between attitudes and behavioral intentions has obvious implications for the measurement of these variables. Less obviously, however, the evidence suggests an important conceptual distinction, namely that behaviors at different levels of specificity really are different behaviors and should be considered as such. Not only are attitudes towards behaviors different from attitudes towards objects but attitudes towards behaviors to be performed at one time or context are different from those to be performed at another time or context. In addition, behaviors to be performed at one time or context differ from behaviors to be performed in an unspecified time or context. As an example, although many people who are couch potatoes might have a positive attitude towards their exercising, they do not have a positive attitude towards their exercising at a specific time (especially not at the present time or in the near future) and consequently they do not exercise. As another example, I have a good friend who has a positive attitude towards his quitting smoking and he has had this attitude for the past decade. Nevertheless, he still smokes because he does not have, and has never had, a positive attitude towards his quitting smoking now!

Behavioral Beliefs—How Many Matter?

Given that attitude is a strong predictor of intention, it is important to know what determines attitude. According to the theory of reasoned action, beliefs and evaluations of beliefs determine attitude (see Equation 1). For example, a person who believes that using a condom will prevent AIDS should have a more positive attitude towards doing so than a person who does not believe this, all else being equal. In fact, numerous studies (e.g., Martin & Newman, 1990; Pryor, 1990; Solomon & Annis, 1989; Stasson & Fishbein, 1990; Trafimow & Miller, 1996; see Ajzen & Fishbein, 1980 for a review) have demonstrated that attitude is well predicted from beliefs and evaluations ($\Sigma b_i e_i$). Nevertheless, the fact that beliefs and evaluations determine attitudes and behavioral intentions leaves open the question of how many beliefs people actually use to form attitudes and behavioral intentions.

To answer this question, van der Pligt and de Vries (1998a) elicited 15 beliefs about smoking from their participants and found that although an attitude measure based on the 3 most important beliefs was highly correlated with smoking status ($r = .52$), a measure based on all 15 beliefs was less correlated with smoking status ($r = .37$), and a measure based on the remaining 12 was practically uncorrelated with smoking status ($r = .06$). These data (also see Budd, 1986; van der Pligt & de Vries, 1998b) suggest that people only use a small number of most important beliefs to form an attitude about a behavior. In addition, this research suggests that Fishbein and Ajzen were wrong in assuming that there are many (as opposed to a small number of) salient beliefs that help to determine attitudes. However, an elicitation study was not conducted to ensure that all 15 beliefs used were salient to the participants, and so it is difficult to draw a firm conclusion from the findings.

Trafimow, McDonald, and Brown (2006) obtained some data bearing on both the issue about whether people use only a small or large number of salient beliefs to form an attitude about a behavior and about summation after the three most important items. These researchers presented participants with 1, 3, or 5 positive or negative statements about a political candidate and then elicited attitudes, intentions, behavioral beliefs, and evaluations about their voting for the candidate (note that the dependent variables pertain to a behavior rather than a person). Consistent with Fishbein and Hunter (1964) and Anderson and Fishbein (1965), Trafimow et al. obtained a significant 2-way interaction between the number and valence of the presented beliefs on both attitudes and intentions. In essence, attitudes and intentions were more positive when participants had been presented with more positive statements and they were more negative when participants had been presented with more negative statements. Because the fourth and fifth beliefs were less extreme than the first, second, or third ones, an averaging hypothesis or a hypothesis that the fourth and fifth beliefs do not count would suggest that these latter beliefs should not have increased voting intentions above and beyond those formed on the basis of the first three beliefs. In fact, however, the fourth and fifth beliefs did increase the extremity of voting intentions, thereby providing support for the summation hypothesis.[1] Interestingly, despite the clear evidence that 5 belief statements resulted in more extreme attitudes and intentions than 1 or 3 belief statements, the prediction of attitudes from the best 3 beliefs was just as good as from all of the beliefs. Thus, the data support the argument by van der Pligt and de Vries (1998) that the best 3 beliefs and evaluations are all that is necessary to gain optimal prediction of attitudes. However, because all 5 statements were clearly important in determining attitudes, Fishbein and Ajzen were clearly correct that several salient beliefs can determine attitudes. These data suggest that future researchers will have to distinguish between the issues of how many beliefs *determine* attitudes versus how many are necessary to *predict* attitudes.

Do 2 Negatives Equal a Positive?

If one looks carefully at Equation 1, a curious phenomenon quickly becomes apparent. Suppose a person is deciding whether or not to use a condom during sexual intercourse and considers various beliefs and evaluations on a scale from −3 to +3. For example, this person believes it is very unlikely (−3) that the behavior will result in contracting AIDS, which is a very negatively (−3) evaluated consequence. Thus, the belief-evaluation product would be −3 × −3 = +9, thereby providing quite a good reason to use a condom. In this case, as Fishbein (e.g., 1980)

---

[1]These data also contradict a potential alternative possibility that the negative statements did not cause participants to have corresponding beliefs about the target person. If this were so, then the manipulation should have been ineffective. Whether the effect of the beliefs was direct or whether people used these statements to form further beliefs is less clear.

anticipated, a low probability of a very negative consequence appropriately implies a very positive reason for performing the behavior.

But consider another scenario where a person is considering beliefs and evaluations about whether or not to eat a chocolate bar on a scale from –3 to +3. Suppose the person believes it is very unlikely (–3) that eating a chocolate bar would result in contracting AIDS, an extremely negative consequence (–3). Computing the product (–3 × –3 = +9) suggests that this belief should strongly contribute to the person's attitude to perform the behavior—a conclusion that seems intuitively implausible. Possibly this example is a bad one because this belief might be unlikely to be salient, but considering a more plausible example does not help matters very much. A person might consider it extremely unlikely (–3) that eating raw broccoli will result in more body fat (an extremely negative consequence to the type of person who would be considering eating raw broccoli!—evaluation = –3), for a product of +9. Nevertheless, it seems intuitively unlikely that this person will have an extremely positive attitude towards eating raw broccoli even if he or she is neutral with regard to other aspects of broccoli eating such as taste, cost of buying broccoli, and so on. Thus, some researchers have argued that there are behaviors for which a low probability of an extremely negative consequence is more likely to be a non-factor than a strong determinant of attitude (e.g., Bagozzi, 1984).

On the other hand, the psychological validity of the logic of the double negative is supported by Sparks et al. (1991), who reviewed 7 studies where both bipolar (allows double-negatives) and unipolar (does not allow double-negatives) scoring were used. Sparks et al. were able to make 13 comparisons between the two methodologies and 10 comparisons revealed that bipolar scoring resulted in significantly better correlations between $\Sigma b_i e_i$ and attitude (2 were nonsignificant and 1 resulted in a significantly better correlation with unipolar scoring). Thus, this research supports the psychological validity of the logic of the double negative. (The reader should note that similar logic is not assumed to apply to the formation of subjective norms.)

Trafimow and Finlay (2002) performed an experimental test of the psychological validity of the logic of the double negative by presenting participants with beliefs about three pleasant and three unpleasant consequences pertaining to each of four behaviors. They manipulated whether the beliefs were framed in a positive direction or a negative one. For example, some positively framed beliefs are "getting a tattoo is fashionable" and "getting a tattoo is painful." (Note that "positive" framing refers to the mention of the consequence, as opposed to its negation, and not to its valence.) These beliefs can be negatively framed by placing the word *not* in appropriate places, thereby rendering them as "getting a tattoo is not fashionable" and "getting a tattoo is not painful." Relevant evaluations were consistent with the belief framing; positively and negatively framed examples are "it is good/bad to be fashionable" and "it is good/bad to not be fashionable." According to the logic of the double negative, the prediction of attitudes from $\Sigma b_i e_i$ should be equally good in both the positive and negative framing conditions. To see this, consider again the positive framing example that getting a tattoo is fashionable. A person who considers this to be extremely likely (+3) and also evaluates being fashionable as extremely positive (+3) should be pushed by this belief-evaluation product (+9) in the direction of a positive attitude. The same should also be true in the negative framing condition. Our hypothetical person should consider it extremely unlikely that getting a tattoo is not fashionable (–3) and that it is extremely negative to not be fashionable (–3) for a similar belief-evaluation product as in the positive framing condition (+9).[2] In contrast to this reasoning, correlations between $\Sigma b_i e_i$ and attitude were significantly larger in the positive than negative framing conditions for all four of the behaviors tested, thereby providing a compelling case against the psychological validity of the logic of the double negative. Stated more generally, processes involving negative framing should be distinguished from those involving positive framing.

Are Evaluations Cognitive or Affective?

If one takes seriously the idea that $\Sigma b_i e_i$ is a "cognitive structure" underlying an evaluation (i.e., attitude) toward the behavior (e.g., Fishbein, 1980, p. 93), then it would seem that the attitude is "cognitive" rather than "affective."[3] In contrast, however, several researchers have performed factor analyses of items making up attitude measures and have obtained two factors rather than one, and have concluded that there is both a cognitive and affective factor (Abelson et al., 1982; Breckler, 1984; Breckler & Wiggins, 1989; Crites, Fabrigar, & Petty, 1994; Triandis, 1980). Interestingly, Fishbein (1980) anticipated this research and made an elegant argument against such an interpretation. The argument is based on three issues. Firstly, factors obtained from factor analyses have to be named, and it is debatable whether the names "affective" and "cognitive" should be used or whether the names "attitude" and "something else" should be used for the two factors. Secondly, if it could be shown that one of the factors is strongly correlated with $\Sigma b_i e_i$ and intention, whereas the other factor is not (or less so), then there is no reason to prefer an "affective/cognitive" interpretation over an "attitude/something else" interpretation; in fact, the reverse would be true. Thirdly, Fishbein actually presented a case where what seemed like an "affective" and a "cognitive" factor based on the types of items that loaded on those factors, respectively, could be more validly described as an "attitude" and "health" factor based on correlations of the factors with $\Sigma b_i e_i$ and intention.

Although Fishbein's (1980) argument is compelling, it only deals with one kind of evidence. Fishbein is clearly correct that factor analytic and correlational approaches are insufficient to demonstrate that attitudes can have both an affec-

---

[2]Of course, it is possible to assume that double negatives are generally weaker than double positives, in which case the experiment could be argued to be unfair. However, if this is assumed, then the logic of the double negative does not work, by definition, thereby rendering an experimental test to be unnecessary.

[3]Possibly the strongest argument for a single component attitude construct was made by Fishbein (1980). However, some more recent research allows for two components (e.g., Ajzen & Fishbein, 2005).

tive and cognitive component but Trafimow and Sheeran (1998) showed that an additional approach is possible. They pointed out that even if it were possible to have beliefs that were purely affective or purely cognitive, matters would not remain so very long (also see Eagly, Mladinic, & Otto, 1994). Nevertheless, they suggested that it is reasonable to assume that some beliefs are "more affective" and some are "more cognitive," which can be referred to as *affective* or *cognitive* beliefs, respectively. Trafimow and Sheeran then proposed the following *associative hypothesis* (pp. 379–380):

Suppose that a person has some affective and cognitive beliefs and has to make a decision regarding the attitude object. It should be easier to compare beliefs to each other if they are on the same dimension (e.g., affective with affective or cognitive with cognitive) than if they are on different dimensions (e.g., affective with cognitive). Consequently, people should be more likely to consider affective beliefs in relation to other affective beliefs than to consider them in relation to cognitive beliefs; and they should be more likely to consider cognitive beliefs in relation to each other than to consider them in relation to affective beliefs. In terms of associations between beliefs, the implication is that more associations should be formed between affective and other affective beliefs, and between cognitive and other cognitive beliefs, than between affective and cognitive beliefs.

In addition, Trafimow and Sheeran (1998) suggested that the associative hypothesis could apply to beliefs about behaviors as well as about objects and that there are implications of the associative hypothesis for how beliefs are retrieved. Specifically, if people write down their beliefs about a behavior, then after retrieving an affective belief they should be likely to traverse an associative pathway to activate other affective beliefs; and after retrieving a cognitive belief they should be likely to traverse an associative pathway to activate other cognitive beliefs. However, the retrieval of an affective belief should not be likely to cause the activation of a cognitive belief, nor should the retrieval of a cognitive belief be likely to cause the activation of an affective belief. Three experiments supported these predictions. Experiment 3 demonstrated that when people considered experimenter-provided beliefs in order to form a behavioral intention, they tended to retrieve affective beliefs adjacently to each other and cognitive beliefs adjacently to each other; however, this "clustering" of recalled beliefs did not happen in various control conditions where people considered the beliefs with alternative processing objectives. This finding is consistent with their argument that it is the process of forming a behavioral intention that stimulates the formation of inter-belief associations in the manner described above. Experiments 4 and 5 demonstrated that belief clustering could also be obtained when people generate their own beliefs towards a behavior with which they are familiar, when they are allowed to decide themselves which beliefs are affective or cognitive, and even when they are primed not to retrieve beliefs in this manner. Thus, the data strongly support the distinction between affective and cognitive beliefs, and therefore by implication, that attitude has an affective and cognitive component.

THE ATTITUDE-SUBJECTIVE NORM DISTINCTION

Researchers such as Miniard and Cohen (1981) and Liska (1984) have questioned whether attitudes and subjective norms are really different constructs. The evidence against and in favor of the attitude-subjective norm distinction are reviewed in the following subsections (also see Trafimow, 1998, 2000 for reviews).

Evidence Against the Attitude-Subjective Norm Distinction

Miniard and Cohen (1981) proposed an argument based on the behavioral and normative beliefs that are the presumed determinants of attitude and subjective norm, respectively. For example, consider the normative belief (belief about what a specific referent thinks I should do) that "My father thinks that I should not perform the behavior" and the behavioral belief (belief about a consequence of performing the behavior) that "Performing the behavior will cause my father to say I was wrong to perform it." Intuitively, it may seem that these beliefs are very similar to each other. Thus, if behavioral and normative beliefs are the same, then the attitude and subjective norm formed from these beliefs, respectively, must also be the same.

A second argument is based on the empirical fact that attitude and subjective norm have often been found to be highly correlated. This suggests that the attitude and subjective norm measures are really tapping into the same construct (but see Fishbein & Ajzen, 1981).

A third argument stems from findings of "crossover" effects between attitudes and subjective norms (Grube, Morgan, and McGree, 1986; Oliver & Bearden, 1985; Shimp & Kavas, 1984; Vallerand, Deshaies, Cuerrier, Pelletier, & Mongeau, 1992), which refer to the fact that paths connecting atitudes and subjective norms to each other often result from "causal modeling" approaches. One interpretation of these crossover effects is that attitudes and subjective norms affect each other (or that whatever affects attitudes affects subjective norms and/or vice versa). In contradiction to the distinction between attitude and subjective norm, however, an alternative explanation is that attitude and subjective norm are different names for the same construct. Consequently, they are correlated with each other even when other variables are taken into account.

Finally, Budd (1987) found that the strengths of the relationships between attitude, subjective norm, and other variables they are supposed to predict, change depending on the order in which they are measured. Thus, previously obtained support for the distinction might be eliminated simply by changing the order of the measures.

Evidence in Favor of the Attitude-Subjective Norm Distinction

As Fishbein and Ajzen (1981) noted, the attitude-subjective norm distinction is supported by correlations involving other variables. For example, Bowman and Fishbein (1978) and Jaccard and Davidson (1972) found that attitude and subjective norm tend to correlate more highly with intention than with each other, and sometimes predict intention independently of each other (Shepherd, 1987). Furthermore, attitude is generally more highly correlated with $\Sigma b_i e_i$ than is subjective norm, and subjective norm is generally more highly correlated with $\Sigma n_i m_i$ than is attitude (Fishbein, 1980; Fishbein & Ajzen, 1975; Trafimow & Miller, 1996). Finally, for some behaviors, intention has been shown to be positively associated with attitude but negatively associated with subjective norm (Taylor & Todd, 1995). An assertion that attitude and subjective norm are different names for the same construct does not easily explain these patterns of correlations.

A second line of evidence concerns variations in the size of attitude-intention and subjective norm-intention correlations as a function of individual differences. In research that will be discussed later in more detail, several findings suggest that the pattern of attitude-intention and subjective-norm intention correlations changes differentially depending on a variety of individual difference measures (e.g., Arie, Durand, & Bearden, 1979; Bagozzi, Baumgartner, & Yi, 1992; Miller & Grush, 1986; Trafimow & Finlay, 1996). If attitudes and subjective norms were merely different names for the same construct, then any individual difference variable that moderates the attitude-intention correlation should similarly moderate the subjective norm-intention correlation.

A third kind of evidence involves experimental manipulations of variables that affect the relations between attitudes, subjective norms, and behavioral intentions. If it could be shown that some behaviors are under attitudinal control (AC behaviors) and some are under normative control (NC behaviors), then the attitude-subjective norm distinction would receive strong support. In fact, researchers have been using multiple regression paradigms for decades where attitudes and subjective norms were used to predict behavioral intentions. In those cases where attitudes acquired large beta weights the behaviors were assumed to be mostly under attitudinal control and in those cases where subjective norms acquired large beta weights the behaviors were assumed to be mostly under normative control. However, it was not until recently that the distinction between AC and NC behaviors was demonstrated experimentally. Trafimow and Fishbein (1994a) primed or manipulated attitudes (in three experiments) towards behaviors that had, on the basis of previous multiple regression studies, been determined to be of the AC or NC variety. They predicted that priming or manipulating attitudes should have a large effect on intentions to perform AC behaviors but that the effect should be significantly attenuated when the attitudes pertained to NC behaviors. The results from all three experiments confirmed the distinction between AC and NC behaviors. Furthermore, they (Trafimow & Fishbein, 1994b) performed an analogous set of experiments showing that manipulations designed to affect subjective norms had a significantly greater effect on intentions to perform NC than AC behaviors.

Finally, Trafimow and Fishbein (1995) tested explicitly the organization of behavioral and normative beliefs presumed to underlie the formation of attitudes and subjective norms, respectively. They argued that if behavioral beliefs are compared to each other to form an attitude, and normative beliefs are compared to each other to form a subjective norm, then behavioral beliefs should become associated with each other and normative beliefs should become associated with each other. However, because behavioral and normative beliefs are not necessarily compared to each other, there is less reason for associations between behavioral and normative beliefs to develop. When people later retrieve their beliefs, the retrieval process should be a function of the pattern of associations that previously had been forged. They should be able to traverse associative pathways from behavioral beliefs to other behavioral beliefs and from normative beliefs to other normative beliefs; but not as easily from behavioral beliefs to normative beliefs nor from normative beliefs to behavioral beliefs. Consequently, behavioral beliefs should tend to be retrieved together, normative beliefs should tend to be retrieved together, and so people's recall protocols should be clustered by belief type. Three experiments resulted in findings that supported the hypothesis.

Overall, then, the evidence favors the attitude-subjective norm distinction. Although there is correlational evidence both for and against the distinction, the experimental evidence is clearly in support of the distinction. To be sure, the distinction between behavioral and normative beliefs may be philosophically untenable (Miniard & Cohen, 1981 but see Fishbein & Ajzen, 1981 for a response) but the simple fact of the matter is that people make the distinction anyway. In addition, several other variables have been shown to affect whether attitudes or subjective norms are the primary determinants of behaviors, and these will be discussed in a later section.

WEIGHTING THE DETERMINANTS OF BEHAVIORAL INTENTIONS

Given that attitudes and subjective norms jointly determine behavioral intentions, what influences their relative importance? This section explores the effects of behavior type, person type, and self-accessibility on how attitude and subjective norm are weighted.

Behavior Type

Stasson and Fishbein (1990) measured attitudes, subjective norms, and behavioral intentions to wear seat belts in either relatively safe or risky driving conditions. Under safe conditions, attitudes were a much better predictor of intentions than were subjective norms. However, under risky conditions, the reverse was true. Therefore, one variable that affects how predictors of intentions are weighted is the type of behavior under investigation; it is useful to distinguish between attitudinally versus normatively controlled behaviors. Consistent with the earlier discussion of the components of a behavior, two behaviors with the same action (wearing), target (seat belts), and time (unspecified) were nevertheless very different in terms of what variables best predicted them; a difference in context (safe versus risky context) was sufficient to completely reverse whether attitudes or subjective norms were the best predictor. Countless other studies have also shown that the relative ability of attitudes versus subjective norms to predict behavioral intentions varies widely across behaviors (e.g., Finlay, Trafimow, & Jones, 1997; Finlay, Trafimow, & Moroi, 1999; Trafimow & Finlay, 1996).

Person Type

Meta-analyses (Farley et al., 1981; Kraus, 1995) have demonstrated repeatedly that greater attitude beta weights than subjective norm beta weights are obtained for the vast majority of behaviors, though the unique contribution of subjective norms to behavioral intentions is usually statistically significant. Trafimow and Finlay (1996) suggested that there were at least two explanations for the small but significant normative effect. One possibility is that most behaviors are primarily under attitudinal control and only slightly under normative control. However, a second possibility is that the majority of *people* are attitudinally controlled across a wide range of behaviors but there is an important minority of people who are under normative control across a wide range of behaviors. It is the presence of these normatively controlled people in most participant samples that causes the small but significant normative effects that are usually obtained. Although the distinction between different types of behaviors has been demonstrated clearly (see previous section), Trafimow and Finlay also wanted to validate the second hypothesis that people, as well as behaviors, could be under attitudinal or normative control. To do this, they attempted to meet three criteria. First, it was important to demonstrate that attitudes and/or subjective norms could predict intentions for a wide variety of behaviors using within-participants analyses. Otherwise it makes no sense to attempt to distinguish whether people are attitudinally or normatively controlled across a set of behaviors. Secondly, there must be a subset of the participant sample for whom subjective norms are a better predictor than attitudes of intentions. Finally, the relationship between subjective norms and intentions should vary predictably with some other individual difference variable.

To meet these criteria, Trafimow and Finlay measured attitudes, subjective norms, and intentions to perform 30 behaviors. Consistent with previous research, traditional between-participants analyses showed that intentions were predicted well from attitudes and subjective norms (median $R = .69$) and larger attitude than subjective norm beta weights were obtained for 29 of the 30 behaviors. Attitudes and subjective norms were also excellent within-participants predictors of intentions (median $R = .82$). However, subjective norms were better within-participants predictors than were attitudes for 21% of the sample. When these normatively controlled people were removed from the sample, and traditional between-participants analyses were again performed, the median unique effect of subjective norms on intentions dropped to .00. Finally, the tendency for people to be under normative control across the set of behaviors (indicated by within-participants normative regression weights) correlated with an outside variable—namely, the tendency for people to be interdependent as opposed to independent (Singelis, 1994). In summary, all of the criteria were met, and the findings were replicated in additional studies (Finlay, Trafimow, & Jones, 1997; Finlay, Trafimow, & Moroi, 1999).

Other individual differences also have been shown to be associated with whether attitudes or subjective norms are better predictors of intentions. Miller and Grush (1986) found that people who were both high in private self-consciousness and low in self-monitoring displayed high attitude-behavior correspondence but people with other combinations of these traits displayed high subjective norm-behavior correspondence. Arie, Durand, and Bearden (1979) found that opinion leaders' (those whose opinions others seek for advice about products and services) intentions to patronize credit unions were under attitudinal control, but non-leaders' intentions were under normative control. Finally, Bagozzi, Baumgartner, and Yi (1992) found a greater attitude-intention than subjective norm-intention correlation for action-oriented people but the reverse was true for state-oriented people. In summary, although attitudinal versus normative control has been studied less in the context of individual difference variables than in the context of different types of behaviors, a great deal of support has accumulated showing that both categories of variables can have important effects on the relative weights of attitudes and subjective norms.

The Accessibility of the Private and Collective Selves

Before explaining how the accessibility of the private and collective selves influence relative weights of attitudes and subjective norms, a brief description of the distinction between these two selves is necessary. Trafimow, Triandis, and Goto (1991) argued that there are at least two ways of interpreting previous findings that people from individualistic cultures tend to describe themselves in terms of traits, states, and behaviors (private self-cognitions) whereas people from collectivist cultures are more likely than individualists to describe themselves in terms of group memberships (collective self-cognitions) (see Triandis, 1989 for a review). Firstly, people may have only one location in memory where self-cognitions are stored, but culture affects the relative number of private versus collective self-cognitions stored there. Secondly, people may have a *private self* where private self-cognitions are stored and a *collective self* where collective self-cognitions are stored; culture affects the relative accessibility of the private self versus the collective self. They also suggested two paradigms for distinguishing between these two possibilities, which they termed the "one-basket" and "two-baskets" theories, respectively.

One paradigm makes use of priming manipulations to increase the accessibility of the private or collective self. The one-basket theory would predict that because self-cognitions are not organized by type of self-concept, such a manipulation should not differentially affect the retrieval of private and collective self-cognitions. In contrast, according to the two-baskets theory, priming the private self should increase the retrieval of private self-cognitions whereas priming the collective self should increase the retrieval of collective self-cognitions.

Secondly, conditional probability analyses could be performed. According to the one-basket theory, each self-cognition is retrieved independently. Thus, the probability of retrieving a self-cognition of a particular type does not depend upon which type of self-cognition was previously retrieved. In contrast, according to the two-baskets theory, self-cognitions are *not* retrieved independently. Suppose someone retrieves a private self-cognition. This private self-cognition must have been stored in the private self, which means that this self must have been accessible. But if the private self was accessible, then the next self-cognition retrieved should have been another private self-cognition. In general, this theory predicts that the probability of someone retrieving a particular type of self-cognition, given that a similar type was retrieved previously, should be greater than if a different type of self-cognition had been retrieved previously. In fact, both predictions were confirmed in two experiments (Trafimow, Triandis, & Goto, 1991): (a) priming the private self increased the proportion of private self-cognitions retrieved whereas priming the collective self increased the proportion of collective self-cognitions retrieved and (b) the probability of retrieval of a private self-cognition was greater following another private self-cognition than a collective self-cognition, and the probability of retrieval of a collective self-cognition was greater following another collective self-cognition than a private self-cognition. Similar findings were obtained in a study performed in Hong Kong (Trafimow, Silverman, Fan, & Law, 1997) and using Native American participants (Trafimow & Smith, 1998). There is now a large literature in support of the two-baskets theory that includes evidence from a variety of paradigms (see Triandis & Trafimow, 2001 for a review).

Let us now consider the relations between the private and collective selves on the one hand, and how attitudes and subjective norms are weighted on the other. As I pointed out in the previous section, Trafimow and Finlay (1996) found that the tendency for participants to use subjective norms was related to their scores on a measure of interdependence. They suggested that having a strong (or accessible) collective self causes people to give subjective norms more weight. Conversely, having an accessible private self should cause attitudes to gain more weight. Ybarra and Trafimow (1998) tested this idea by priming the private or collective self in three experiments. In each experiment priming the private self caused attitudes to acquire a larger beta weight than subjective norms whereas priming the collective self reversed these beta weights. Thus, the accessibility of the private or collective self can have a powerful effect on the extent to which attitudes or subjective norms determine behaviors.

CONCLUSION

The contributions of theory of reasoned action research to social psychology are clear, distinctive, and unmistakable. Because of these contributions, social psychologists can do a much better job of measuring attitudinal variables, they can predict behavior at a level that used to be unthinkable, and this thinking continues to generate a great deal of research as investigators continue to look for variables that account for additional variance in behavioral intentions or behaviors. Less obvious, but equally important, this work has paved the way for researchers to discern some important distinctions that otherwise would be likely to have remained undiscovered. Some of these distinctions, such as the attitude-subjective norm distinction, come directly from the theory of reasoned action. Other distinctions are implied by the measurement model that Fishbein and Ajzen included in the theory. For example, behaviors with the same action may nevertheless differ with regard to target, time, or context and they should consequently be considered to be different behaviors. Yet other distinctions come out of a critical evaluation of the theory and even contradict the theory. One such distinction is between the affective and cognitive components of attitudes. A second distinction is between positively or negatively framed beliefs; because positive framing results in better attitude prediction than does negative framing, this distinction implies that there is a problem with the logic of the double negative. Thus, although many of the distinctions that pertain to the theory support it, some of them may cause a problem for the theory.

Ironically, in evaluating the extent of the theory of reasoned action's contribution, perhaps the best argument for its heuristic value is provided by the distinctions that contradict it. Here is why. Some of the most publicized criticisms of the theory feature the idea that it is not falsifiable (see Greve, 2001 for a recent example). The fact that some empirically verified distinctions actually go against the theory provides the best refutation of this criticism. What better evidence could there be that the theory of reasoned action is falsifiable than the fact that some aspects of it have actually been falsified?

In response to this argument, one might claim that if the theory has been falsified, then it is simply wrong, and therefore not an important contribution. But this argument misses an important point about where the value of theories resides. Few, if any, of the important theories in the history of science are completely true. Physicists, for example, are well aware that Newton's theory of motion is inaccurate in several ways yet Newton is widely considered to be the greatest physicist in history. For another example, consider Darwin's theory of evolution. Because the existence of genes was unknown at the time, Darwin failed to include genetics in his theory, and yet biologists continue to look upon his theory with reverence. Notwithstanding the distinctions that they failed to make, Newton's and Darwin's theories dominated their areas for a long time, and generated a great deal of research. Thus, the heuristic value of these theories is exemplified by research that disconfirmed their predictions as well as by research that confirmed them. Judged in this light, the theory of reasoned action was the beginning of a program of research that has been demonstrated to be one of the most successful in the history of social psychology.

REFERENCES

Abelson, R. P., Kinder, D. R., Peters, M. D., & Fiske, S. T. (1982). Affective and semantic components in political person perception. *Journal of Personality and Social Psychology, 42*, 619–630.

Ajzen, I., & Fishbein, M. (1970). The prediction of behavior from attitudinal and normative variables. *Journal of Experimental Social Psychology, 6*, 466–487.

Ajzen, I., & Fishbein, M. (1977). Attitude-behavior relations: A theoretical analysis and review of empirical research. *Psychological Bulletin, 84*, 888–918.

Ajzen, I., & Fishbein, M. (1980). *Understanding attitudes and predicting social behavior.* Englewood Cliffs, NJ: Prentice-Hall.

Ajzen, I., & Fishbein, M. (2005). The influence of attitudes on behavior. In D. Albarracin, B. T. Johnson, & M. P. Zanna (Eds.), *The handbook of attitudes* (pp. 173–221). Mahwah, NJ: Erlbaum.

Albrecht, S. L., & Carpenter, K. E. (1976). Attitudes as predictors of behavior versus behavior intentions: A convergence of research traditions. *Sociometry, 39*, 1–10.

Anderson, L. R., & Fishbein, M. (1965). Prediction of attitude from the number, strength, and evaluative aspect of beliefs about the attitude object: A comparison of summation and congruity theories. *Journal of Personality and Social Psychology, 2,* 437–443.

Arie, O. G., Durand, R. M., & Bearden, W. O. (1979). Attitudinal and normative dimensions of opinion leaders and nonleaders. *The Journal of Psychology, 101,* 305–312.

Bagozzi, R. P. (1984). Expectancy-value attitude models: An analysis of critical measurement issues. *International Journal of Research in Marketing 1,* 295–310.

Bagozzi, R. P., Baumgartner, H., & Yi, Y. (1992). State versus action orientation and the theory of reasoned action: An application to coupon usage. *Journal of Consumer Research, 18,* 505–518.

Bowman, C. H., & Fishbein, M. (1978). Understanding public reactions to energy proposals: An application of the Fishbein Model. *Journal of Applied Social Psychology, 8,* 319–340.

Breckler, S. J. (1984). Empirical validation of affect, behavior, and cognition as distinct components of attitude. *Journal of Personality and Social Psychology, 47,* 1191–1205.

Breckler, S. J., & Wiggins, E. C. (1989). Affect versus evaluation in the structure of attitudes. *Journal of Experimental Social Psychology, 25,* 253–271.

Budd, R. J. (1986). Predicting cigarette use: The need to incorporate measures of salience in the theory of reasoned action. *Journal of Applied Social Psychology, 16,* 663–685.

Budd, R. J. (1987). Response bias and the action. *Social Cognition, 5,* 95–107.

Calder, B. J., & Ross, M. (1973). *Attitudes and behavior.* Morristown, NJ.: General Learning Press.

Campbell, D. T. (1963). Social attitudes and other acquired behavioral dispositions. In S. Koch (Ed.), *Psychology: A study of a science* (Vol. 6). New York: McGraw-Hill.

Courneya, K. S. (1994). Predicting repeated behavior from intention: The issue of scale correspondence. *Journal of Applied Social Psychology, 24,* 580–594.

Crites, S. L., Fabrigar, L. R., & Petty, R. E. (1994). Measuring the affective and cognitive properties of attitudes: Conceptual and methodological issues. *Personality and Social Psychology Bulletin, 20,* 619–634.

Davidson, A. R., & Jaccard, J. J. (1975). Population psychology: A new look at an old problem. *Journal of Personality and Social Psychology, 31,* 1073–1082.

DeFleur, M. L., & Westie, F. R. (1958). Verbal attitudes and overt acts: An experiment on the salience of attitudes. *American Sociological Review, 23,* 667–673.

DeFleur, M. L., & Westie, F. R. (1963). Attitude as a scientific concept. *Social Forces, 42,* 17–31.

Deutscher, I. (1966). Words and deeds. *Social Problems, 13,* 235–254.

Deutscher, I. (1969). Looking backward: Case studies on the progress of methodology in sociological research. *American Sociologist, 4,* 35–41.

Eagly, A. H., Mladinic, A., & Otto, S. (1994). Cognitive and affective bases of attitudes toward social groups and social policies. *Journal of Experimental Social Psychology, 30,* 113–137.

Ehrlich, H. J. (1969). Attitudes, behavior, and the intervening variables. *American Sociologist, 4,* 29–34.

Farley, J. U., Lehmann, D. R., & Ryan, M. J. (1981). Generalizing from "imperfect" replication. *Journal of Business, 54,* 597–610.

Finlay, K. A., Trafimow, D., & Jones, D. (1997). Predicting health behaviors: Between-subjects and within-subjects analyses. *Journal of Applied Social Psychology, 27,* 2015–2031.

Finlay, K. A., Trafimow, D., & Moroi, E. (1999). The importance of subjective norms on intentions to perform health behaviors. *Journal of Applied Social Psychology.*

Fishbein, M. (1963). An investigation of the relationships between beliefs about an object and the attitude toward that object. *Human Relations, 16,* 233–239.

Fishbein, M. (1967). Attitude and the prediction of behavior. In M. Fishbein (Ed.), *Readings in attitude theory and measurement* (pp. 477–492). New York: John Wiley.

Fishbein, M. (1980). Theory of reasoned action: Some applications and implications. In H. Howe and M. Page (Eds.), *Nebraska Symposium on Motivation, 1979* (pp. 65–116). Lincoln, NE: University of Nebraska Press.

Fishbein, M., & Ajzen, I. (1975). *Belief, attitude, intention and behavior: An introduction to theory and research.* Reading, MA: Addison-Wesley.

Fishbein, M., & Ajzen, I. (1981). On construct validity: A critique of Miniard and Cohen's paper. *Journal of Experimental Social Psychology, 17,* 340–350.

Fishbein, M., & Hunter, R. (1964). Summation versus balance in attitude organization and change. *Journal of Abnormal and Social Psychology, 69,* 505–510.

Fishbein, M., & Raven, B. H. (1962). The AB scales: An operational definition of belief and atitude. *Human Relations, 15,* 35–44.

Greve, W. (2001). Traps and gaps in action explanation: Theoretical problems of a psychology of human action. *Psychology Review, 108,* 435–451.

Grube, J. W., Morgan, M., & McGree, S.T. (1986). Attitudes and normative beliefs as predictors of smoking intentions and behaviours: A test of three models. *British Journal of Social Psychology, 25,* 81–93.

Jaccard, J. J., & Davidson, A. R. (1972). Toward an understanding of family planning behaviors: An initial investigation. *Journal of Applied Social Psychology, 2,* 228–235.

Kelman, H. C. (1974). Attitudes are alive and well and gainfully employed in the sphere of action. *American Psychologist, 29,* 310–324.

Kim, M., & Hunter, J. E. (1993). Relationships among attitudes, behavioral intentions, and behavior: A meta-analysis of past research: II. *Communication Research, 20,* 331–364.

Kraus, S. J. (1995). Attitudes and the prediction of behavior: A meta-analysis of the empirical literature. *Personality and Social Psychology Bulletin, 21,* 58–75.

Liska, A. E. (1984). A critical examination of the causal structure of the Fishbein/Ajzen model. *Social Psychology Quarterly, 47,* 61–74.

Manstead, A. S. R., & van der Pligt, J. (1998). Should we expect more from expectancy-value models of attitude and behavior? *Journal of Applied Social Psychology, 28,* 131–1316.

Martin, G. L., Newman, I. M. (1990). Women as motivators in the use of safety belts. *Health Values, Health Behavior, Education and Promotion, 14,* 37–47.

McClenney, L., & Neiss, R. (1989). Psychological responses to the threat of nuclear war. *Journal of Applied Social Psychology, 19,* 1239–1267.

Miller, L. E., & Grush, J. E. (1986). Individual differences in attitudinal versus normative determination of behavior. *Journal of Experimental Social Psychology, 22,* 190–202.

Miniard, L. E., & Cohen, J. B. (1981). An examination of the Fishbein behavioral intentions model's concept and measures. *Journal of Experimental Social Psychology, 17,* 309–329.

Mischel, W. (1968). *Personality and assessment.* New York: John Wiley & Sons.

Oliver, R. L., & Bearden, W. O. (1985). Crossover effects in the theory of reasoned action: A moderating influence attempt. *Journal of Consumer Research, 12,* 324–340.

Pryor, B. W. (1990). Predicting and explaining intentions to participate in continuing education: An application of the theory of reasoned action. *Adult Education Quarterly, 40,* 146–157.

Rokeach, M. (1967). Attitude change and behavior change. *Public Opinion Quarterly, 30,* 529–550.

Rokeach, M., & Kliejunas, P. (1972). Behavior as a function of attitude-toward-object and attitude-toward-situation. *Journal of Personality and Social Psychology, 22,* 194–201.

Schlegel, R. P., Crawford, C. A., & Sanborn, M. D. (1977). Correspondence and mediational properties of the Fishbein model: An application to adolescent alcohol use. *Journal of Experimental Social Psychology, 13,* 421–430.

Shepherd, G. J. (1987). Individual differences in the relationship between attitudinal and normative determinants of behavioral intent. *Communication Monographs, 54,* 221–230.

Shimp, T. A., & Kavas, A. (1984). The theory of reasoned action applied to coupon usage.

Journal of Consumer Research, 11, 795–809.

Singelis, T.M. (1994). The measurement of independent and interdependent self-construals. *Personality and Social Psychology Bulletin, 20*, 580–591.

Solomon, K. E., & Annis, H. M. (1989). Development of a scale to measure outcome expectancy in alcoholics. *Cognitive Therapy and Research, 13*, 409–421.

Sparks, P., Hedderley, D., & Shepherd, R. (1991). Expectancy-value models of attitudes: a note on the relationship between theory and methodology. *European Journal of Social Psychology, 21*, 261–271.

Stasson, M., & Fishbein, M. (1990). The relation between perceived risk and preventive action: Within-subjects analysis of perceived driving risk and intentions to wear seat belts. *Journal of Applied Social Psychology, 20*, 1541–1557.

Taylor, S., & Todd, P. (1995). An integrated model of waste management behavior: A test of household recycling and composting intentions. *Environment and Behavior, 27*, 603–630.

Tittle, C. R., & Hill, R. J. (1967). Attitude measurement and prediction of behavior: An evaluation of conditions and measurement techniques. *Sociometry, 30*, 1999–213.

Trafimow, D. (1996). The importance of attitudes in the prediction of college students' intentions to drink. *Journal of Applied Social Psychology, 26*, 2167–2188.

Trafimow, D. (1998). Attitudinal and normative processes in health behavior. *Psychology and Health, 13*, 307–317.

Trafimow, D. (2000). A theory of attitudes, subjective norms, and private versus collective self-concepts. In D. J. Terry and M. A. Hogg (Eds.), *Attitudes, behavior, and social context: The role of norms and group membership*. Lawrence Erlbaum Associates.

Trafimow, D., & Fitlay, K.A. (2002). The prediction of attitudes from beliefs and evaluation: The logic of the double negative. *British Journal of Social Psychology, 41*, 77–86.

Trafimow, D., & Finlay, K. (1996). The importance of subjective norms for a minority of people. *Personality and Social Psychology Bulletin, 22*, 820–828.

Trafimow, D., & Fishbein, M. (1994a). The importance of risk in determining the extent to which attitudes affect intentions to wear seat belts. *Journal of Applied Social Psychology, 24*, 1–11.

Trafimow, D., & Fishbein, M. (1994b). The moderating effect of behavior type on the subjective norm-behavior relationship. *Journal of Social Psychology, 134*, 755–763.

Trafimow, D., & Fishbein, M. (1995). Do people really distinguish between behavioural and normative beliefs? *British Journal of Social Psychology, 34*, 257–266.

Trafimow, D., McDonald, J., Brown, J., Castro, J., & Frank, R. (2006). The importance of consistency in evaluating beliefs: A feedback effect of attitudes on evaluations of beliefs. Submitted Manuscript.

Trafimow, D., & Miller, A. (1996). Predicting and understanding mental practice. *The Journal of Social Psychology, 136*, 173–180.

Trafimow, D., & Sheeran, P. (1998). Some tests of the distinction between cognitive and affective beliefs. *Journal of Experimental Social Psychology, 34*, 378–397.

Trafimow, D., Silverman, E. S., Fan, R. M., and Law, J. S. F. (1997). The effects of language and priming on the relative accessibility of the private self and the collective self. *Journal of Cross-Cultural Psychology, 28*, 107–123.

Trafimow, D., & Smith, M.D. (1998). An extension of the two-baskets theory to Native Americans. *European Journal of Social Psychology, 28*, 1015–1019.

Trafimow, D., Triandis, H. C., & Goto, S. G. (1991). Some tests of the distinction between the private self and the collective self. *Journal of Personality and Social Psychology, 60*, 649–655.

Triandis, H. C. (1980). Values, attitudes, and interpersonal behavior. In H. Howe & M. Page (Eds.), *Nebraska symposium on motivation, 1979*, Lincoln, NE: University of Nebraska Press.

Triandis, H. C. (1989). The self and social behavior in differing cultural contexts. *Psychological Review, 96*, 269–289.

Triandis, H. C., & Trafimow, D. (2001). Cross-national prevalence of collectivism. In Constantine Sedikides & Marilynn Brewer (Eds.), *Individual self, relational self, and collective self.* Philadelphia: Taylor & Francis.

Vallerand, R. J., Deshaies, P., Cuerrier, J. R., Pelletier, L. G., & Mongeau, C. (1992). Ajzen and Fishbein's theory of reasoned action as applied to moral behavior: A confirmatory analysis. *Journal of Personality and Social Psychology, 62,* 98–109.

van der Pligt, J., & de Vries, N. K. (1998a). Belief importance in expectancy-value models of attitudes. *Journal of Applied Social Psychology, 28,* 1339–1354.

van der Pligt, J., & de Vries, N. K. (1998b). Expectancy-value models of health behaviour: the role of salience and anticipated affect. *Psychology and Health, 13,* 298–305.

Wicker, A. W. (1969). Attitudes versus actions: The relationship of verbal and overt behavioral responses to attitude objects. *Journal of Social Issues, 25,* 41–78.

Wicker, A. W., & Pomazal, R. J. (1971). The relationship between attitudes and behavior as a function of specificity of attitude object and presence of a significant person during assessment conditions. *Representative Research in Social Psychology, 2,* 26–31.

Ybarra, O., & Trafimow, D. (1998). How priming the private self or collective self affects the relative weights of attitudes or subjective norms. *Personality and Social Psychology Bulletin, 24,* 362–370.

CHAPTER 3

The Role of Discrete Emotions in the Theory of Reasoned Action and Its Successors: Quitting Smoking in Young Adults

Joseph N. Cappella

University of Pennsylvania

The Theory or Reasoned Action and its successors, the Theory of Planned Behavior (TPB; Ajzen, 1991, 2002) and the Integrated Model (IM) of behavior change (Fishbein et al., 2002) have spawned a wide array of research in advertising, politics, health, and other arenas. Although the application of these theories has been primarily to model the routes to behavior and behavior change, they have invited important thinking about the selection of interventions as well (Fishbein & Cappella, 2006; Hornik & Wolf, 1999). The application of the IM to select interventions depends in large measure on the routes to intention and behavior identified by the theory and formative research identifying which routes are the strongest predictors of intention and behavior. If an important route to intention and behavior is absent from the theory, then that route cannot be selected as a route to intervene to achieve a particular change.

In this chapter, I argue that models, such as the IM, have downplayed the direct role of discrete emotions in accounting for intention and behavior. Both conceptual arguments and some evidence for rethinking this conclusion are offered. The implications of including emotions for the development of interventions are considered.

THE ROLE OF DISCRETE EMOTIONS

Research on risk information and its impact on health decisions has been criticized on a variety of grounds, including its ineffectiveness in predicting behavior change. Positive and negative consequences that are typically employed as predictors of behavioral intention and behavior are derived through procedures that often produce deliberative, rational consequences of a behavioral action rather than specific emotional consequences.

This view has guided our research in profitable ways, but it has limits. In this section the argument is made that specific, anticipated emotions can also function like consequences. Emotional consequences of a behavior, when treated as anticipated emotions associated with the behavior, have the capacity to make independent contributions to behavioral intentions. The emotional consequences of an action may be as important a set of predictors of behavioral intentions as more deliberative consequences in some circumstances. This is true even though the emotional consequences are not typically produced during the elicitation stage of research on consequences associated with healthy and unhealthy behaviors.

Conceptualizing risk in terms of positive and negative discrete emotional consequences associated with healthy and unhealthy behaviors can add substantial variance explained to models of behavior change and open routes to persuasion that models based only on rational, deliberative consequences cannot.

Work by Loewenstein, Weber, Hsee, and Welch (2001) considers the role of emotional and rational processes in decision making. They identify two broad views of emotion in decision making: one called *consequentialist* and the other *emotion-as-feeling*.

The consequentialist view implies that behavioral intentions result from cognitive evaluations in just the way they are described in theories such as reasoned action (Fishbein & Ajzen, 1975) and its extensions (Fishbein et al., 1992)—that is, anticipated outcomes and the subjective probabilities that those anticipated outcomes are going to actually take place combine to produce a disposition toward action. Emotion is a component in all consequentialist views, but emotion simply attends to or goes hand in hand with the consequentialist or more cognitive points of view. Emotions in this view are seen as both a consequence of consideration of

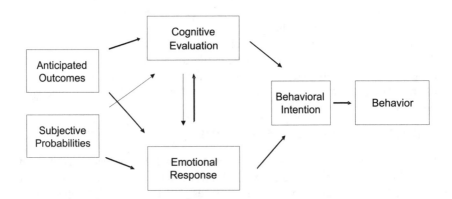

FIGURE 3–1. The typical role of emotion in consequentialist theories according to Loewenstein et al. (2001).

other expected outcomes and of the attitude that is formed by them, as well as a contributor to that attitude. However, emotions per se have no independent, direct effect on intentions or behavior. This is the old argument that cognitions and emotions are inseparable and that when people activate cognitive dispositions, they are also activating emotional dispositions as well. Emotions attend cognitions but exert no distinctive causal force on consequences such as intentions or behaviors, as is illustrated in Figure 3–1.

The feeling as emotion viewpoint goes beyond this claim, suggesting that it is not just the cognitive evaluation that has an effect on behavioral intention with emotion an associate of cognition, but rather that there is a wholly separate path through which emotions work to predict behavioral intention. This emotional path would either support the cognitive evaluation or oppose it, providing a causal force in an opposite direction.

The hypothesis is that there are two distinct routes to behavioral intention, one through emotion and one through cognitive consequences. The relevant emotions for this argument are anticipated emotions—what emotional consequence one would expect if one engaged in a recommended behavior. This hypothesis assumes that anticipated emotions matter, not just emotions that are contemporaneous with the behavior or even the behavioral intention. One argument for positing alternative pathways is based on studies from brain physiology (LeDoux & Phelps, 2000). A second is that anticipated emotion and rational consequences have separate, distinct predictors (Lowenstein et al., 2001).

This hypothesis was tested using standard predictors from the IM (and other consequentialist theories) on quitting smoking. Previous research indicates that social normative approval, personal efficacy, past smoking history, and behavioral beliefs and attitudes should affect smoking intentions (Skara, Sussman, & Dent, 2001; Choi, Gilpin, Farkas, & Pierce, 2001 Hennrikus, Jeffrey, & Lando, 1995). Our study extended these predictions to quitting intentions. To test the emotion-as-feeling prediction, anticipated emotional reactions to quitting were added. We hypothesized that unique variance would be added to the intention to quit once typical predictors such as attitude, social normative pressure, personal efficacy, and past smoking history were taken into account.

DATA

Data come from a nationally representative sample of smokers. The sample was obtained via Random Digital Dialing (RDD) telephone survey conducted May–June 2002 by Schulman, Ronca & Bucuvalas, Inc. on behalf of the University of Pennsylvania. The sample included 450 young adults, ages 18 to 25, who had smoked at least one whole cigarette in the previous six months.

MEASURES

Two measures of *intention* were obtained. Intention to *try* to quit smoking completely and permanently in the next three months was assessed, and a similar question asked how likely it is that the person *will* quit smoking completely and permanently in the next three months. Only the first is discussed in this chapter.

Attitude towards trying to quit smoking completely and permanently in the next three months was measured by the average of three semantic differential items, ranging from –2 as "very bad/harmful/foolish" to +2 as "very good/ beneficial/wise."

Behavioral beliefs are the positive and negative consequences that a person thinks will occur as a result of trying to quit smoking. Behavioral beliefs were assessed by asking respondents to indicate the extent to which they thought that their trying to quit smoking would lead to 13 outcomes, such as "I would have better health" and "I would be more tense."

Subjective norms toward trying to quit smoking were measured by responses to the item, "How do you think most people important to you would feel if you quit smoking completely and permanently in the next three months?"

Self-efficacy was measured by the question, "How sure are you that you can quit smoking cigarettes completely and permanently in the next three months if you really wanted to?"

Smoking behaviors were assessed by 5 items that measured whether respondents smoked at least 100 cigarettes in their lifetime, whether they ever smoked a cigarette every day for at least a month, whether in the last 30 days they smoked at least one cigarette daily, and whether they consider themselves smokers and addicted to smoking. All items were coded either 1 for an affirmative answer or 0 for a negative one. The items were averaged into a scale (Cronbach's *alpha* = .87).[1]

Emotions toward current levels of smoking were measured by the statement, "I am going to read a list of words that some people use to describe how they feel about smoking cigarettes. Please tell me if the word describes how YOU feel about your current level of smoking." The emotion items used were *proud*, *disgusted, angry, apprehensive*, and *hopeful*. Each item was coded on a 4-point scale, ranging from 0 as "not [proud] at all" to 3 as "extremely [proud]."

Emotions toward quitting smoking were measured by the statement, "Please tell me if the word describes how YOU feel about your intention to quit smoking." The emotion items used were *proud, disgusted, angry, apprehensive*, and *hopeful*. Each item was coded on a 4-point scale, ranging from 0 as "not [proud] at all" to 3 as "extremely [proud]."

This operational definition of emotion towards quitting smoking places emotion between Lowenstein et al.'s (2001) *anticipated* and *anticipatory* (that is, concurrent) conceptualizations. If we had asked the smokers how they would feel if they quit smoking, then we would have operationalized an anticipated emotion. If

---

[1]All analyses were also run with an index made up of smoking behaviors only, excluding the perceptual measures of smoking status and smoking addiction. The three item behavioral measure had an alpha of .81. The scale of smoking behaviors produced no significant differences from those reported here using the more general scale of smoking behaviors and smoking perceptions.

we had asked smokers how they were feeling during a period of quitting, then we would have evidence about concurrent emotions. Lowenstein et al. (2001) argue that concurrent emotions are more likely to create conditions where the emotions experienced are at odds with the anticipated consequences (emotional or otherwise). In a sense, concurrent emotions have the capacity to hijack behavior, driving it in a direction that is different from the more deliberative forces of anticipated consequences.

Operationalizing emotion toward quitting as emotion about one's intention to quit is an emotional state. Certainly it is not a state that can be considered equivalent to emotions experienced while trying to stay off cigarettes during a quit attempt, but it is a state that is less hypothetical than would be produced with a question about what emotions one is likely to experience in some hypothetical quitting scenario at some future undefined time point. The result of this operational maneuver, as odd as it might seem, would be to create an independent emotional path to intention to quit over and above the more deliberative paths that are typically found in research using the TRA and its extensions.

This reasoning produces the major hypothesis. Emotions about quitting intentions will add unique variance explained to intentions to quit smoking over and above that accounted for by cognitive and normative factors, self-efficacy, and past smoking history.

RESULTS

A complete set of findings is available in Cappella, Romantan, Patterson, and Lerman (2006), but a representative set of findings is found in Table 3–1 that is not reported in their article. The key outcome is that anticipated emotions about quitting add substantial variance to the intention to quit smoking permanently in the next three months. In the specific test presented in Table 3–1, 13 behavioral beliefs are included as well as demographics, social normative pressure, self-efficacy, past smoking behavior, and sensation-seeking. Those variables account for 25% of the variance in quitting intentions. When emotions toward quitting are added, an additional 16% of the variance is explained. Pride and hope about quitting are the major predictors, and their effects remain significant even after emotions toward current smoking are entered as a block of predictors. Positive emotions that are anticipated are significant factors in intentions to quit.[2]

CONCLUSION

In this test, the conventional IM variables mattered but so did emotions about the intention to quit, and their effects were independent and substantial. These results are important because they argue for an extension of the IM model and the inclusion of anticipated emotions along with other anticipated outcomes. They also have important implications for the construction of persuasive campaigns.

---

[2]We also followed up the intention to quit a year later with the same sample. Intention was a significant predictor of reports of quitting with stronger reported intentions predicting successful quitting for the three-month period of the summer following the initial survey (see Cappella et al., 2006).

TABLE 3–1

Intention to Try to Quit: Bs, Betas, and R^2 Change for Three Blocks of Predictors (Controls, Behavioral Beliefs, and Quitting- and Smoking-Related Emotions)

DV: Intention "Try to Quit Smoking"	Model 1		Model 2	
	B	Beta	B	Beta
Constant	2.096***		2.046***	
1. Controls				
		R^2 Change .025		
2. Behavioral beliefs				
Have a good time with one's non-smoking friends	-.041	-.056	-.037	-.051
Have a good time with one's smoking friends	.003	.005	.003	.005
Do less harm to people around	.039	.069	.038	.066
Have trouble keeping one's weight down	-.013	-.022	-.000	-.001
Be more tense	-.049#	-.086	-.057#	-.099
Easier to exercise or play sports	.046	.073	.039	.062
Have better health	.028	.031	.039	.043
Decrease one's chances of getting heart disease	.038	.049	.046	.059
Decrease one's chances of getting cancer	-.005	-.006	-.037	-.041
Show one's independence	.167	.026	010	.017
Show one cannot be manipulated by tobacco companies	-.024	-.042	-.013	-.023
Have nothing to do when bored	.027	.048	.029	.051
Respect oneself more	.038	.060	.027	.043
Self-Efficacy	.123**	.145	.120**	.141
Perceived Social Norms	.040	.044	.059	.065
Sensation Seeking	-.051	-.030	-.037	-.022
Smoking Behavior Index	-.281**	-.124	-.276*	-.119
		R^2 Change .252***		
3. Quitting-Related Emotions				
Proud	.195***	.305	.183***	.287
Disgusted	.089	.076	.039	.033
Angry	-.034	-.023	.005	.004
Apprehensive	.031	.035	.047	.053
Hopeful	.182***	.249	.176***	.241
		R^2 Change .165***		
4. Smoking-Related Emotions				
Proud			.079	.056
Disgusted			.069#	.090
Angry			-.027	-.026
Apprehensive			-.078#	.099
Hopeful			.019	.019
		R^2 Change .111		
R^2	.442		.450	
N	374		356	

#p<.1; *p<.05; **p<.01; ***p<.001

Note: The above models enter the following controls as the first block, but do not report them: age, race (Black), education, marital status (married), religion (Protestant), and income. Standardized and unstandardized coefficients are reported for the full models only.

The anticipated positive emotions are as readily exploitable in persuasion campaigns as any other consequence is. These data invite the interpretation that emotions are consequences and that as consequences they can be exploited as the basis for appeals to the negative emotional consequences of continued smoking and the positive emotional consequences of quit attempts and actual quitting. For example, these analyses suggest that appeals to pride and hope, the positive emotional consequences of quitting, can be emphasized as opposed to emphasizing the negative health consequences of failing to quit. Unlike the more cognitively based consequences, emotional ones may be able to be activated through emotional appeals. Given their apparent predictive power in our cross sectional data, such appeals may be especially effective.

Although we believe that a sound test of the role of discrete emotion in adding to the predictive adequacy of the IM has been conducted, limitations of various kinds invite subsequent, more comprehensive testing. First, a limited range of discrete emotions has been employed. Limitations of the survey allowed only five discrete emotions to be included. Other emotions such as regret have received a fair amount of attention, especially given the high likelihood of failure linked to attempts to quit smoking. Second, at least three versions of emotions toward quitting smoking could have been included in our survey—emotions about current intention, emotions anticipated during attempts to quit smoking, and emotions experienced during the various stages of quitting. With all three, it would be possible to disambiguate the role of emotion in the behavior of quitting. For example, is the anticipation of particular emotions during quitting a better predictor of intention to quit than emotions about the intention? Or, will successful quitting depend on accuracy in anticipating emotional responses during successful and unsuccessful quit attempts? The psychological function of emotion about an intention may be redundant with other measures of emotion or independent of them. Third, the semantic differential items employed in the test reported in this chapter have limited scope. Items tapping more directly into emotional valence, for example, pleasant-unpleasant, might account for more of the variance in intention to quit than the more cognitive pairs such as wise-foolish.

One counterargument that might be raised to the incorporation of emotional anticipated consequences to the IM is that elicitation studies, which are the recommended approach for generating the sets of anticipated outcomes, typically do not produce emotional anticipated outcomes as high priority. In a typical application of the IM, formative research is done to elicit positive and negative consequences associated with the target behavior. Although participants can provide considerations such as feeling proud, hopeful, or disgusted, these are uncommon responses, perhaps because people do not use emotional language about themselves to describe considerations that are otherwise central to behavior change (Planalp, 1999). Instead, they think in terms of more tangible consequences such as improved health, control of stress, sharing with friends, and so on. With some modifications in the elicitation procedure, participants could be invited to provide not only tangible consequences of the behavior but also less tangible, but just as consequential, emotional consequences.

In summary, emotions, as a conceptually distinct determinant of intention, have not typically been granted a prominent role in theories such as IM. Instead, theories that have been regarded as having the greatest potential for guiding behavior change interventions are those that have identified and communicated the target behavior's positive and negative behavioral consequences (Cappella, Yzer, & Fishbein, 2003; Fishbein et al., 1992; Fishbein et al., 2002; Rothman & Kiviniemi, 1999). The current data showing the predictive role of positive anticipated emotions on quitting intention suggest that the anticipated emotional consequences of an action may be as important a set of predictors of behavioral intentions as the more deliberative consequences. As such, conceptualizing risk in terms of positive and negative discrete emotional consequences associated with behaviors can add substantial variance explained to models of behavior change. In turn, this may open routes to persuasion that models based only on consequentialist assumptions cannot.

The role of anticipated emotional consequences in the IM can be seen as an extension of its scope rather than as a challenge to the IM's core principles and predictions. Just as some recent theories of attitude change have invited researchers to think about emotional responses to persuasive messages as "information" equivalent to the information provided by evidence and reason (Albarracín & Kumkale, 2003; Kruglanski, Thompson, & Spiegel, 1999), so too can the consequences of a behavior be extended to include emotional responses as consequences.

ACKNOWLEDGMENTS

This research was supported by the Annenberg Public Policy Center and a grant from the National Cancer Institute P50 CA095856.

REFERENCES

Ajzen, I. (1991). The theory of planned behavior. *Organizational Behavior and Human Decision Processes, 50*, 179–211.

Ajzen, I. (2002). Perceived behavioral control, self-efficacy, locus of control, and the theory of planned behavior. *Journal of Applied Social Psychology, 32*, 665–683.

Albarracín, D., & Kumkale, G. T. (2003). Affect as information in persuasion: A model of affect identification and discounting. *Journal of Personality and Social Psychology, 84*(3), 453–469.

Cappella, J. N., Romantan, A., Patterson, F., & Lerman, C. (2006). *The emotional bases for quitting smoking: Anticipated emotions as predictors of intention and behavior.* Unpublished manuscript, Annenberg School for Communication, University of Pennsylvania, Philadelphia.

Cappella, J. N., Yzer, M., & Fishbein, M. (2003). Using beliefs about positive and negative consequences as the basis for designing message interventions for lowering risky behavior. In D. Romer (Ed.), *Reducing Adolescent Risk* (pp. 210–219). Thousand Oaks, CA: Sage.

Choi, W, Gilpin, E., Farkas, A., & Pierce, J. (2001). Determining the probability of future smoking among adolescents. *Addiction, 96*, 313–23.

Fishbein, M., & Ajzen, I. (1975). *Belief, attitude, intention, and behavior: An introduction to theory and research.* Reading, MA: Addison-Wesley.

Fishbein, M., Bandura, A., Triandis, H. C., Kanfer, F. H., Becker, M. H., & Middlestadt, S. E. (1992). *Factors Influencing Behavior and Behavior Change: Final Report–Theorist's Workshop.* Rockville, MD: National Institute of Mental Health.

Fishbein, M., & Cappella, J. N. (2006). The role of theory in developing effective health communications. *Journal of Communication, 56,* S1–S17.

Fishbein, M., Cappella, J. N., Hornik, R., Sayeed, S., Yzer, M., & Ahern, R. K. (2002). The role of theory in developing effective anti-drug public service announcements. In W. Crano & M. Burgoon (Eds.), *Mass media and drug prevention: Classic and contemporary theories and research* (pp. 89–118). Mahwah, NJ: Lawrence Erlbaum Associates.

Hennrikus, D., Jeffrey, R. W., & Lando, H. (1995). The smoking cessation process: Longitudinal observations in a working population. *Preventive Medicine, 24,* 235–44.

Hornik, R., & Wolf, K. D. (1999). Using cross-sectional surveys to plan message strategies. *Social Marketing Quarterly, 5,* 34–41.

Kruglanski, A. W., Thompson, E. P., & Spiegel, S. (1999). Separate or equal? Bimodal notions of persuasion and a single-process "unimodel." In S. Chaiken & Y. Trope (Eds.), *Dual-process theories in social psychology* (pp. 293–313). New York: Guilford Press.

LeDoux, J. E., & Phelps, E. A. (2000). Emotional networks and the brain. In M. Lewis & J. M. Haviland-Jones (Eds.), *Handbook of emotions* (2nd ed., pp. 157–172). New York: Guilford.

Loewenstein, G. F., Weber, E. U., Hsee, C. K., & Welch, N. (2001). Risk as feelings. *Psychological Bulletin, 127,* 267–286.

Planalp, S. (1999). *Communicating emotion: Social, moral, and cultural processes.* New York: Cambridge University Press.

Rothman, A. J., & Kiviniemi, M. T. (1999). Treating people with information: An analysis and review of approaches to communicating health risk information. *Journal of the National Cancer Institute Monographs, 25,* 44–51.

Skara, S., Sussman, S., & Dent, C. (2001). Predicting regular cigarette use among continuation high school students. *American Journal of Health Behavior, 25*(2), 147–156.

CHAPTER 4

An Extension of the Theory of Reasoned Action and Its Successors to Multiple Behavior Interventions

Robert Hornik

University of Pennsylvania

The Theory of Reasoned Action (TRA; Fishbein and Ajzen, 1975 and its successor models, the Theory of Planned Behavior (Ajzen, 1991, 2002; Ajzen and Albarracín, this volume) and the Integrated Model (Fishbein et al, 2002; Fishbein et al., 1992) are central theories of behavior, and in particular, have been widely applied to health behavior. They have been important to the development of interventions to change such behaviors. Once interventionists understand the possible influences on behavior, they are in a stronger position to choose strategies for interventions, including promising messages to emphasize, confidence in skills to enhance, and sources of normative pressure to address. Thus as a theoretical framework, and as a guide to applications, these theories have had great importance.

Fishbein and Ajzen have insisted that their model is meant to account for behavior, not for behavioral categories or for behavioral goals (Ajzen and Fishbein, 1980; Fishbein and Ajzen, 1975). This approach works well when there are specifiable behaviors with large effects on health-relevant outcomes and thus which justify large investments in research and implementation of behavior change programs. For example, the model does not address reduction of HIV transmission (a goal) or safer sex (a behavioral category). However, it is well designed for planning interventions to affect condom use with casual partners, and that makes it valuable indeed, because increases in condom use with casual partners may substantially limit transmission of sexually transmitted infections including HIV. Similarly, interventions focusing on avoiding first cigarette use, or preparing a living will find it straightforward to make use of TRA and its successors. However, there are some important goals which are not substantially related to any single behavior; it does not appear that they can justify the required research and intervention investments required by these models.

Two examples of such goals often on current social change agendas include preventing or reducing obesity and encouraging pro-environmental behaviors. Obesity results from actions within two behavioral categories—energy consumption and energy expenditures. However, there are many actions one can take to reduce consumption of energy and many ways to increase energy expenditure. While popular books sometimes encourage single foci for diets (no simple carbohydrates; lots of grapefruits or cabbage), most authorities seem to expect calorie reduction from the combination of many discrete behaviors. Similarly energy expenditure can come from many different possible exercise behaviors. In both cases, success may not reflect adoption by many people of a single behavior, but adoption by single individuals of a set of new behaviors and/or adoption by different individuals of different single behaviors. The theory recommends that each of these behaviors be addressed separately and for each segment of the target audience. In practice this is unlikely to be feasible as a basis for intervention development. This suggests that by insisting on focusing on single behaviors the models may be sidelined in the context of these sorts of problems.

So the issue to be addressed in this chapter is the relevance of TRA and, by extension, its successors (Theory of Planned Behavior and the Integrated Model) to the development of interventions for behavioral categories. Are they simply irrelevant to the issues of developing interventions to address childhood obesity, for example, or is it possible that some alternative framing of the issues will permit productive application of these models to these types of problems as well? The chapter develops an argument that there are productive ways to think about the application of these models.

The chapter presents five approaches to interventions which suggest that these TRA-related models, designed for individual behaviors, might be relevant for behavioral categories. Each of them describes a type of intervention path which might exploit or change a commitment to a broad value which bears on multiple outcomes:

1. Single behavior interventions that diffuse to *like* behaviors.
2. Interventions that encourage increased commitment to a broad behavioral category and produce change in many sub-behaviors.
3. Interventions that focus on changing a belief about the desirability of an outcome and affect willingness to engage in all behaviors that are perceived to be related to that outcome.
4. Interventions that focus on *priming* thinking about a particular outcome in making related behavioral decisions.
5. Interventions that focus on changing the desire to conform to expectations of a particular member (or category of members) of a social network, where that person is likely to support many behaviors that lead to the desired outcome.

In the following section these approaches are developed conceptually, elaborating their explicit implications for the equations which underpin the TRA and its successor models, and through examples.

The basic argument of the Theory of Reasoned Action has been summarized in a series of arguments:

1. that behavior is the result of intentions,
2. that intentions are the result of attitudes and subjective norms,
3. that attitudes are the result of the sum of the product of expected outcomes of engaging in behavior with the evaluation of those behaviors,
4. that subjective norms are the result of the sum of the product of expected response of important sources to an individual's undertaking of a behavior with the desire to conform to those important sources.

Figure 4–1 portrays these relationships. The Theory of Planned Behavior and the Integrated Model add additional constructs, but they do not affect the following arguments, so Figure 1 is an adequate starting point.

For the purposes of this discussion it is helpful to formalize the equations for the last two relationships:

$$A = b_1(E_1V_1) + b_2(E_2V_2) + \ldots + b_n(E_nV_n) + e_1 . \tag{1}$$

$$SN = b_1{}'(SN_1DC_1) + b_2{}'(SN_2DC_2) + \ldots + b_n{}'(SN_nDC_n) + e_1{}'. \tag{2}$$

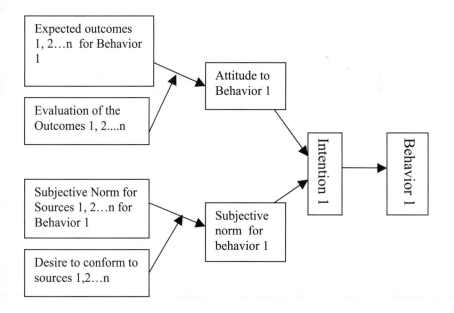

FIGURE 4–1. The Basic TRA Model.

Where, A = Attitude, SN = Subjective Norm. E_n = an Expected Outcome of the Behavior, V_n = the evaluation of that expected outcome, SN_n = the extent to which a particular member of a social network expects the respondent to engage in the behavior, and DC_n = the desire to conform to the expectations of that person. The coefficients b_n and $b_n{'}$ represent the relative weights of each of those cross products in affecting, respectively, attitude and subjective norm.[1]

The usual versions of the TRA simply sum the cross products in these equations to predict the overall norm or attitude, but it will be helpful for the purpose of this analysis to recognize that the cross product [(E,V) or (SN,DC)] couplets may vary in their influence on attitudes and subjective norms. Thus in this version of the TRA, the use of the b coefficients allows each couplet to contribute to a different degree to the attitude or norm outcome.

The rest of the chapter considers each of the paths through which an intervention might affect multiple relevant behaviors consistent with TRA ideas.

1. *Single behavior interventions diffuse to like behaviors.* One environmental example would be a campaign (or other intervention) to encourage a specific driving behavior which reduces fuel consumption (e.g., combining errands into a single trip). That campaign might focus on a message that says that an expected outcome of this behavior, combining errands, is the protection of the environment. A side effect of this campaign might be that it enhances a commitment to that protection of the environment value; it increases the evaluation of that outcome. The increased commitment to that protection of the environment affects other behaviors that share a link to that outcome evaluation, and thus that fall in that behavioral category. The effects might then generalize to avoiding rapid acceleration while driving, avoiding purchase of gas-guzzling cars, or even to reducing energy consumption in household use, and to increasing recycling behavior, if each of those was seen as protecting the environment.

This approach argues for the following elaboration of the TRA:

Assume there are two behaviors whose attitude components are a function of some common values. For simplicity's sake one can assume that each one is a function of two expectancy outcome couplets, and that one evaluation of an outcome (V_1, e.g., protection of the environment) is common to one couplet for each attitude.

$$\text{Attitude} B_1, \text{ or } A_1 = b_1(E_1{*}V_1) + b_2(E_2{*}V_2) \tag{3}$$

$$\text{Attitude} B_2, \text{ or } A_2 = b_3(E_3{*}V_1) + b_4(E_4{*}V_4). \tag{4}$$

---

[1]The Integrated Model adds self-efficacy as an influence in the Intentions equation; the Theory of Planned Behavior adds Perceived Behavioral Control as an influence in the Behavior equation. However, neither of these additions affects the structure of the analysis here, which focuses on the attitude and subjective norm equations, so they are not incorporated. Also, there has been some recent discussion of the possible role for descriptive norms alongside of subjective norms in affecting the normative pressures. However, almost any part of the argument that follows for strategy five can be generalized to that situation.

Then, assume that a successful intervention affects belief in the likelihood of Expected Outcome1 (E_1) if the behavior is performed: Intervention$\rightarrow E_1$.

Then the novel part of the argument is that if a behavior is performed as a function of a newly learned belief that the behavior achieves an outcome, and that behavior is rewarding, it also reinforces the perceived evaluation of that outcome, as illustrated in Figure 4–2.

If the campaign affects E_1 and $(E_1 * V_1) \rightarrow A_1 \rightarrow B_1$, then one would expect a change in B_1. If the change in B_1 is rewarding, then the change in B_1 and E_1 will produce a corresponding change in V_1, as well. The campaign then has affected E1, and that in turn affects B1 and also V_1. There is some speculation following as to why a change in E_1 might be expected to affect V_1. However, assume for the moment that this claim for a resulting change in V_1 is correct.

Then, given Figure 4–2, AttitudeB_2 would be affected also by the change in V_1 since V_1 is a component of one of the determining couplets for A_2. Then given the standard assumptions of the TRA, behavior B_2 would also be affected. The crucial and novel assumption here, $E_1 \rightarrow V_1$, is that performing a behavior successfully because of the influence of an E,V couplet enhances the V component of the couplet.

A mechanism that might support this path of effect is Kanfer's self-image hypothesis (Kanfer, 1970). By engaging in the behavior because it protects the environment, a person comes to see him or herself as a protector of the environment. This enhanced self-image as an environmentalist affects the value placed on protecting the environment, and that then influences all other behaviors perceived as affecting the environment. Thus C$\rightarrow$E1, (E1V1)$\rightarrow$A1$\rightarrow$B1, B1$\rightarrow$Self Image$\rightarrow$V1. Another example: a campaign which affects regular outside walking during good weather leads a person to see him or herself as a regular walker, and reinforces the idea that walking is valuable. That self-image as a regular walker stimulates consideration of other ways to realize that self-image, whether walking

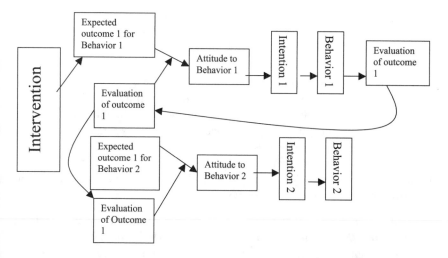

FIGURE 4–2.   Single behavior interventions diffuse to *like* behaviors.

in malls or making use of a treadmill at home, that might be necessary in bad weather. In a larger leap, regular exercise reinforces a self-image as someone concerned about a healthy lifestyle; that self-image, in turn, stimulates the decision to reduce calories through specific dietary changes. In this argument, the campaign to affect an expected outcome of a behavior leads to the valuing of that outcome, and the valuing of an outcome leads to increasing all other behaviors that are already understood to affect that outcome.

A quite different explanation for why performance of one behavior might lead to performance of other behaviors underpins *gateway* campaigns. The argument is made that some behaviors are necessary predecessors to others (marijuana use precedes heavier drug use) so a campaign is mounted to address the predecessor behavior in order to limit the more worrisome successor behavior. One logic underpinning the gateway hypothesis suggests that the prior behavior, entailing a smaller challenge to societal expectations and with milder risks, builds a foundation for sharper challenges and bigger risks. Another logic focuses on the concrete opportunities for a second behavior associated with engaging in a first behavior: exposure to marijuana dealers may provide access to those who also deal harder drugs; or, smoking of cigarettes develops a skill helpful for smoking marijuana. The implication of both of these gateway arguments is that preventing the first behavior will reduce the likelihood of the follow-on behavior. The second example is beyond the reach of TRA (although it does bear on perceived behavioral control from TPB.) However the first gateway mechanism can be addressed within this model.

Thus engaging in behavior$_1$ (using marijuana) leads to beliefs about an expected outcome (whether there will be bad consequences for using marijuana). Then the crucial assumption is that the belief about that expected outcome, at first specific to marijuana, then generalizes to the larger class of illegal substances.

Returning to equation 3 and a revised version of equation 4 formalizes this argument:

$$A_1 = b_1(E_1*V_1) + b_2(E_2*V_2) \tag{5}$$

$$A_2 = b_3(E_3*V_3) + b_4(E_4*V_4) \tag{6}$$

This pair of equations, in contrast to the previous 3) and 4), assumes that the two attitudes need not share value determinants. However, if a Campaign affects an important expectancy value (e.g., E1: increases the perception that there will be bad consequences for using marijuana), and E1→E3 (the generalized perception that there will be bad consequences to the use of any drugs like marijuana, or drugs "worse" than marijuana) then one would expect that a Campaign to affect E1 would also affect E3, which would then affect AttitudeB2 (given equation 4b.) So the novel argument here is that E1→E3.

2. An intervention encourages increased commitment to a broad behavioral category and that produces change in many sub-behaviors. For example, a campaign to encourage calorie restriction (because it affects desired outcomes) expects to produce adoption of a variety of diets which restrict calories. A campaign to encourage moderate exercise three times per week produces adoption of many different behaviors which satisfy that behavioral category. The intervention would first link the behavioral category to the already desirable outcome, and then either assume preexisting knowledge, or provide examples of behaviors which satisfy that valued consequence. Thus an intervention might focus on the idea that calorie restriction produces a variety of good outcomes (weight loss, alertness, fewer stains on shirts…). It might assume that audiences are already aware of many behaviors that lead to calorie restriction, or it can mention some of the specific behaviors. It assumes that an increase in commitment to calorie restriction will affect any behaviors which are in that category.

This path appears to contradict directly the assumption of the TRA that it does not deal with behavioral categories. So how might this strategy work within the model?

The crucial assumption is that there is an existing set of behaviors that the population already knows belong to a behavioral category. If they have a positive attitude towards the behavioral category, they increase their likelihood of performing all of the behaviors seen as belonging to that category. The intervention focuses on increasing beliefs in the shared expected outcomes for the behavioral category. This is expected to influence the attitude towards the behavioral category. The preexisting link between the behavioral category and the specific behaviors (even if the campaign does not name them) is expected to produce the generalization across behaviors. The entire intervention model is pictured in Figure 4–3.

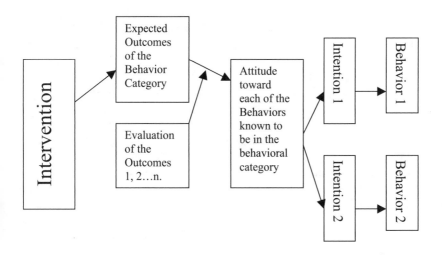

FIGURE 4–3.   An intervention encourages increased commitment to a broad behavioral category and that produces change in many sub-behaviors.

Formally:

B (the behavioral category) includes B_1, B_2,...B_n.

The campaign affects one or more of the expected outcomes of the behavioral category:

Intervention→ E_{1B}; Intervention→E_{2B}; Intervention→E_{nB}.

This affects the resulting attitude towards that behavioral category, given the usual attitude equation.

$$\text{AttitudeB, or } A_B = b_1(E_{1B}*V_1) + b_2(E_{2B}*V_2) +...+ b_2(E_{nB}*V_n) \quad (7)$$

Then either because the attitude towards the category affects the attitudes towards each of the specific behaviors within the category:

$$A_n = b_1 A_B \quad (8)$$

or, because the specific behaviors are influenced directly by (some of) the expected outcomes of the behavioral category:

$$A_n = b_1(E_{1B}*V_1) + b_2(E_{2B}*V_2) +...+ b_2(E_{nB}*V_n) \quad (9)$$

the attitude towards each of the specific behaviors (and the resulting intentions and behaviors) are affected as well.

The crucial modification of the theory is the argument that the expected values associated with a behavioral category will affect the likelihood of performing specific behaviors in that category. It requires an assumption that people know what fits into the category, and that if they increase their beliefs in the expected outcomes of the category it will translate into positive attitudes towards specific (albeit unnamed) behaviors.

In practice this would only be relevant if (a) the relationship between a behavioral category and its good outcomes was not well known, so an audience might learn about the association from a campaign, and (b) it can also be assumed that people know or can easily find out what falls into the behavioral category. Thus some family planning campaigns do advocate for a category of behaviors (use of modern contraception) and describe benefits that accrue to the entire category (healthier children, better economic lives). They assume that once people accept this linkage they can choose the specific contraceptive technique that fits their needs (pills, IUDs, condoms, etc.). While family planners may not assume that all potential users understand the range of specific techniques, they assume (and recommend) that intenders go to clinics to get that information as well as to obtain the services. It is probably worth noting that in the area of environmental behaviors, the evidence that one pro-environmental behavior is associated with another is not strong; this may undermine the persuasiveness of the idea of a behavioral category (cf. Oskamp et al., 1991.)

3. *Interventions focus on changing a belief about the desirability of an outcome and affect willingness to engage in all behaviors that are perceived to be related to that outcome.* For example, an intervention argues that improving physical fitness is valuable. If the audience already believed that particular behaviors (for example, walking 30 minutes a day) increased physical fitness, and the new intervention increased the value placed on physical fitness, then the likelihood of adopting all particular behaviors known to increase physical fitness would increase (although the intervention did not mention, for example, walking 30 minutes per day).

This formal presentation begins with equations 3 and 4 from the first strategy:

$$A_1 = b_1(E_1{}^*V_1) + b_2(E_2{}^*V_2) \tag{10}$$

$$A_2 = b_3(E_3{}^*V_1) + b_4(E_4{}^*V_4). \tag{11}$$

As in the first case, the model assumes that attitudes towards both behaviors are a function of two common values and two distinct values. However, in the first example the intervention strategy focused on affecting the E_1 component. Here the path to the effect would be simpler, by having a campaign directly address the V_1 component. Figure 4 illustrates this model. If the value placed on a particular outcome increases (even if the expected outcome of a behavior is unchanged), the TRA model says the attitude towards that behavior should become more positive. In this example, if physical fitness is the outcome and a campaign increases the perceived worth of being physically fit, then any behavior already linked to that outcome ought to be affected. In contrast to the previous strategies, this approach

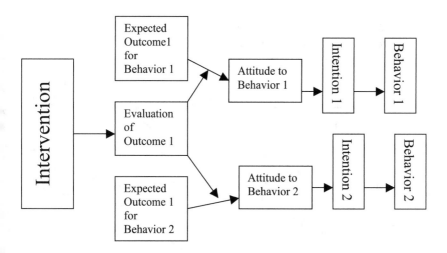

FIGURE 4–4. Interventions focus on changing a belief about the desirability of an outcome and affect willingness to engage in all behaviors that are perceived to be related to that outcome.

requires no modification of the TRA. It does require locating an outcome which is not already highly valued, which is relevant to a number of behaviors, and whose value an intervention might enhance.

4. *Interventions that focus on priming thinking about a particular outcome in making related behavioral decisions.*   Building on the previous example, it is possible that individuals already believe that improving physical fitness is valuable and they may already believe that a variety of specific behaviors affect that outcome. However, a campaign that talks about the value of physical fitness (even if it might not increase the degree to which someone valued physical fitness) might affect the cognitive accessibility of that valued outcome. This increase in cognitive accessibility is called *priming*. It encourages people to take physical fitness into account in their own behavioral choices. So when an individual begins to consider adopting new behaviors, including behaviors not mentioned in an intervention, physical fitness looms more substantially as an influence on behavioral choices.

This example is very close to the previous one and is presented in Figure 5. It begins with the same two equations:

$$A_1 = b_1(E_1*V_1) + b_2(E_2*V_2) \tag{12}$$

$$A_2 = b_3(E_3*V_1) + b_4(E_4*V_4). \tag{13}$$

In this case, the campaign might look a lot like an intervention for the previous example. It might involve, for example, making sure that people were frequently

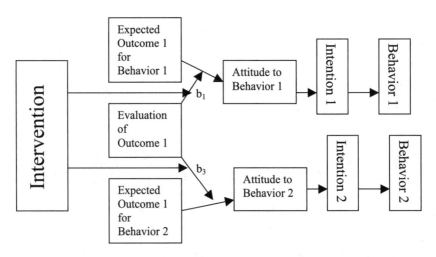

FIGURE 4–5. Interventions that focus on priming thinking about a particular outcome in making related behavioral decisions.

exposed to commentary about the value of physical fitness, even though that value was already widely accepted. One might not then expect any increase in the mean acceptance of that value—the mean of the various E_n and V_n would not change in equations 3 or 4. However, the public attention to the idea of physical fitness might be expected to influence how much a couplet (E_1V_1 in equation 3 or E_3V_1 in equation 4, if V1 is the value placed on physical fitness) would influence their respective attitudes towards behaviors 1 and 2. Specifically, a priming campaign would attempt to increase the size of the coefficients b_1 and b_3 in Figure 4–5. If the coefficients were positive and increased as the result of priming, then the model suggests that the attitude towards the behavior would become more positive as well. The likelihood of adopting the behavior would have increased without any increase in the expected outcomes for the behavior or in the values placed on the outcome. So this would lead one to expect that (a) if a campaign paid attention to the importance of physical activity, and (b) physical activity was already an important value associated with an attitude towards a behavior, for example regular walking, then the campaign by paying attention to physical fitness might influence the likelihood of adopting regular walking (or any other behavior seen as enhancing physical fitness). This would be expected to happen even if none of the specific behaviors were mentioned or there was no mean change in the expected outcome or evaluation of the outcome. One implication of this strategy is "increase exposure to the issue in any form" as long as both the expected outcome and the evaluation have the same sign (both positive or both negative) in their relationship to the attitude.

5. *Interventions that focus on changing the desire to conform to expectations of a particular member (or category of members) of a social network, where that member is likely to support many behaviors that lead to the desired outcome.* For example, an intervention might encourage trust in, and dependence on, medical sources in choosing behaviors to produce weight loss. It might recommend avoidance of sources which recommend magic bullet solutions to weight loss. If it can be assumed that medical sources will consistently recommend productive calorie restriction behaviors, the model suggests that an increasing reliance on medical sources will increase the intention to engage in any specific behavior recommended by that source.

The logic of this path to intervention is similar to the third approach; however it operates through the subjective norm equation rather than the attitude equation most relevant to the previous paths.

Using and simplifying the subjective norm equation, in the same way as was done for the attitude equation, and focusing on the simple case of two normative influence sources and considering two subjective norm outcomes for different behaviors, the equations would be:

$$\text{SubjectiveNormB}_1, \text{ or } S_1 = b_1(SN_1{*}DC_1) + b_2(SN_2{*}DC_2) \tag{14}$$

$$\text{SubjectiveNormB}_2, \text{ or } S_2 = b_3(SN_3{*}DC_1) + b_4(SN_4{*}DC_2). \tag{15}$$

The model is presented in Figure 4–6. A campaign might try to increase the perceived desire to conform to the expectations of medical sources for the broad area of weight loss strategies. Assume equation 6 dealt with the adoption of a balanced calorie restricting diet, and equation 7 dealt with the adoption of a magic bullet diet (low carbohydrate diet, for example). SN_1 would be the degree to which medical sources expect a person to adopt a balanced diet, SN_3 would be the degree to which medical sources expect a person to adopt a magic bullet diet. DC_1 in both equations reflects the desire to conform to the advice of medical sources. SN_2 and SN_4 refer to the expectations of other possible influence sources (perhaps from friends) with regard to the two diets, with DC_2 capturing the desire to conform with friends' expectations. (DC_2 related influences are not pictured in Figure 4–6.). Given this, a campaign to increase the desire to do what medical sources say (assuming that SN_1 was favorable and the b_1 coefficient in equation 6 was positive) would be expected to increase the overall subjective norm for that diet. At the same time, assuming medical advice was against the magic bullet diet, an increased reliance on medical sources would make the subjective norm less supportive towards that diet. This approach would translate into a particular campaign influencing a wide rage of potential behaviors without those behaviors being specifically addressed. As long as (a) the campaign was successful in affecting desire to conform to a particular source in a behavioral category, and (b) that source's expectation on each of the target behaviors was known and favorable, one would expect influence of a single campaign on all the behaviors that were in the category.

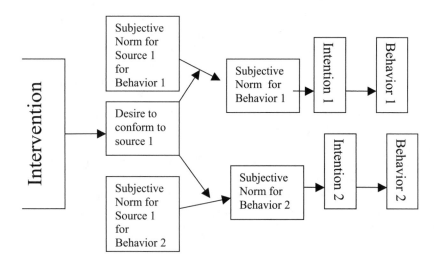

FIGURE 4–6. Interventions that focus on changing the desire to conform to expectations of a particular member (or category of members) of a social network, where that member is likely to support many behaviors that lead to the desired outcome.

CONCLUSION

TRA and its successor models, taken explicitly, are unable to support developing interventions that cannot choose single behaviors for their focus. Nonetheless, both by formal analysis of the theory, along with some extensions of the theory, and by offering some examples, an argument can be made for the relevance of those theories to health outcomes which require multiple behavior changes. Some interventions may hope to affect multiple behaviors within a behavioral category, even while they rely mostly on the TRA to describe the behavior. The paths included: the idea that adoption of one behavior consistent with an outcome expectancy might lead to adoption of other behaviors similarly related; the idea that a general attitude towards a class of behaviors might influence the sub-behaviors within it; the idea that a campaign to change a value that related to a variety of behaviors might affect them all; the idea that a campaign to *prime* a value related to a variety of behaviors might affect them all; and the idea that an intervention which encouraged reliance on a particular source for normative values might affect all behaviors relevant to that source. In each case, the suggested paths accept TRA as the core, but either show how a campaign focused on one particular component, or relying on an extension of the model without contradicting it, can allow it to deal with the issue of affecting multiple behaviors.

This analysis, however, has important limitations. First, the TRA is not about doing interventions; it is about explaining behaviors. The need to extend it to deal with this issue of behavioral categories is a practical one reflecting the need to develop relevant interventions. It is not an argument against the validity of the theory, only a struggle to adapt it for a purpose it does not now address.

Second, the magnitude of expected effects through each of these ideas is uncertain, theoretically. In some cases, given that interventions as described here may affect only small components of the influence equations, or work indirectly, the expected effects may be small. Each of the models presents a way that some influence might be realized on a variety of behaviors through a single campaign. However the actual extent to which such influence should occur depends on observed levels for variables and for coefficients, and for how important the focus components are in the influence model for each behavior.

One example and one path of effect illustrate this issue. Assume a campaign tries to increase the mean acceptance of one value (e.g., the value placed on physical fitness: through path #3 above). Accepting all of the model assumptions, the amount of influence will depend on the product of (a) the size of the change in the value placed on physical fitness, and (b) the extent to which it is an expected outcome of a variety of behaviors, and (c) the extent to which the expectancy value couplets involving the physical fitness outcome are themselves major predictors of the attitude towards the behavior, relative to other outcome couplets. If this product is small, or if attitude is not a major factor in determining the intention to act, this campaign might have a small or even an undetectable effect on these outcomes. Each of these five paths represents an indirect approach to influence on the behaviors. They contrast with the direct approaches that would be the subject of campaigns that adapt to the TRA but are specific to a single behavior. Campaigns that must rely on indirect paths, or on paths that address only one component of the influence model, may be expected to be weaker than single behavior focused interventions. Whether their possibility for influencing a range of behaviors counterbalances their lesser expected influence on any one behavior is only to be seen in a specific case.

A third concern with these approaches is that they might not be as logistically efficient in addressing multiple behaviors as intended. Their entire justification is that they can address multiple behaviors more efficiently than can applying the TRA one behavior at a time. If there are 5 or 10 distinct behaviors to be addressed, then the conventional form of TRA requires an equal number of formative TRA models. However, do these new approaches require less foundational research? Don't they require parallel knowledge about which common value or which common source is likely to be influential across behaviors? Thus wouldn't this approach produce little of the savings in foundational research that is its justification? So the question is not whether this approach can work; the question is whether it can work more efficiently than the single behavior approach. This is a legitimate concern; but there are two responses:

It should be possible to establish the role of a particular core value, or core source across behaviors without the sort of full-scale research effort typical of TRA work for every behavior. The formative investigation would focus, for example, on the role of only one or two values hypothesized, a priori, to be important across a behavioral domain. If there was evidence for their relevance across behaviors, this research would provide support for exploiting them in a campaign, without needing to know what else might be influential with regard to particular behaviors.

Also, even if one needed to do the full measure of TRA research for each potential behavior, there would still be some savings in the construction of a persuasive intervention. The analysis of the research would be focused on locating the common value or source that promised to unlock multiple behaviors, rather than on specifying a different approach for each behavior. That ought to produce a savings on the campaign itself, since messages would be focused on affecting beliefs (or sources) whose effects involved multiple behaviors. That focus would permit less expense on exposure to messages.

There is a fourth limitation of this presentation, and this one has no counter-arguments. In contrast to the discussions in other chapters in this book, there are no data here to support the models. There is a need for evidence, whether from experiments that try to vary levels of exposure to targeted messages, or from observational research on interventions that follow one or another of these strategies. They will test whether interventions making use of these strategies can affect acceptance of multiple related behaviors. They should also be designed to test what theoretical mechanisms explain any influences that are seen. Some studies need to see whether the proposed mechanisms work theoretically; some studies are needed to see whether the suggested intervention paths produce influence on multiple outcomes, in real settings.

This chapter has tried to extend the TRA and its successor models. An argument was presented, with examples but no data, that the models can be applied to the problem of outcomes attributable to many individual behaviors. These ideas are meant to extend the application of TRA and its successor models to new applied circumstances. The test of the usefulness of these ideas will be their actual utility, whether they actually respond to the current demands of interventionists.

REFERENCES

Ajzen, I. (1991). The theory of planned behavior. *Organizational Behavior and Human Decision Processes, 50*, 179–211.

Ajzen, I. (2002). Perceived behavioral control, self-efficacy, locus of control, and the theory of planned behavior. *Journal of Applied Social Psychology, 32*, 665–683.

Ajzen, I., & Fishbein, M. (1980). *Understanding attitudes and predicting social behavior.* Englewood Cliffs, NJ: Prentice Hall.

Fishbein, M., & Ajzen, I. (1975). *Belief, attitude, intention, and behavior: An introduction to theory and research.* Reading, MA: Addison-Wesley.

Fishbein, M., Bandura, A., Triandis, H. C., Kanfer, F. H., Becker, M. H. & Middlestadt, S. E. (1992). *Factors Influencing Behavior and Behavior Change: Final Report—Theorist's Workshop.* Rockville, MD: National Institute of Mental Health.

Fishbein, M., Cappella, J., Hornik, R., Sayeed, S., Yzer, M. & Ahern, R. K. (2002). The role of theory in developing effective anti-drug public service announcements. In W. Crano & M. Burgoon (Eds.), *Mass Media and Drug Prevention: Classic and Contemporary Theories and Research* (pp. 89–118). Mahwah, NJ: Lawrence Erlbaum Associates.

Kanfer, F. H. (1970). Self-regulation: Research issues, and speculations. In C. Neuringer & J. L. Michael (Eds.), Behavior modification in clinical psychology. East Norwalk, CT: Appleton.

Oskamp, S., Harrington, M., Edwards, T., Sherwood, D., Okuda, S., & Swanson, D. (1991, July). Factors influencing household recycling behavior. *Environment and Behavior, 23*, 494–519.

CHAPTER 5

A Theory of Implicit Reasoned Action: The Role of Implicit and Explicit Attitudes in the Prediction of Behavior

James Jaccard

Florida International University

Hart Blanton

Texas A&M University

The relationship between attitudes and behavior has been at the forefront of research on attitudes for decades. Ever since early studies observed low correlations between attitudes and behaviors, social psychologists have tried to determine why this is the case and under what conditions attitudes impact behavior. One of the most influential theorists by far in this area has been Martin Fishbein who, coupled with his collaborative efforts with Icek Ajzen, has provided major insights into the relationship between attitudes and behavior. Grounded in the Theory of Reasoned Action (TRA) and the Theory of Planned Behavior (TPB), fundamental principles of the attitude-behavior relationship have emerged that have been the basis for influential reviews of diverse literatures in the social sciences and that have led to the development of important applied intervention programs to improve society.

During the past 10 years, there has been a resurgence of interest in non-conscious influences on behavior in social psychology and this work has managed to find its way into the literature on the attitude-behavior relationship. One construct that has received a great deal of attention is that of implicit attitudes, with the most recognizable research program being that of Greenwald and associates on the Implicit Association Test (e.g., Greenwald, et al., 2002). Another important area of research has been on automaticity, which has focused on the effects of priming and attitude accessibility on the attitude-behavior relationship (e.g., Bargh, 1996;

Fazio, 1990). This research has emerged independent of the TRA and the TPB and the field would benefit from a theoretical integration of the different streams of research. In a recent chapter, Ajzen and Fishbein (2000) thoughtfully describe how research on automatic processes complements and fits within the Theory of Reasoned Action and the Theory of Planned Behavior. They also briefly discuss the role of implicit attitudes relative to the attitudinal constructs in their theories in Ajzen & Fishbein (2005). Given how popular research on implicit attitudes has become, it is important to examine this literature critically and to place it in the context of the more traditional and influential attitude theories of Fishbein and Ajzen. This chapter does so.

We begin by presenting a brief summary of features of the Theory of Reasoned Action and the Theory of Planned Behavior relevant to the analysis of the attitude-behavior relationship. We then consider the conceptual definition of an implicit attitude and how this differs from traditional definitions of attitude. We next describe the most popular methodology used to measure implicit attitudes, the Implicit Association Test (IAT). We examine the conceptual and measurement underpinnings of the IAT and map these onto basic principles derived from the TRA and the TPB about the attitude-behavior relationship. We suggest possible mechanisms through which implicit constructs may impact behavior using the TRA and the TPB as an organizing framework. Finally, we discuss directions for future research on the attitude-behavior relationship using implicit constructs.

These issues are, of course, of critical importance to applied health researchers. If health-related behavior is impacted independently by implicit health attitudes relative to explicit attitudes, then a whole new set of attitudinal constructs are on the table for health interventions to address. Behavior change strategies might take on very different forms than is currently the case, as the science documenting how to change implicit attitudes emerges. For example, are subliminal messages that are outside the range of human awareness (such as those used in subliminal advertising) more effective in changing implicit attitudes than explicit messages are? Are there specialized ways of enhancing or accentuating the impact of implicit attitudes or, by the same token, weakening their impact on behavior? What ethical issues must be taken into account, as one attempts to influence health attitudes outside the conscious awareness of people? Although we do not address such issues here, the matters we address are stepping stones to them. For if implicit attitudes are shown to be viable and measurable constructs that are independently predictive of behavior more generally, then this opens the door for their application in the health domain.

A SUMMARY OF THE TRA AND THE TPB RELEVANT TO THE ATTITUDE-BEHAVIOR RELATIONSHIP

The Theory of Reasoned Action states that a major determinant of many behaviors is a person's intention to perform that behavior: If a person intends to do something, he or she probably will do it, and if the person does not intend to do something, he or she probably will not do it. Despite the obvious strong connection between intentions and behavior, the Theory of Reasoned Action explicitly recognizes that intentions will not always guide behavior, and it specifies a number of factors that can block or facilitate the translation of behavioral intentions into behavior. For example, a person's intention to perform a behavior may not translate into behavior if the person lacks the knowledge, ability, and skills to perform the behavior, if behavioral performance is dependent on other people or events, or if habitual processes override the intention. For a discussion of specific examples of these conditions and elaboration of other factors that impact the intention-behavior relationship, see Fishbein and Ajzen (1975) and Ajzen and Fishbein (1980).

In a now classic paper, Ajzen and Fishbein (1977) identified methodological reasons why intentions may not predict behavior independent of facilitating and constraining conditions. They argued that a given behavior has different core elements, including the action itself, the setting in which the action takes place, the timing of the action, and the object that the action is directed towards. For an intention to predict behavior optimally, the core facets of the measured behavior must be correspondent with the core facets of the behavioral intention. For example, if one is trying to predict if a man will use condoms with his regular partner during the next month, then the measured intention should be the intent to use condoms with one's regular partner in the next month. As a measure of intent deviates from this correspondence (e.g., if one measures the intention to use condoms in general), then behavioral predictability can be adversely affected.

According to the Theory of Planned Behavior, a person's intention to perform a behavior is impacted by three core variables, (1) the attitude toward performing the behavior (A_B), (2) the subjective norm reflecting the normative pressure to perform or not perform the behavior (SN), and (3) one's perceived control over behavioral performance (PC). The impact of these variables on intention is represented in the form of a linear model such that

$$BI = \alpha + w_1 A_B + w_2 SN + w_3 PC + \varepsilon \qquad (1)$$

where α is a scaling constant, w_1, w_2 and w_3 represent regression weights or numerical constants that indicate how much change in intention will result from a one unit change in the predictor variable associated with the regression weight, and ε is an error term reflecting minor random departures from the basic linear function (i.e., noise). For elaboration of the individual components of this theory, see Fishbein and Ajzen (1975), Ajzen and Fishbein (1980), and Ajzen (1991).

As with the relationship between behavioral intentions and behavior, it is important that the core facets of each predictor be correspondent with those of the intention for optimal prediction of behavioral intention to occur. For example, if one is trying to predict if a man intends to use condoms with his regular partner during the next month, then the measured attitude should be the attitude toward using condoms with one's regular partner in the next month. As the measure of attitude, subjective norm, or perceived control deviates from this correspondence, then predictability of behavioral intent can be adversely affected.

The previous description of TRA and TPB sets the stage for elucidating three major reasons why studies of the attitude-behavior relationship may not have observed strong relationships between attitudes and behaviors. These include:

1. The facets of the measure of attitude used may not be correspondent with the facets of the behavioral criterion being predicted.
2. Attitudes may impact someone's intention to perform an action, but facilitating or constraining conditions can prevent that intention from being translated into behavior. It is only when attitudes are taken into account multivariately in conjunction with the facilitating and constraining conditions that one can understand how attitudes translate into behavior.
3. Attitudes may be but one factor impacting behavior and factors such as norms and perceived control also must be taken into account.

We return to these three central points later when discussing the prediction of behavior from implicit and explicit attitudes.

WHAT IS AN IMPLICIT ATTITUDE?

Implicit attitudes typically have been measured using response latencies. The latencies are timed in terms of how long it takes someone to answer a question on a survey or how long it takes them to classify stimuli into different categories. These methods are distinct from the more traditional measures of attitudes that tend to rely on self-reports as measured on paper-and-pencil inventories. The latter are often called *explicit attitudes*. An important question is whether implicit attitudes simply reflect a different methodological strategy for assessing the same underlying attitudinal construct, or if they represent something that is conceptually distinct from what has traditionally been called an attitude. Theorists working with the implicit attitude construct have been somewhat lax in addressing this issue and seem to suggest that both phenomena are operating. In this section, we first consider the traditional definition of an attitude and then elucidate conceptual definitions of implicit attitudes relative to it. This leads us to a two-component view of attitudes that seems to capture the spirit of theories of implicit attitudes.

The Traditional Definition of an Attitude

Although the definition of *attitude* varies from theory to theory (Eagly & Chaiken, 1993; Fishbein & Ajzen, 1975; Petty, Wegener & Fabrigar, 1997), there are commonalities across theories that are worth noting. First, most theories conceptualize an attitude in terms of a bipolar, evaluative, affective dimension that results in favorable or unfavorable evaluations of an attitude object. Second, most theories agree that an attitude always has a referent, or an *attitude object*. An attitude object is simply an entity that the individual can perceive or cognitively make note of. Attitude objects can refer to concrete objects (e.g., a motorcycle) or abstract concepts (e.g., enthusiasm), to social categories (e.g., motorcycle enthusiasts) or to non-social categories (e.g., British motorcycles). Any perceptual unit that can be discerned from the physical or social environment can be the object of an attitude, but it is meaningless to refer to attitudes in the absence of an object referent. Third, most theories conceptualize attitudes as latent variables or hypothetical constructs that cannot be observed directly. Rather, one must infer a person's attitude based on observable actions that are influenced by attitudes, such as the person's responses to a questionnaire, his or her facial expressions, or the person's vocalizations. A psychometric theory linking measures of observable behavior (e.g., responses to a questionnaire) to the unobserved latent construct is fundamental to standard attitude scaling methods, such as Thurstone scales, Guttman scales or Likert scales (Edwards, 1957; Fishbein & Ajzen, 1975). Finally, most theories characterize attitudes as predisposing individuals toward behavior. As an example, a negative attitude toward the attitude object "people who are African American" might increase the likelihood that an individual will express some form of disapproval toward African Americans in the future.[1]

The Conceptualization of an Implicit Attitude

As noted, one plausible way of thinking about the relationship between the scores obtained via self-report measures and those obtained via implicit measures of attitudes such as the IAT is to assume that both types of measures reflect the same psychological construct and that differences that emerge are due to method variance. Based on the finding that IAT scores typically have weak correlations with corresponding self-report measures of attitudes, many researchers have instead concluded that the two approaches assess distinct but related constructs (e.g., Cunningham, Preacher, & Banaji, 2001; Greenwald and Farnham, 2000; Greenwald, McGhee & Schwartz, 1998). Explicit attitudes as measured by traditional self-reports are thought to be attitudes or evaluations that are consciously accessible and, hence, amenable to assessment via self-reflection. By contrast, implicit attitudes are thought to be attitudes and evaluations that are not consciously accessible and that must therefore be measured via other methods, such as the IAT. As the distinction between implicit attitudes and explicit attitudes has taken hold, researchers have suggested that parallel assessment of both implicit and explicit attitudes may improve our ability to predict behavior. In essence, a new psychological construct has been added to our theoretical repertoire: For every *explicit* attitude that has been the focus of theorizing in attitudinal research, there also exists an *implicit* attitude that can be integrated into one's theoretical framework to add insight and predictive utility to important behavioral outcomes.

The two components of an attitude according to implicit attitude theory.   As noted previously, an attitude has traditionally been defined as a hypothetical construct that reflects the positive or negative affect associated with an attitude object. This definition stands independent of any particular method used to assess the construct. Attitude constructs have a long history of being measured by paper-and-pencil methods, physiological methods, behavioral and environmental traces,

---

[1]Componential definitions of attitude also have been popular, where the attitude construct is seen as consisting of a cognitive component, an affective component, and a behavioral component. However, most current day research views affect and evaluation as the defining feature of an attitude.

as well as a variety of clever and innovative disguised methods that do not involve responses to questions about the attitude object on a questionnaire (e.g., Fishbein & Ajzen, 1975). There is nothing in the traditional definition of an attitude that equates it with affect in conscious awareness or that states that it resides in declarative memory.

Greenwald and his associates (Greenwald, Nosek, & Banaji, 2003) elaborate a theory of implicit attitudes and define an attitude similarly to traditional definitions but draw on the concept of nodes from network models of memory. Specifically, they conceptualize an attitude as the totality of associational nodes linking an attitude object to valenced concepts (which is analogous to the totality of one's beliefs about an attitude object in the TRA and TPB), but they further argue that implicit measures like the IAT tap into associations that more traditional explicit attitude measures miss:

The predictions of the theory presented here can be tested in studies that use self-report measures of the types widely used in social psychology for the last several decades. However, for two reasons, self-report measures are not necessarily preferred for tests of the present theory. First, some of the associative links…may not be available to introspection and may therefore not permit accurate assessment by self-report measures (cf. Greenwald & Banaji, 1995). Second, self-report measures are susceptible to artifacts (such as impression management and demand characteristics) that can distort reporting even of associations that are introspectively available. Consequently, in the experiments reported here the unified theory's predictions have been tested not only with self-report measures, but also with a recently developed indirect measurement method, the IAT (Greenwald et al., 2003, p. 8).

In some respects, an attitude is seen as having parts that are accessible to declarative memory and parts that are not. The IAT is supposedly sensitive to the latter, but traditional attitude measures are not.

This two-component view of attitude (one part that is accessible to declarative memory and one part that is not) raises numerous conceptual and measurement questions. Does the IAT measure only those aspects of attitude that are not accessible to declarative memory or does it reflect the entire attitude construct, thereby encompassing both accessible and inaccessible associations? Can the implicit component of attitudes influence and shape what is accessible in declarative memory with respect to the attitude object, that is, does the implicit component of attitudes influence the explicit component of attitudes? Can the type of implicit associations that a person has be uncorrelated or even negatively correlated with the type of associations that are accessible in memory? No matter how one chooses to answer such questions, the central idea is that the reliance of the TRA and the TPB on traditional self-report measures of attitude means that tests of these theories have overlooked an important component of attitudes, namely the implicit component. Implicit attitude theorists would argue that if such components of the attitude can be tapped into, then better prediction of behavior might result. The key is (1) devising a measure that is sensitive to the implicit component of attitudes and (2) testing if these measures add explained variance in behavior over and above the more traditional measures of the TRA and TPB.

THE MEASUREMENT OF IMPLICIT ATTITUDES

The Implicit Association Test.   Probably the most popular method for assessing implicit attitudes is the Implicit Association Test (IAT). The IAT is believed to measure implicit attitudes by assessing individuals' reaction times on two cognitive tasks. In a given IAT task, participants are presented with a set of stimulus words or pictures on the computer, which they then classify into one of two categories through the use of a key press. The two categories are created by superimposing two concept labels with two evaluative anchors. As an example, Greenwald et al., (1998) developed an IAT to measure a relative preference for European Americans versus African Americans by assessing the ease with which people could classify stimulus words into categories created from the concepts, African American and European American, with the evaluative anchors, Pleasant and Unpleasant. Following what have now become the conventions in the field, they created one discrimination task in which participants placed words shown on a computer screen into one of two categories. If they judged the word to be either an African American name or an unpleasant word, they pressed a certain key on the keyboard to reflect the category *African American or Unpleasant*. If they judged the word to be either a European American name or a pleasant word, they would press a different key on the keyboard to reflect the category *European American or Pleasant*. This task can be symbolized as African American + Unpleasant vs. European American + Pleasant. In a second discrimination task, they had participants place the same words into either the category *African American or Pleasant* or *European American or Unpleasant*. This task can be symbolized as African American + Pleasant vs. European American + Unpleasant). Greenwald et al. then interpreted the difference in the response latencies for the two tasks as a measure of prejudice. Specifically, participants who categorized words faster during the African American + Unpleasant versus European American + Pleasant task than in the African American + Pleasant versus European American + Unpleasant task were viewed as having an evaluative preference for European Americans over African Americans (see also Dasgupta, McGhee, Greenwald & Banaji, 2000; McConnell & Leibold, 2001). Central to the IAT measure is the differencing of the two response latencies.

In the IAT, one of the two tasks traditionally is called the *compatible task (CT)* and it is thought to be easy for people who are high on the construct of interest. The other task is called the *incompatible task (IT)* and it is thought to be hard for people who are high on the construct of interest. If one were measuring the implicit preference for European Americans over African Americans using the race IAT just described, the compatible task would be the one that asks participants to categorize the different stimuli presented on the computer screen into the two categories *European American and Pleasant* and *African American and Unpleasant* and the incompatible task would be the one asking participants to use the categories *European American and Unpleasant* and *African American and Unpleasant*. The logic is that it is easier for someone who prefers European Americans to African Americans to associate European Americans with Pleasant and African Americans with Unpleasant than it is to associate European Americans with Unpleasant and African Americans with Pleasant. This should result in faster response times for the compatible task as opposed to the incompatible task. The IAT score, which in this case reflects a preference for European Americans over African Americans is defined as

$$\text{Implicit Attitude} = \text{IAT Score} = \text{IT} - \text{CT} \qquad (2)$$

where IT is the response latency for the incompatible task and CT is the response latency for the compatible task. Higher IAT scores reflect an increasing preference for European Americans over African Americans.

THE CONCEPTUAL MODEL UNDERLYING THE IAT

Two Attitudes, Not One

Although researchers fail to emphasize it, the IAT framework imposes a different theoretical approach to relating attitudes to behavior than is the convention in traditional attitude theory. This difference can have consequences for behavioral prediction. Whereas traditional attitude researchers focus on attitudes towards a single attitude object, IAT researchers instead focus on *relative attitudes*. Relative attitudes represent the difference in how two attitude objects are evaluated (e.g., the difference in the implicit evaluation of African Americans versus the implicit evaluation of European Americans). Greenwald and Farnham (2000) acknowledged that the IAT is designed to measure a relative construct and suggested that "the IAT can nevertheless be effectively used because many socially significant categories form complementary pairs, such as positive-negative (valence), self-other, male-female, Jewish-Christian, young-old, weak-strong, warm-cold, liberal-conservative, aggressive-peaceful, etc." (p. 1023). The very nature of the IAT task is such that researchers must study two attitude objects and their relative difference. In this respect, the conceptual approach of the IAT is distinct from that of TRA and TPB and the implications of this have not been fully appreciated. Researchers have tended to focus attention on the supposed difference in how conscious versus non-conscious attitudes affect behavior rather than other fundamental differences between the approaches.

The two attitudes combine additively to impact behavior. Although IAT theorists have been somewhat vague about it, discussions of the IAT strongly suggest that the two attitudes being measured by the IAT are thought to combine additively to impact behavior. More specifically, the construct the IAT measures represents the difference between the implicit attitude towards one object minus the implicit attitude toward the other object. As examples, Greenwald et al.,

(1998) often refer to attitudinal differences when summarizing results for IAT analyses:

> *"In Experiment 2, the expected correlation was in the relationship of an IAT measure of attitude difference between Korean and Japanese ethnicities and subjects' self-described ethnic identities."* (p. 1476, italics added)
>
> *"The data of Experiment 3... clearly revealed patterns consistent with the expectation that White subjects would display an implicit attitude difference between the Black and White racial categories."* (p.1474, italics added)
>
> *"Findings of three experiments consistently confirmed the usefulness of the IAT (implicit association test) for assessing differences in evaluative associations between pairs of semantic or social categories."* (p. 1478, italics added).

In addition, when IAT researchers compare the IAT to explicit attitudes, they measure the explicit attitude by computing a simple difference score for two self-reported single-attitude measures (e.g., by subtracting the explicit attitude towards African Americans from the explicit attitude towards European Americans). These difference scores are then correlated with IAT scores (see Greenwald et al., 1998) and behavior to assess the relationship between them.

The choice of a function for describing the disparity between the two implicit attitudes at the conceptual level is not trivial and has implications for criterion prediction. For example, let the true (unmeasured and unobservable) relative implicit attitude (RIA) of interest be represented as

$$RIA = IA_{EA} - IA_{AA} \qquad (3)$$

where IA_{EA} is the true (unmeasured and unobservable) implicit attitude toward European Americans and IA_{AA} is the true (unmeasured and unobservable) implicit attitude toward African Americans. Suppose that an investigator wants to predict a behavioral criterion, Y, from the relative implicit attitude. If the researcher applies a traditional linear model vis-à-vis correlation or regression, then the relationship between the variables is:

$$Y = \alpha + \beta\, RIA + \varepsilon \qquad (4)$$

where α represents an intercept, β represents a slope (i.e., the predicted change in Y given a one unit change in RIA), and ε is a residual term. If we substitute the right-hand side of Equation 3 for RIA in the above model and expand the products, the investigator is found to be modeling:

$$Y = \alpha + \beta IA_{EA} - \beta\, IA_{AA} + \varepsilon \qquad (5)$$

Equation 5 reveals a model that is restrictive in form. It asserts that the impact of the two implicit attitudes on the criterion is additive and that the effects of each implicit attitude (as reflected by β) are equal in magnitude but opposite in sign. To the extent that this causal structure is not operating, Equation 4 can provide suboptimal prediction of the criterion, Y, and can yield inappropriate causal inferences.

Consider as an example investigators who want to predict racist actions in a sample of European American participants as a function of their implicit evaluations of European Americans and their implicit evaluations of African Americans. It may be that racist actions of these individuals are driven more by implicit evaluations of African Americans (IA_{AA}) than by implicit evaluations of European Americans (IA_{EA}). This suggests that the regression coefficient for IA_{AA} will be larger than the regression coefficient for IA_{EA}. In this case, the regression coefficient one obtains from regressing racist actions onto the IAT will be an intermediate value between the (relatively large) coefficient one would have obtained from a valid measure of IA_{AA} and the (relatively small) coefficient one would have obtained from a valid measure of IA_{EA}. As another example, suppose that negative evaluations of African Americans lead to more racist actions the more positively participants evaluate other European Americans. This implies an interaction between IA_{EA} and IA_{AA}. This causal dynamic cannot be detected with the IAT.

Although difference scores are one way of representing attitudinal disparities, other functions are possible. For example, one might use a ratio function instead

$$RIA = IA_{EA} / IA_{AA} \qquad (6)$$

with equal attitudes yielding a value of 1.0 and non-equal values departing increasingly from 1.0. To predict a criterion with this function, we again use a simple linear model:

$$Y = \alpha + \beta \, (IA_{EA} / IA_{AA}) + \varepsilon \qquad (7)$$

which is the same as

$$Y = \alpha + \beta \, (IA_{EA})(1 / IA_{AA}) + \varepsilon \qquad (8)$$

In contrast to the differencing function, the multiplicative term in this model implies an interaction between IA_{EA} and IA_{AA} when predicting Y. Stated another way, in the difference model, the effect of variations in IA_{AA} on Y will be the same no matter what the value of IA_{EA} whereas for the ratio model, the effect of variations in IA_{AA} on Y will differ depending on the value of IA_{EA}.

The lack of a clear statement by IAT researchers about the nature of the relative attitude is problematic. As illustrated herein, different conceptualizations of the term *relative* invoke different causal models. The most common orientation seems to view the IAT as an index of the difference between two attitudes. When using IAT scores to predict behavior, IAT researchers thus (knowingly or unknowingly) invoke the assumption that the two attitude objects have additive influences on the criterion that are equal in magnitude but opposite in sign. Whether this function occurs in practice is unknown.

THE PSYCHOMETRIC PROPERTIES OF THE IAT

As noted previously, IAT researchers view the IAT as methodologically advantageous to explicit measures of attitude because self-report measures are susceptible to artifacts such as impression management and demand characteristics. However, response latency measures carry with them a host of potential artifacts and these need to be dealt with in research on implicit attitudes. The IAT is constructed in such a way that it introduces artifacts that typically are avoided when researchers design explicit measures. These different artifacts may be sufficiently prevalent that they render causal inferences from the IAT ambiguous. In this section, we briefly review some of these artifacts.

The IAT Is Inherently Double Barreled

It is well known in traditional attitude research that the use of double-barreled question formats can be problematic. Double-barreled questions assess two beliefs or two attitudes simultaneously, often making it difficult for individuals to accurately report their attitudes (e.g., to what extent do you agree that European Americans are honest and African Americans are athletic?). The IAT supposedly measures four association strengths (described later) but uses only two items to do so, namely the CT and the IT (which are differenced to yield a single index of attitude). Unfortunately, the four associations' strengths may not be related in ways that make it meaningful to represent them all with a single score.

To illustrate, consider the IAT that measures relative implicit preferences for African and European Americans. According to Greenwald et al. (2002), the IAT taps into the association strength of four crucial associations: (1) the association strength between European Americans and positive valenced attributes or constructs, (2) the association strength between European Americans and negative valenced attributes or constructs, (3) the association strength between African Americans and positive valenced attributes or constructs, and (4) the association strength between African Americans and negative valenced attributes or constructs. The strength of these four associations is reflected in the two response latencies of the IAT. The compatible task of the IAT asks individuals to categorize stimuli presented on the computer screen into the categories of *European American or Pleasant* versus *African American or Unpleasant*. Presumably, if individuals have a strong association between "European Americans and positive valenced constructs" as well as a strong association between "African Americans and negatively valenced constructs," then they will be able to do this task much faster than if these linkages are weak. As such, a single response latency reflects the combination of two association strengths, although the nature of the combinatorial function is unknown. For example, the response latency could be a function of the sum of the two association strengths, a weighted sum of the two association strengths, an average of the two association strengths, a weighted average of the two association strengths, a product of the two association strengths, or some other function.

The incompatible task of the IAT asks individuals to categorize stimuli presented on the computer screen into the categories of *European American or Unpleasant* versus *African American or Pleasant.* Again, if individuals have a strong association between "European Americans and negatively valenced constructs" as well as a strong association between "African Americans and positively valenced constructs," then they will be able to do this task much faster than if these linkages are weak. The single response latency for this task also reflects the combination of two association strengths, although, again, the nature of the combinatorial function is unknown.

In some sense, the response latency for an IAT task is double barreled because it must reflect two different association strengths with a single number, that is, the latency. This double barreled nature of the IAT coupled with an unknown function relating the component association strengths to the response latency makes it difficult to know what the IAT truly reflects.

The IAT Is Contaminated by General Processing Speed

Because the measures yielded by the two IAT tasks are based on reaction times, they are each influenced by a person's ability to respond quickly to cognitive tasks in general, independent of implicit attitudes. We refer to this ability as a person's general processing speed, and we view it as a psychological resource that may be imperfectly representative of such general attributes as cognitive efficiency, general intelligence, and attention span. It also may reflect such skills as finger dexterity and hand-eye coordination and more transitory states such as mood, drug use, and the like. There can be little doubt that this source of method variance impacts performance on each of the IAT tasks. Indeed, across a wide range of studies, the compatible and incompatible response latencies show a moderate to strong positive correlation when, in their purest form, one would expect negative correlations between them because the associations they reflect are polar opposites. The strong positive correlation between them suggests that general processing speed exerts a greater systematic influence on the two component scores of the IAT than do the implicit attitudes and the associations that these responses are thought to measure.

The desire to expunge general processing speed from IAT scores is implied by the traditional reliance on difference coding, but IAT researchers were not explicit about this goal in their published papers. More recent scoring strategies have directly stated this goal. A scoring algorithm for the IAT recently has been introduced that supposedly removes the influence of general processing speed from IAT scores (Greenwald et al., 2003; Nosek, Greenwald & Banaji, 2005). This method incorporates a difference score, but it also uses new data elimination procedures and new data transformations. Even if this method is successful at removing general processing speed (and we do not think that it is), the entire enterprise of finding ways to expunge the IAT of processing speed confounds has shortcomings.

One problem is that general processing speed can have a meaningful relationship to the theoretical constructs one wishes to represent. Suppose, for instance, that general processing speed is reflective of intelligence, more or less. Suppose also that intelligence is related to implicit racist attitudes, such that people with higher intelligence are less likely to have racist attitudes. In this case, one would expect general processing speed to be correlated with the latent construct of implicit racist attitudes and this correlation has a conceptually meaningful basis. If a scoring algorithm removes the influence of general processing speed on the IAT measure, it then would remove some of the true variation in the implicit attitude, namely that portion that covaries with intelligence. The result is a distorted index of the implicit attitude.

The heart of the problem is that a researcher may not know if the source of the correlation between the IAT score and general processing speed should be treated as artifactual, as conceptually meaningful, or as a combination of both. It would be better if the measure was simply not susceptible to method artifacts of this nature, but such is a fact of life of latency-based indicators.

Numerous researchers have noted the contaminating influence of general processing speed in the IAT, although they have either labeled it differently (e.g., the *cognitive skill confound, reliable contamination*) or focused on a more narrow feature of it, such as task-switching ability (e.g., Back, Schmuckle & Egloff, 2005; McFarland & Crouch, 2002; Mierke & Klauer, 2003). Research has affirmed the complicating effects of these variables in studying individual difference variables, such as attitudes, and this source of method variance represents a major obstacle to theory construction with implicit attitudes that rely on the IAT.

Scores on the IAT Are Impacted by Measurement Context

Several studies have examined if scores on the IAT are impacted by the context in which the measures are taken when the focus is on constructs that are assumed to be relatively stable in character. For example, Schmuckle and Egloff (2005) used latent trait-state techniques to document contextual shifts in the IAT over a one-week test-retest period. They found that the IAT showed larger context effects than did explicit measures. These effects were manifest across a range of different IAT tasks, suggesting that the contextual changes in IAT scores are inherent in the general IAT procedure and are not specific to the type of attitude assessed with the IAT. De Houwer, Geldof and De Bruycker (2005) found the IAT to be susceptible to manipulations of salience of irrelevant dimensions (see also Mierke & Klauer, 2003). Context effects also have been noted by Devine (1993). Strategies need to be developed to remove the influence of such extraneous factors on the IAT.

The IAT Reflects Meaningful Phenomena Other Than Attitudes

Numerous studies have suggested that the IAT may reflect socially meaningful factors other than attitudes. For example, several scientists have suggested that the IAT measures the similarity between objects rather than evaluations of them (De Houwer, Geldof & De Bruycker, 2005). Kinoshita and Peek-O'Leary (2005) argue that IAT scores reflect familiarity with the group categories activated by the IAT rather than their attitudes towards the groups. Brendl, Markman & Messner (2001) also raise this possibility invoking a figure-ground analysis of the IAT. Rothermund, Wentura and De Houwer (2005) emphasize and convincingly argue for the effects of salience asymmetry on the IAT. As an example, the category *Black* is less familiar than *White* to most White participants, and *Unpleasant* is less familiar than *Pleasant* to most people (see Skowronski & Carlston, 1989). Black and Unpleasant thus become cognitively salient for many White participants when they take the race IAT, and this can impact IAT scores and contribute to correlations between IAT measures and other criteria.

The IAT Has Borderline Reliability Properties

Numerous studies have evaluated the reliability of the IAT, primarily using test-retest paradigms. Overall, estimates of reliability have been low. For example, Steffens & Buchner (2003) assessed test-retest reliability of IAT measures using a paradigm where the IAT retest was an immediate replication of the just-measured implicit attitude. The test-retest correlations ranged from 0.50 to 0.62. Greenwald et al. (2006) note that the average test-retest reliability of the IAT across a wide range of studies is 0.56. Overall, the IAT as a measure of implicit attitudes tends to yield suboptimal reliability levels.

In sum, there appears to still be much work that needs to be done on the measurement of implicit attitudes. Just as it has taken many years, elegant scaling models, and numerous methodological studies to evolve reliable and valid measures of explicit attitudes, the same will probably be necessary for the development of adequate measures of implicit attitudes. Without such measures, research on implicit attitudes and their relationship to behavior is limited in terms of what it can contribute theoretically.

DO IMPLICIT ATTITUDES PREDICT BEHAVIOR OVER AND ABOVE EXPLICIT ATTITUDES?

The Typical Research Paradigm

Numerous studies have explored the relationship between implicit attitudes and behavior. In this section, we describe these studies and consider the empirical evidence that implicit attitudes as measured by the IAT predict behavior over and above measures of explicit attitudes. The typical IAT paradigm used for testing the relationship between an IAT measure and behavior is to obtain a measure of implicit attitude (which actually is a measure of the difference between two implicit attitudes, as discussed above) as well as a self-report rating of how favorable or unfavorable the research participant feels about each of the two attitude objects being studied. For example, in the race IAT, one might obtain a self-report rating of how favorable or unfavorable a person feels about African Americans, and a separate rating of how favorable or unfavorable the person feels about European Americans. The measure of *explicit attitudes* that is used to predict behavior is the difference between these two ratings, and the correlation of this difference score with behavior is compared with the correlation between the IAT score and behavior.

A meta-analysis. Poehlman, Uhlmann, Greenwald and Banaji (2006) conducted a meta-analysis examining the predictive validity of a wide variety of IAT measures. This meta-analysis was not restricted to implicit attitudes (it also included implicit personality constructs and implicit self-concepts), nor were the

TABLE 5-1

Summary of Studies Measuring Implicit and Explicit Attitudes Predicting Behavior

Study	Criterion	N	Imp	Exp	Inter
Ashburn-Nardo et al. (2003)	Black/White partner choice	77	0.25	0.15	0.19
Bane et al. (2004) [a]	Voting	110	0.45	0.64	0.58
Brunel et al. (1999)	Usage of IBM/Apple computers	50	0.54	0.64	0.50
Czopp et al (2006)	Condom use	132	0.16	0.22	0.25
Florack (2004, sample 1) [a]	Fruit/chocolate choice	48	0.46	0.46	0.51
Florack (2004, sample 2) [a]	Fruit/chocolate choice	48	0.09	0.31	0.51
Jellison et al. (2004)	Pro-gay activities	39	0.26	0.25	
Karpinski (2004) [a]	Voting behavior	194	0.39	0.77	
Karpinski & Hilton (2001)	Choice of apple vs. candy bar	65	-.05	0.40	0.04
Lemm & Banaji (2000) [a]	Interaction with gay man	47	0.38	0.16	0.23
Maison et al. (2001, Study 1)	Juice vs. soda drinking	71	0.27	0.46	0.28
Maison et al. (2004, Study 1)	Yogurt versus fast food	38	0.43	0.80	0.52
Maison et al. (2004, Study 1)	Drinking Coke vs. Pepsi	102	0.45	0.80	0.42
Marsh et al. (2001)	Condom use	80	-.01	0.27	
McConnell & Leibold (2001)	Non-verbal behaviors towards a Black confederate	41	0.21	0.05	0.42
Neumann et al. (2004)	Avoiding person with AIDS	37	0.16	0.24	0.19
Nosek et al. (2002)	Math SAT performance	227	0.38	0.49	0.41
Perugini (2006, Sample 1)	Smoking	48	0.48	0.64	0.48
Perugini (2006, Sample 2)	Candy bar/fruit choices	109	0.19	0.28	0.09
Rudman et al. (2000, Study 1) [a]	Funding of Jewish organizations	89	0.40	0.35	0.35
Rudman et al. (2000, Study 2) [a]	Funding of Japanese organizations	116	0.26	0.11	0.10
Rudman et al. (2000, Study 3) [a]	Funding of Black organizations	64	0.13	0.04	0.19
Sekaquaptewa, et al (2003)	Friendliness towards Black person	79	0.03	0.01	0.16
Swanson et al. (2001)	Smoking	70	0.36	0.49	0.22
Wiers et al. (2002)	Alcohol use	48	0.34	0.29	0.06
Median		70	0.27	0.31	0.25

Notes: Imp = Correlation of implicit measure with criterion, Exp = Correlation of explicit measure with the criterion, Inter = Correlation between explicit attitude measure and implicit attitude measure.

[a] Unpublished, raw data that is analyzed but not written up, is reported in Poehlman et al. (2004) but not referenced.

criteria that were predicted restricted to behavior (other criteria included beliefs, other attitudes, electrical brain activity, and a wide range of social judgments). Table 5–1 presents an abridged table from their report that focuses only on studies that (1) measured attitudes, (2) used a measure of behavior as a criterion, and (3) obtained a measure of both implicit attitudes and explicit attitudes. About one third of the studies in our table were unpublished, were reports of data that were informally analyzed but not written up, or were cited in the meta-analytic table of Poehlman et al. but were not included in their reference section. These studies are superscripted in our table. They should be judged as not having yet passed peer review in terms of their methodological standards or theoretical contribution.

The behaviors that have been predicted in the studies depicted in Table 5–1 are diverse, but for the most part they have tended to be inconsequential and/or socially trivial behaviors that occur in laboratory settings. Across the studies, the median correlation of the IAT measure with behavior was 0.27 and for the explicit attitude it was 0.31. Poehlman et al. noted that few studies examined the question of whether the IAT added incremental variance to the prediction of behavior over and above the measures of explicit attitudes. Of the studies listed in Table 5–1 that did so, only one of the four of them observed a statistically significant increment in predictability (Nosek et al., 2002).

Comparisons with an Outdated Attitude Model

Even if significant incremental explained variance for attitude measures had been more pervasive for the IAT, it would not have meant much. The approach taken in these studies for predicting behavior from explicit attitudes violates all of the well-known attitude-behavior principles that have evolved from the influential work of Fishbein and Ajzen in the attitude area. Specifically, the focus in the IAT research has not been on attitudes towards behaviors but has instead focused on more general attitude objects. The facets of the measures of attitude have not been correspondent with the facets of the behavioral criteria. Furthermore, the IAT invoked two attitudes, not one, which introduces additional complications, as discussed later. In short, the IAT has not been tested relative to its ability to add incremental explained variance to the Theory of Reasoned Action or the Theory of Planned Behavior. Instead, it has been tested relative to an approach to attitude-behavior prediction that was long ago shown to be inadequate and that has been abandoned by modern day attitude theorists. Even with this outdated attitude model, the IAT has accounted for significant incremental explained variance in only a single study focused on attitude constructs.

TOWARDS A THEORETICAL INTEGRATION

Although the concept of implicit attitudes has become very popular in social psychology, a closer look at the construct and the leading measure of it (the IAT) suggests that there is a long way to go before one can conclude that the concept and measure are viable. In this section, we first integrate the concept of implicit attitudes with the Theory of Reasoned Action and the Theory of Planned Behavior, and then we consider directions for future research in light of this.

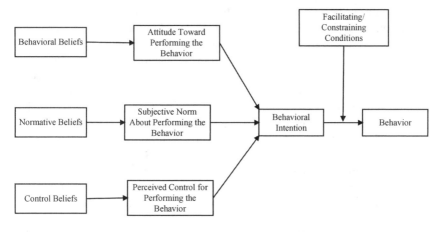

FIGURE 5–1.   Core constructs in the Theory of Reasoned Action/
Theory of Planned Behavior.

Integration with the TRA/TPB

Implicit attitudes have a home in the Theory of Reasoned Action and the Theory of Planned Behavior, and that home is where many other variables reside, namely, as a distal variable that impacts behavior through the core variables of the theories. Figure 5–1 presents the full version of the Theory of Planned Behavior, which we use to organize the present discussion. According to the theory, a distal variable can impact behavior in many ways. First, it can influence behavioral beliefs which impact behavior through attitudes, and, in turn, behavioral intentions (see Figure 5–1). In the TRA and the TPB, a given behavioral belief has two components, (1) a subjective probability that performing the behavior will lead to some consequence, and (2) the judged favorability or unfavorability of that consequence. Consider the subjective probability component, which we label SP. The subjective probabilities that people hold with respect to a given behavioral belief can derive from many different sources. For example, a subjective probability might be based, in part, on what other people tell us (e.g., a woman is told by a health professional that if she has unprotected sex, she will have a good chance of contracting a sexually transmitted disease). Or, a subjective probability might be based, in part, on direct experience (e.g., a woman knows people who engaged in unprotected sex and who contracted an STD). A subjective probability also may be colored by a basic personality disposition, such as the tendency to perceive oneself as invincible to negative consequences or by an internal or external locus of control. Or, it can be a result of the rationalization of a desired goal (e.g., a woman may want to have a relationship with an attractive man who does not like using condoms, so the woman rationalizes that the likelihood of her contracting an STD if she has unprotected sex with him is low). A subjective probability can be influenced by one's mood (e.g., people often see desirable events as more likely if they are in a good mood and undesirable events as more likely if they are in a bad mood) and it can be influenced by events that serve as primes (e.g., reading a story in the newspaper that morning about a person with AIDS). A subjective probability can be influenced by the physical context in which the belief is thought about (e.g., if a room is uncomfortably hot, then the probability of an undesirable consequence occurring might be perceived as being higher because of the effect of room temperature on mood). And, a subjective probability can be influenced by residues of experience that are not accessible in memory but which nonetheless exert an influence on it, that is, by an implicit attitude. The meta-analysis presented by Poehlman et al. (2006) reviewed several studies that linked implicit attitudes to behavioral beliefs, so it is not unreasonable to suggest that implicit attitudes may impact behavior through their impact on beliefs within the TRA and the TPB. Indeed there is a long tradition in many theories in psychology about unconscious and subconscious influences on behavioral beliefs.

Along these same lines, it is entirely possible that implicit attitudes influence other core components of the TRA and the TPB, such as how favorable or unfavorable one judges a consequence to be, how much a particular referent is perceived as approving or disapproving of a behavior, one's motivation to comply with a referent, and one's perceptions about the obstacles that stand in the way of performing a behavior and his or her perceived ability to overcome those obstacles. In short, an implicit attitude is like any other distal variable that can impact behavior through the many core components of the TRA and the TPB.

Mediation is not the only mechanism relevant for distal variables impacting behavior in the TRA and the TPB. Distal variables also can serve as moderators to impact (1) the importance of a behavioral belief in influencing an attitude, (2) the importance of a normative belief in influencing a subjective norm, (3) the importance of a control belief in influencing perceived control, (4) the importance of an attitude in influencing a behavioral intention, (5) the importance of subjective norms in influencing a behavioral intention, (6) the importance of perceived control in influencing a behavioral intention, (7) the importance of a behavioral intention in influencing behavior, and (8) they can even play a role in higher-order interaction effects that qualify the effect of a facilitating or constraining condition on the intention-behavior relationship. Another mechanism through which implicit attitudes may impact behavior is through any of these channels as well.

In our opinion, it is hard to imagine a case where an implicit attitude would impact behavior directly without having any impact at all on some aspect of how one construes that behavior in terms of the components of the TRA and the TPB or in serving as a moderating influence of some aspect of these models. Despite this, interlinkages between implicit attitudes and the components of the TRA and the TPB have not been the subject of investigation in IAT oriented research. Instead, the most common focus has been on demonstrating a correlation between implicit attitudes and other beliefs, attitudes, or behaviors while ignoring the potential integrative possibilities with the TRA and the TPB through the analysis of behavioral mediators and moderators. We believe the field can benefit from such integrative research and analysis.

This comment should not be taken to imply that we endorse the two-component view of attitude that IAT theorists often espouse (i.e., a component that is accessible to declarative memory and a component that is inaccessible). We personally believe that there are many conceptual and psychometric ambiguities with such an orientation. However, if theorists choose to go down this path, then more integrative work with the dominant paradigms of attitude-behavior analysis will be more useful than focusing on approaches with explicit attitude measures that have long ago been rejected as being viable. Viewing implicit attitudes as a distal variable impacting behavior through the components of the TRA and the TPB promises to yield more informative perspectives on behavior, presuming that the measurement challenges associated with the measurement of implicit attitudes can be overcome.

Moving from Two Attitudes to One Attitude

Use of the IAT requires that *complementary* attitude objects be studied because the methodology requires the use of two attitude objects in a discrimination task. Yet in many behavioral prediction situations, only a single attitude object is relevant and, according to modern day attitude theory, this is the attitude towards performing the behavior in question. Another direction for future research using the IAT is to try to alter the IAT task so that it can measure an implicit attitude towards performing a behavior rather than measuring the relative difference between two attitudes. There is a straightforward strategy that can be used to isolate a single attitude, and we now discuss it.

The strategy involves the use of a *control category* in the IAT in conjunction with the attitude object one is interested in. A control category represents an attitude object that has no psychological relevance for the criterion or the problem at hand. As an example, Swanson, Rudman and Greenwald (2001) investigated cigarette smoking using an IAT that assessed the relative implicit attitudes for *smoking* versus *sweets*. The attitude object *sweets* was seen as being irrelevant to smoking so that the attitude towards sweets should bear no relationship to smoking behavior. If, in theory, one regresses an index of smoking behavior onto the two implicit evaluations separately, we would get

$$Y = \alpha + \beta_1 \, IA_{\text{SMOKING}} - \beta_2 \, IA_{\text{SWEETS}} + \varepsilon \qquad (9)$$

where β_2 should be zero. Given that β_2 is zero, the equation becomes

$$Y = \alpha + \beta_1 \, IA_{\text{SMOKING}} + \varepsilon \qquad (10)$$

and smoking is a simple linear function of the implicit attitude toward smoking.

There is a complication, however. Recall that the most common conceptualization of the IAT seems to imply attitude differencing, leading to the assumption that β_1 and β_2 are of equal value but opposite in sign:

$$Y = \alpha + \beta \, RIA + \varepsilon$$
$$= \alpha + \beta \, IA_{\text{SMOKING}} - \beta \, IA_{\text{SWEETS}} + \varepsilon \qquad (11)$$

The estimate of β in this case necessarily will be an intermediate value between 0 (the true value of β_2) and the true value of β_1. As such, the standard technique of regressing criteria onto IAT scores will mischaracterize both β_1 and β_2 rendering the use of a control category problematic (at least as it was used by Swanson et al., 2001).

There are conditions, however, where the use of a control category can isolate a single attitude without the above problem. If one assumes that the evaluation of the control category is constant for all study participants, then the IAT may be viable as an indicator of a single attitude. More specifically, if

$$RIA = IA_{SMOKING} - IA_{SWEETS} \tag{12}$$

and IA_{SWEETS} is a constant, k, then we obtain

$$Y = \alpha + \beta (IA_{SMOKING} - k) + \varepsilon \tag{13}$$

and the value of β is identical to that of the equation

$$Y = \alpha + \beta \, IA_{SMOKING} + \varepsilon \tag{14}$$

because subtracting a constant from a predictor does not alter the regression coefficient for that predictor.

In sum, it is possible to isolate a single implicit attitude using the IAT if one uses a control category that acts as a near constant (e.g., a bland and likely neutral attitude object, such as *furniture*, or one that is uniformly seen as being very positive). The strategy also requires that one remove the impact of artificial effects of general processing speed (which can be accomplished in some cases by obtaining an independent measure of processing speed and then statistically controlling for it in the modeling effort), as well as contextual influences. If people vary in their evaluations of the control category, then the use of a control category can be problematic. However, if the implicit evaluation of the control category is constant, then the implicit relative attitude reflects a single implicit attitude. The key is choosing a control category whose implicit attitude is (near) constant.

Assuming that a single attitude can be isolated using the IAT, the next problem is to ensure that the primary facets of the single attitude are correspondent with the behavioral criterion of interest. Because the IAT measures attitudes that are general in nature, one strategy is to use the IAT to predict broad behavioral criteria. For instance, one might predict the aggregate of tendencies to use racial slurs, to tell racist jokes, to discriminate against Black job applicants, to avoid activities where Blacks will be encountered and so forth. Research of this type typically has not been a concern to IAT researchers. Instead, studies have used the IAT to predict such specific behavioral criteria as the funding of Black organizations (Rudman, Feinberg, & Rey, 2000) and the friendliness expressed towards a

Black person (McConnell & Leibold, 2001; Sekaquaptewa, Espinoza, Thompson, Vargas, & von Hippel, 2003). To focus on specific outcomes such as these, better behavioral prediction typically will result if one measures more specific implicit attitude towards performing these behaviors, rather than the more global attitudes. In its current format, there is no easy way of using an IAT to accomplish this task.

The need for a single-attitude IAT and an IAT that allows for correspondence with specific behavior criteria point to two fundamental limitations of current IAT conceptualizations. Outside of scenarios where one expects two global attitudes to predict a broad set of criterion outcomes, one would expect the additional predictive power of the IAT over and above traditional attitude constructs to be limited.

Behavioral Decision Making and Behavioral Alternatives

One area where the IAT's focus on two attitude objects may be advantageous is situations that involve a choice among multiple behavioral options. For example, when faced with four different behavioral options from which to choose, decision theorists often are interested in examining beliefs, norms, perceived control, attitudes, and intentions with respect to each option and then conducting a comparative analysis between all possible pairs of options on those variables. In the IAT, one could document how relative implicit attitudes differ for all possible pairs of decision options, with each pair of options being explored in the context of the two-object IAT. Thus, there is a potentially natural application of the concept of relative attitudes in decision-making contexts, and this probably can be explored effectively with implicit concepts using the IAT (providing that the rather substantial measurement artifacts detailed earlier can be overcome). These implicit concepts would then be used in conjunction with the TRA and the TPB as applied to each decision option to gain a broader understanding of behavioral decision making.

AN IMPLICIT THEORY OF REASONED ACTION AND THEORY OF PLANNED BEHAVIOR

Just as IAT theorists have defined the notion of implicit attitudes, it is not a large conceptual leap to also think about implicit norms and implicit behavioral control. Another avenue for IAT researchers might be to develop parallel implicit concepts for all components of the TRA and the TPB and then explore how these distal variables operate through the traditional TRA and TPB variables to impact behavior. In essence, one can form an *explicit* TPB and an *implicit* TPB and then work with these constructs in an integrative way to better understand the bases of behavior.

The Need for a Scaling Theory

Another important direction for future research using the IAT is to elaborate a viable psychometric model with respect to it. At present, no such model has been articulated, at least in the manner that is typical in psychometrics. We develop this idea further by presenting one plausible psychometric model that is consistent with a large number of scaling applications in psychology. This model assumes that the measured variables are a linear function of the theoretical construct that one is trying to assess. To import this logic to the IAT, we assume that each response latency is a linear function of the relative implicit attitude, RIA:

$$IT = \alpha_1 + \lambda_1 \, RIA + \varepsilon_1$$
$$CT = \alpha_2 + \lambda_2 \, RIA + \varepsilon_2 \tag{15}$$

where the α are intercepts, the λ are slopes or regression coefficients, and the ε represent random measurement error. The question of interest to IAT researchers is how they might take the two IAT responses, IT and CT, and obtain the best single estimate of RIA. As already noted, the method settled upon has been to calculate a difference between CT and IT. This method in conjunction with the equations suggests that a single factor model should underlie the two measures, with factor loadings for the IT and CT that are equal in magnitude but opposite in sign. Blanton and Jaccard (2006) tested such a model empirically and found no support for it. This, in part, was due to the large contaminating influence of general processing speed on the two measures, but even when this was taken into account, a single factor model could not account for the observed measures. It appears instead that the IT and CT reflect different constructs (after controlling for processing speed) and that there is little justification for differencing them. More research is needed to isolate a viable scaling model for the IAT.

CONCLUSION

Implicit attitudes have become increasingly popular in social psychology. This chapter considered the role of implicit attitudes in helping us understand the relationship between attitudes and behavior. This was done by analyzing implicit attitude constructs from the perspective of the influential Theory of Reasoned Action and Theory of Planned Behavior.

Implicit attitude theorists have been lax about specifying a conceptual definition of implicit attitudes and distinguishing it from the traditional definition of an attitude. Instead, they have presumed a difference between the two constructs based on the fact that they are traditionally measured by different methods (see also Fazio & Olson, 2003). A careful analysis suggests that most implicit attitude theorists view an attitude as having two components, an explicit component that is accessible to declarative memory and an inaccessible component that exists outside the realm of declarative memory. They are concerned with the latter.

The major method for assessing implicit attitudes is the Implicit Association Test. The test measures the difference between two implicit attitudes and imposes a fairly restrictive model on analyzing the relationship between attitudes and behavior. The psychometric properties of the IAT are somewhat problematic because the instrument is double barreled, it is contaminated by processing speed (which sometimes needs to be controlled but other times should not be controlled), it is impacted by the measurement context in which it is measured, it may reflect familiarity and similarity rather than attitudes, and it has borderline reliability.

We reviewed 25 studies of the relationship between implicit attitudes and behavior based on a meta-analysis of Poehlman et al. (2006). Only a handful of studies evaluated the incremental predictive utility that implicit attitudes added over and above explicit measures of attitude, and the typical finding was that they did not do so. More problematic, however, was that the studies used an outdated model of attitude-behavior relations, thereby setting up a straw-man explicit theory as a standard of comparison. To date, there are no studies that examine the incremental explained variance in behavior that implicit attitudes add over and above the constructs of the Theory of Reasoned Action and the Theory of Planned Behavior.

We described how implicit attitudes can be integrated with the Theory of Reasoned Action and the Theory of Planned Behavior by viewing implicit attitudes as distal variables that impact behavior through the constructs of these models. We then described future research directions that might be pursued using implicit attitudes, including how to measure a single attitude rather than the relative difference between two attitudes, use of the IAT in analyses of behavioral decision making with multiple behavioral options, developing an implicit Theory of Reasoned Action and an implicit Theory of Planned Behavior and integrating these with the current TRA and TPB, and developing a viable scaling model for the IAT. Perhaps based on this research, the construct of implicit attitudes will establish an empirical foundation that is commensurate with the theoretical attention that it is currently receiving.

REFERENCES

Ajzen, I. (1991). The theory of planned behavior. *Organizational Behavior and Human Decision Processes, 50*, 179–211.

Ajzen, I., & Fishbein, M. (1977). Attitude-behavior relations: A theoretical analysis and review of empirical research. *Psychological Bulletin, 84*, 888–918.

Ajzen, I., & Fishbein, M. (1980). *Understanding attitudes and predicting social behavior.* Englewood Cliffs, NJ: Prentice Hall.

Ajzen, I., & Fishbein, M. (2000). Attitudes and the attitude-behavior relation: Reasoned and automatic processes. In W. Stroebe and M. Hewstone (Eds.), *European Review of Social Psychology.* New York: John Wiley & Sons.

Ajzen, I., & Fishbein, M. (2005). The influence of attitudes on behavior. In D. Albarracín, B. T. Johnson, & M. P. Zanna (Eds.), *The handbook of attitudes* (pp. 173–221). Mahwah, NJ: Lawrence Erlbaum Associates.

Ashburn-Nardo, L., Knowles, M. L., & Monteith, M. J. (2003). Black Americans' implicit racial associations and their implications for intergroup judgment. *Social Cognition, 21*, 61–87.

Back, M. D., Schmuckle, S. & Egloff, B. (2005). Measuring task-switching ability in the Implicit Association Test. *Experimental Psychology, 52*, 167–179.

Bargh, J. A. (1996). Automaticity in social psychology. In E. T. Higgins & A. W. Kruglanski (Eds.), *Social psychology: Handbook of basic principles* (pp. 169–183). New York: Guilford Press.

Blanton, H. & Jaccard. J. (2006). Decoding the Implicit Association Test: Perspectives on criterion prediction. *Journal of Experimental Social Psychology* (in press).

Brendl, C. M., Markman, A. & Messner, C. (2001). Evaluating the inference of prejudice in the Implicit Association Test. *Journal of Personality and Social Psychology, 81*, 760–773.

Brunel, F. F., Collins, C. M., Greenwald, A. G. & Tietje, B. C. (1999). Making the public private, accessing the inaccessible: Marketing applications of the implicit association test. *Polish Psychological Bulletin, 32,* 1–9.

Cunningham, W. A., Preacher, K. J., & Banaji, M. R. (2001). Implicit attitude measures: Consistency, stability, and convergent validity. *Psychological Science, 12,* 163–170.

Czopp, A. M., Monteith, M. J., Zimmerman, R. S., & Lynam, D. R. (2006). Implicit attitudes as potential protection from risky sex: Predicting condom use with the IAT. *Basic and Applied Social Psychology.*

Dasgupta, N., McGhee, D. E., Greenwald, A. G., & Banaji, M. R. (2000). Automatic preference for White Americans: Eliminating the familiarity explanation. *Journal of Experimental Social Psychology, 36,* 316–328.

De Houwer, J., Geldof, T. & De Bruycker, E. (2005). The Implicit Association Test as a general measure of similarity. *Canadian Journal of Experimental Psychology, 59,* 228–239.

Devine, P. (1993). Implicit prejudice and stereotyping: How automatic are they? Introduction to the special section. *Journal of Personality and Social Psychology, 81,* 757–767.

Eagly, A., & Chaiken, S. (1993). *Psychology of attitudes.* New York: Harcourt, Brace Jovanovich.

Edwards, A. (1957). *Techniques of attitude scale construction.* New York: Appleton-Century-Crofts.

Fazio, R. H. (1990). Multiple processes by which attitudes guide behavior: The MODE model as an integrative framework. In M. P. Zanna (Ed.), *Advances in experimental social psychology* (Vol. 23, pp. 75–109). San Diego, CA: Academic Press.

Fazio, R. H., & Olson, M. A. (2003). Implicit measures in social cognition research: Their meaning and uses. *Annual Review of Psychology, 54,* 297–327.

Fishbein, M., & Ajzen, I. (1975). *Beliefs, attitudes, intentions and behavior.* Reading, MA: Addison-Wesley.

Greenwald, A. G., Banaji, M., Rudnam, L., Farnham, S., Nosek, B. A. & Mellott, D. (2002). A unified theory of implicit attitudes, stereotypes, self-esteem, and self-concept. *Psychological Review, 109,* 3–25.

Greenwald, A. G, & Farnham, S. D. (2000). Using the implicit association test to measure self-esteem and self-concept. *Journal of Personality and Social Psychology, 79,* 1022–1038.

Greenwald, A. G., McGhee, D. E., & Schwartz, J. L. K. (1998). Measuring individual differences in implicit cognition: The implicit association test. *Journal of Personality and Social Psychology, 74,* 1064–1480.

Greenwald, A. G., Nosek, B. A., & Banaji, M. R. (2003). Scoring procedures to improve implicit association test measures. *Journal of Personality and Social Psychology, 85,* 197–216.

Jellison, W. A., McConnell, A. R., & Gabriel, S. (2004). Implicit and explicit measures of sexual orientation attitudes: In-group preferences and overt behaviors among gay and straight men. *Personality and Social Psychology Bulletin, 30,* 629–642.

Karpinski, A. & Hilton, J.L. (2001). Attitudes and the Implicit Association Test. *Journal of Personality & Social Psychology, 81,* 774–788.

Kinoshita, S. & Peek-O'Leary, M. (2005). Does the compatibility effect in the race IAT reflect familiarity or affect? *Psychometric Bulletin and Review, 32,* 440–448.

Lemm, K.M. (2000). Personal and social motivation to respond without prejudice: Implications for implicit and explicit attitude and behavior. Unpublished doctoral dissertation, Yale University.

Maison, D., Greenwald, A. G., & Bruin, R. H. (2004). Predictive validity of the Implicit Association Test in studies of brands and consumer attitudes and behavior. *Journal of Consumer Psychology. 14,* 405–415.

Maison, D, Greenwald, A. G., & Bruin, R. (2001). The implicit association test as a measure of consumer attitudes. *Polish Psychological Bulletin, 2,* 79.

Marsh, K. L., Johnson, B. T., & Scott-Sheldon, L. A. J. (2001). Heart versus reason in condom use: Implicit vs. explicit attitudinal predictors of sexual behavior. *Zeitschrift fur Experimentelle Psychologie, 48*, 161–175.

McConnell, A. R., & Leibold, J. M. (2001). Relations among the Implicit Association Test, discriminatory behavior, and explicit measures of racial attitudes. *Journal of Experimental Social Psychology, 37*, 435–442.

McFarland, S. G., & Crouch, Z. (2002). A cognitive skills confound on the Implicit Association Test. *Social Cognition, 20*, 481–506.

Mierke, J., & Klauer, K. C. (2003). Method-specific variance in the Implicit Association Test. *Journal of Personality and Social Psychology, 85*, 118–128.

Neumann, R., Hülsenbeck, K. & Seibt, B. (2004). Attitudes towards people with AIDS and avoidance behavior: Automatic and reflective bases of behavior. *Journal of Experimental Social Psychology, 40*, 543–550.

Nosek, B. A. & Banaji, M. R. (2002). [Polish language] (At least) two factors moderate the relationship between implicit and explicit attitudes. In R. K. Ohme & M. Jarymowicz (Eds.), *Natura Automatyzmow* (pp. 49–56). Warszawa: WIP PAN & SWPS.

Nosek, B. A., Greenwald, A. G., & Banaji, M. R. (in press). The Implicit Association Test at age 7: A methodological and conceptual review. In J. A. Bargh (Ed.), *Automatic processes in social thinking and behavior*. New York: Psychology Press.

Perugini, M. (2006). Predictive models of implicit and explicit attitudes. *British Journal of Social Psychology*.

Petty, R. E., Wegener, D. T., & Fabrigar, L. R. (1997). Attitudes and attitude change. *Annual Review of Psychology, 48*, 609–647.

Poehlman, T., Uhlmann, E., Greenwald, A. & Banaji, M. (2006). *Understanding and using the Implicit Association Test: III. Meta-analysis of predictive validity.* Unpublished manuscript, Department of Psychology, Yale University.

Rothermund, K., Wentura, D. & De Houwer, J. (2005) Validity of the salience asymmetry account of the Implicit Association Test: Reply to Greenwald, Nosek, Banaji, and Klauer (2005). *Journal of Experimental Psychology: General, 134*, 426–430.

Rudman, L., Feinberg, J., & Rey, A. (2000). *Minority members' implicit stereotypes and attitudes.* Unpublished manuscript, Rutgers University.

Schmuckle, S. C. & Egloff, B. (2005). A latent state-trait analysis of implicit and explicit personality measures. *European Journal of Psychological Assessment, 21*, 100–107.

Sekaquaptewa, D., Espinoza, P., Thompson, M., Vargas, P., & von Hippel, W. (2003). Stereotypic explanatory bias: Implicit stereotyping as a predictor of discrimination. *Journal of Experimental Social Psychology, 39*, 75–82.

Skowronski, J.J., & Carlston, D.E. (1989). Negativity and extremity biases in impression formation: A review of explanations. *Psychological Bulletin, 105*, 131–142.

Steffens, M. & Buchner, A. (2003). Implicit Association Test: Separating transsituationally stable and variable components of attitudes toward gay men, *Experimental Psychology, 33*, 45–57.

Swanson, J. E., Rudman, L. A., & Greenwald, A. G. (2001). Using the Implicit Association Test to investigate attitude-behavior consistency for stigmatized behavior. *Cognition and Emotion, 15*, 207–230.

Wiers, R. W., Woerden, N. V., Smulders F. T. Y. & de Jong, P. T. (2002). Implicit and explicit alcohol-related cognitions in heavy and light drinkers. *Journal of Abnormal Psychology, 111*, 648–658.

CHAPTER 6

Commentary on Attitudes and Behavior

Harry C. Triandis

University of Illinois

The chapters of this section are excellent, so I will first point to the particular strengths of each chapter, and then comment on some themes that cut across the chapters.

The Ajzen and Albarracín chapter has a good discussion of the advantages of specific constructs, as opposed to global dispositions. It does an excellent job of reviewing studies of the relationship of intentions and behavior, and summarizes both meta-analyses and behavioral predictions concerning a diverse set of behaviors. It contrasts the pessimism about the relationship of attitudes and behavior found in the 1960s (e.g., Wicker, 1969) with the more recent results where the multiple Rs are impressive. Especially notable are the results of the relationship of training efforts to change condom use, as reflected in Figure 1–2. It presents several complex relationships showing that distraction can have different effects on the variables of the Fishbein–Ajzen theory. Some of the attitude change findings are consistent with those of the Hovland program some 60 years ago, but others are not.

The Trafimow chapter is a scholarly discussion of the distinctions that were introduced by Fishbein's theorizing. He comments on the distinction between attitude and subjective norm, and the need to distinguish the same behavior when it occurs in different contexts, toward a different target, or at different times. He sees some problems, however, with the distinction between the affective and cognitive components of attitudes, and between positively and negatively framed beliefs. He argues convincingly that the value of the theory has been great exactly because some aspects of it were falsified. He makes the correct point that no theory in the history of science is true under all conditions. For instance, Einstein showed the limitations of Newton's theoretical views when an object's velocity approaches that of the speed of light. He concludes that Fishbein's theory has been one of the most successful in the history of social psychology.

One of Trafimow's points is that in some cases 3 beliefs do a better job in predicting behavior than do 15 beliefs. Here, I think, it is important to extend the research to examine if there are interactions between the number of beliefs needed and cognitive complexity, which is an important individual differences variable. It may be that for cognitively simple people (the majority) this finding holds, but it is not correct for cognitively complex people. This is worth investigating. Another point is more technical. The more constructs are used the more measurement error there is likely to be in the data. The measurement errors are likely to be additive, so that the sum of 15 beliefs may have more measurement error than the sum of 3 beliefs.

The Hornick and Cappella chapters have two foci. Cappella discusses the role of emotion and shows increased predictive utility, when predicting behavior, if emotions are included as an independent variable. Hornick outlines how behavioral outcomes that are a function of many small behaviors can be investigated using the Fishbein-Ajzen theory. He outlines five strategies for exploiting the framework when multiple behaviors must be considered.

The role of emotion is stressed similarly in research by Westen (1998). Westen, Blagov, Feit, Arkowitz & Thagard (2004) argue that humans process emotional stimuli unconsciously. They slant the representation of those they like and care about in positive directions, and those they dislike in negative directions. Their judgments are influenced by several emotions simultaneously, which pull their cognitions in different directions. They process cognitions and emotions in parallel (like two computers set to work in parallel, one processing the emotions and the other processing the cognitions), and at some point the two computers "talk to each other," and the emotions often overwhelm the cognitions. Westen et al. presented several empirical studies of decision making that show that emotions often overwhelm cognitions. For example, a community sample was asked to judge whether an Abu Ghraib prison keeper accused of mistreating prisoners should be able to subpoena Secretary of Defense Rumsfeld and President Bush to obtain exculpatory evidence. Their judgments did not reflect legal reasoning but were simply determined by the way they *felt* about the issue (i.e., their party affiliation, attitudes toward human rights, and toward the military).

The Jaccard and Blanton chapter provides an extensive, critical examination of implicit attitudes and integrates this research area with the Fishbein-Ajzen theory. It explores several important questions about implicit attitudes, and is particularly good in pointing to ambiguities and unsettled issues. In my opinion they might also consider the role or measurement error. When constructs are subtracted, the measurement errors are likely to be additive, and that may be the explanation for the low test-retest reliabilities of implicit measures. Perhaps implicit attitude theorists should use simpler ways of measurement, such as the difference in reaction time between "X / pleasant" and "X / unpleasant."

Jaccard and Blanton discuss artifacts that are problematic for implicit methods, but not for explicit measures. Of course, explicit measures have their own problems, such as impression management biases. They provide a sound critique of implicit measures because the double-barrel problem is confounded with general processing speed. They point to the researcher's dilemma of whether to treat general processing speed as an artifact or as conceptually meaningful. They conclude that implicit measures do not impact behavior directly, but their influence is exerted on the key variables of the Fishbein-Ajzen model.

Both the Ajzen-Albarricín and Trafimow chapters discuss the issue of specificity of constructs. I think that this is a point inviting some discussion. There is no doubt that Fishbein's major contribution has been the extension of social psychology in the direction of specificity, which has raised the multiple Rs into the stratosphere. However, one limitation of this strategy needs to be mentioned.

If we think of a hierarchy of levels of abstraction, we have something like this:

All-inclusive constructs (e.g., God)

Dispositions

Values

Attitudes

Beliefs

Beliefs in context, specifying time, target, place

Even within the constructs of this hierarchy there is variability in specificity, with for instance, the *value* of *stimulation* being more specific that the value of *security* simply because there are fewer behaviors that involve stimulation than behaviors that involve security. Again, the more specific the constructs the better the behavioral prediction (Bardi & Schwartz, 2003). But consider the economics of data collection. The specific constructs require data collection for each behavior, specifying the action, target, context, and time, while the abstract constructs are independent of time and context. True, the multiple Rs are dramatically different, since values predict in the .25 to .45 range, depending on the criterion (Bardi & Schwartz, 2003), while the amount of variance accounted by the specific constructs can be several times greater.

In the history of human thought we note that explanations begin with the most general level, such as the behavior is due to "the will of God," which explains everything and predicts nothing. They end with Fishbein, that is, very powerful specific constructs which have immense predictive power. The specific constructs, however, are only useful in a narrow domain. As the constructs become more specific their value increases, but so does the labor needed to measure them. Instead of one construct we need a myriad of constructs to predict a myriad of behaviors.

This issue has been examined by Cronbach and Glaser (1965, chapter 8), in the context of the use of tests. They discuss the *bandwidth* versus *fidelity* problem. Bandwidth corresponds to specificity-generality, while fidelity corresponds to the prediction of some criterion, such as a behavior. They note that the narrower the bandwidth the higher is the fidelity. However, broad bandwidth means that the test applies to a wide range of situations. They propose that the problem be examined over *all* decisions that are to be taken. In our present situation that means predicting all the behaviors that one wishes to predict. They then do a *utility analysis* and examine how investigators might distribute their effort. Since large bandwidth means low fidelity, it is necessary to find the optimal compromise from the point of view of investigator effort. They provide a series of equations that can be helpful in achieving the highest utility for one's effort, taking into account the cost of testing.

Cronbach and Glaser conclude that the optimum distribution of effort is a function of the number of tests, the time that is required to test, the contribution of each test per unity of cost, and the intercorrelations among the units of tests. Their final conclusion is that the benefit from a series of moderately valid tests may be larger than the benefit from a small number of very high fidelity tests.

I suggest that this kind of analysis might be done with respect to the prediction of behavior from attitudes. It would be desirable to find out under what conditions we should spend our energy getting large multiple Rs, or if we might do better by using broader constructs that result in more modest multiple Rs.

Also, as we move around the world, the meaning of specific concepts changes more than the meaning of abstract concepts. Anthropologists have argued that abstract concepts such as language, food habits, art, myths, religious practices, family, economic systems, truth, government, war, kinship, shelter, training systems, hygiene, and incest taboos exist in all cultures (Brown, 1991). Yet the specific meanings of these constructs are quite different from culture to culture. Thus *food habits* means more or less the same thing around the world. But when we look at specific behaviors we need to consider very different patterns. People differ in what they eat, when they eat, where they eat, with whom they eat, how they eat, and so on. Thus, to predict eating behavior we need to measure in each culture a myriad of beliefs at the specific level, while we can get along with few beliefs at the abstract level.

Thus intensive data collection is needed in each culture, and one can legitimately ask: In a study of humans from 100 cultures, is a multiple R of .80 worth a million dollars, when one can get a multiple R of .4 with $100,000 with the use of a broader construct?

This raises issues such as how important is the study of values or roles or norms, or broad attitudes such as *liberalism* as opposed to specific beliefs? How feasible is the extensive data collection? For example, if we wish to study the views of a senator over a six-year period, concerning national defense, would it be feasible to ask hundreds of questions? Perhaps the senator can only be asked to rank the importance of national defense against a dozen other issues, such as preserving the environment, reducing the deficit, and so on. It is unlikely that extensive data collection would be feasible.

Thus, in my view, the optimal strategy depends on the nature of the problem. If one needs to reduce the frequency of AIDS one needs to be specific, but if one is to understand why it is better to invest a million dollars in Scandinavia than in Saudi Arabia, (there is no country "Arabia") then the broader construct may well be optimal. In short, we need to see the issue in the context of what we aim to achieve.

In my view the broader constructs do have a place, and the work of Shalom Schwartz (1992) or Inglehart and Baker (2000) also makes a contribution. I find it interesting, for instance, that around the world the value of *power* is low relative to the other values studied by Schwartz. This indicates that humans are likely to disguise their lust for power, and to tell us that what they are doing is due to some other cause. Thus, for instance, there is a Muslim cleric in Indonesia (Stern, 2003) who told his followers that they would go to hell if they made friends with a Christian. He exerted power over them, but he did not express it in power terms, but instead in theological terms.

A large study by Inglehart & Baker (2000) examined data from several countries and found two dimensions distinguishing countries. One dimension contrasted *traditional authority* with *secular-national authority*. The traditional side emphasized the importance of God. The secular side emphasized permissive attitudes toward sexual and other issues. This contrast, among cultures, is positively related to individualism (more secular) and negatively to power distance (hierarchical cultures give more importance to God). The other dimension contrasted *survival* (emphasis on money, hard work) with *well-being* (leisure, friends, concern for the environment). The Northern European countries were high on both the *secular* and the *well-being* dimensions. The African and Muslim countries were on the *traditional* and the *survival* sides of the two dimensions. The remaining countries were in-between these two sets of countries. Thus the Scandinavian countries are maximally different in values from the African and Muslim countries. This implies that we can expect that Northern Europeans will have considerable difficulties getting along with people from Arab countries. The recent conflict over the Danish cartoons of the prophet Mohammad confirms that the two sets of cultures are very different.

Thus, if what we want to achieve is to reduce AIDS, we need to be very specific; if we want to advise people on where to place their money it may be more economical to collect the data using more abstract constructs.

CONCLUSION

These chapters show that much has been achieved in the prediction of behavior in general, and health behavior in particular. At the same time the work discussed in this book is a living, vibrant research tradition, that can always be improved, expanded, made more sophisticated, and occasionally falsified, so that it is in the best tradition of the history of science.

REFERENCES

Bardi, A & Schwartz, S. H. (2003). Values and behavior: Strength and structure of relations. *Personality and Social Psychology Bulletin, 29,* 1207–1220.

Brown, D. E. (1991) *Human universals.* Philadelphia: Temple University Press.

Cronbach, L. & Glaser, G. C. (1965). *Psychological tests and personnel decisions* (2nd ed.). Urbana: University of Illinois Press.

Inglehart, R. & Baker, W. E. (2000). Modernization, cultural change, and the persistence of traditional values. *American Sociological Review, 65,* 19–51.

Schwartz, S. H. (1992) Universals in the content and structure of values. Theoretical advances and empirical tests in 20 countries. In M. Zanna (Ed.), *Advances in Experimental Social Psychology* (Vol. 25). New York: Academic Press.

Stern, J. (2003). *Terror in the name of God.* New York: Harper Collins.

Westen, D. (1998). The scientific legacy of Sigmund Freud: Toward an informed psychological science. *Psychological Bulletin, 124,* 333–371.

Westen, D., Blagov, P., Feit, A., Arkowitz, J., & Thagard, P. (2004). When reason and passion collide: Emotional constraint in motivated political reasoning. (in preparation, retrieved from dwesten@emory.edu).

Wicker, A. (1969). Attitudes versus actions: The relationship of verbal to behavioral responses to attitude objects. *Journal of Social Issues, 25,* 41–78.

CHAPTER 7

Attitudes and Behavior: Critical Issues

Victor Ottati and Nathaniel D. Krumdick

Loyola University Chicago

The chapters contained within the Attitudes and Behavior section of this volume provide a compelling analysis of Martin Fishbein's contributions to psychology. Trafimow's chapter includes an interesting discussion of factors that influence the relative weight ascribed to normative and attitudinal considerations when individuals form a behavioral intention. Trafimow also addresses important questions regarding the nature and number of beliefs that determine attitudes and behavior. Ajzen and Albarracín summarize a large body of research that examines key assumptions of the reasoned action approach. They also provide a cogent critique of research that violates the principle of correspondence when assessing the attitude-behavior relation. Capella considers an interesting extension of Fishbein's work, one that incorporates *anticipated emotional outcomes* as additional determinants of behavior intentions. Finally, Jaccard and Blanton provide a thought-provoking critique of implicit attitude research that has failed to address fundamental advances associated with the reasoned action tradition.

This commentary focuses on five issues that are directly relevant to the aforementioned chapters. These concern (a) episodic affect and attitude formation, (b) the distinction between *integration at encoding* and *integration at the time of judgment*, (c) direction of causality, (d) the principle of correspondence, and (e) implicit attitudes as determinants of behavior.

EPISODIC AFFECT AND ATTITUDE FORMATION

When considering episodic affect, it is useful to distinguish (a) an emotional reaction to an object (e.g., "Reagan made me feel angry"), (b) affect toward a behavior (e.g., "Smoking is pleasurable"), and (c) the perceived emotional outcome of performing a behavior (e.g., "Smoking will lead me to feel guilty afterwards"). Trafimow (see also Trafimow & Sheeren, 1998) makes a distinction between *cognitive beliefs* (e.g., "My smoking cigarettes is/would be harmful versus beneficial") and *affective beliefs* ("My smoking cigarettes is/would be enjoyable versus unenjoyable). The cognitive beliefs focus on the outcomes of the behavior, and are similar to *behavioral beliefs* measured within the theory of reasoned action (e.g., "My smoking will lead me to get cancer, likely versus unlikely" (Fishbein & Ajzen, 1975). The affective beliefs assess what Triandis (1980) has labeled *affect toward the behavior*. These items assess affective reactions to the actual performance of the behavior, affective reactions that arise concurrent to the act, not outcomes that follow the behavior. In accordance with Triandis's (1980) model, Trafimow finds that cognitive and affective beliefs are represented distinctly, and function as independent predictors of behavior intentions.

Capella makes a theoretical distinction between beliefs that reflect the cognitive consequences of a behavior and beliefs that reflect the emotional outcomes of a behavior. The beliefs that assess the cognitive consequences are similar to behavioral beliefs assessed within the TRA tradition (e.g., "If I try to quit smoking, I would have better health"). However, the items that assess the emotional outcomes assess emotional reactions to an intention ("Describe how you feel about your intention to quit smoking," items labeled *proud*, *disgusted*, etc.). Emotional reactions to an intention may not reflect emotional outcomes that are anticipated to arise subsequent to performing a behavior (e.g., "I don't know how I will feel after I stop smoking. But, my intention to stop smoking next summer currently makes me feel hopeful."). Thus, this affect measure may not assess anticipated outcomes in the same way that the cognitive beliefs do.

Measurement issues aside, it is intriguing to consider the possibility that anticipated emotional outcomes of a behavior determine intentions independent of the anticipated cognitive outcomes. An analogous (although slightly different) stream of research has examined the possibility that beliefs and emotional reactions to an object function as independent determinants of attitude toward the object (e.g., Abelson, Kinder, Peters, & Fiske, 1982). Research in this related area has encountered some methodological difficulties. Specifically, Ottati (1996) has noted that reliance on closed-ended measures to assess beliefs and emotions is problematic. By administering a common set of belief and emotion items to all respondents, it is virtually guaranteed that the researcher will fail to assess beliefs that are emotionally relevant for each individual. When using an open-ended measurement procedure that specifically targets emotionally relevant beliefs, it is found that these beliefs (e.g., "Reagan joked about bombing the Soviets") fully account for the role of emotions (e.g., "Reagan made me angry") when predicting attitudes toward the object (Ottati, 1996). A similar finding might emerge if Capella were to use an open-ended cognitive consequence measure that specifically targets *emotionally relevant cognitive consequences*. These cognitive consequences might fully account for the role of anticipated emotional outcomes when predicting intentions and behavior.

INTEGRATION AT ENCODING VERSUS INTEGRATION AT THE TIME OF JUDGMENT

It might be beneficial for researchers within the Theory of Reasoned Action (TRA) tradition to more explicitly consider the distinction between integration at encoding and integration at the time of judgment (see Hastie & Park, 1986). When integration occurs at the time of judgment, it is presumed that beliefs about the object are formed while the individual encodes (i.e., receives) information about the object, and that these beliefs are stored in memory. When later asked to report an attitude judgment, these specific beliefs are retrieved from memory, and then integrated for purposes of forming and reporting an attitude judgment. When integration occurs at encoding, it is presumed that beliefs are integrated into a *running tally* of the attitude while the individual initially encodes (i.e., receives) information about the object. This summary tally is stored in memory. When later asked to report an attitude judgment, this previously integrated tally (rather than the specific beliefs it was derived from) is retrieved and used as a basis for judgment.

The integration at encoding model assumes that a previously integrated attitude can be retrieved and used as a basis for reporting an attitude at a later point in time. Similarly, a previously integrated intention can be retrieved and used as a basis for reporting an intention at a later point in time. Namely, when faced with an initial opportunity to perform a behavior, an individual might form an integrated behavioral intention and store it in memory. When later faced with a similar opportunity, the individual might retrieve the stored intention (rather than the specific information that it was originally derived from) and use it as a basis for the behavioral decision. For this reason, the TRA does not imply that people form a new intention immediately prior to performing each and every behavior (see Ajzen & Albarracín, this volume).

The integration at encoding model, however, also raises challenges to the TRA tradition. Proponents of this model argue that the beliefs that are initially integrated into the running tally may not be salient when the individual later reports a judgment. Thus, the content and number of beliefs that are salient at the time of judgment may not be identical to the content and number of beliefs that actually determine the attitude (i.e., tally) at encoding. Indeed, beliefs that are salient at the time of judgment might simply justify an attitude that was originally determined by a different set of beliefs. Empirical tests of the TRA approach frequently assess beliefs that are salient at the time of judgment. The integration at encoding model suggests that these may not be the beliefs that actually determine the attitude (i.e., tally) at encoding. Moreover, the number of beliefs that determine the attitude (i.e., tally) at encoding may not be equal to the number of beliefs (assessed at the time of judgment) that best predict the attitude judgment. Thus, to establish the number of beliefs that actually *determine* the attitude, Trafimow might be advised to focus on the number of beliefs that are salient at encoding.

DIRECTION OF CAUSALITY: REASONED OR RATIONALIZED ACTION?

Whereas the TRA approach presumes that beliefs determine attitudes, cognitive consistency theory accommodates a more varied set of causal relations. If one defines "P" as the respondent, "O" as the attitude object, and "X" as an attribute of the object; there is a direct correspondence between the elements of the Fishbein and Ajzen attitude model and the links composing Heider's P–O–X triad (Ottati, Fishbein, & Middlestadt, 1988). Attitude toward the object (A_O), belief about the object (b_i), and evaluation of the belief (e_i) correspond to the P–O, O–X, and P–X links, respectively (see Figure 7–1).

The TRA approach assumes that the belief (b_i, O–X link) and evaluation (e_i, P–X link) combine to determine the attitude (A_O, P–O link). According to balance theory, it is also possible that the attitude (A_O, P–O link) and belief (b_i, O–X link) combine to determine the evaluation (e_i, P–X link). Alternatively, the attitude (A_O, P–O link) and evaluation (e_i, P–X link) can combine to determine the belief (b_i, O–X link). In these later two cases, beliefs and evaluations are not the determinants of the attitude. Rather, they are justifications for an attitude that was originally derived on the basis of other considerations. Importantly, all three of these causal possibilities can account for a positive (cross-sectional) correlation between the sum of $b_i e_i$ and A_O. Analogous concerns arise when considering the determinants of attitude toward a behavior.

A cynic might therefore argue that the beliefs assessed within the TRA tradition are pure rationalizations for attitudes that are based on other factors. Ottati, Fishbein, & Middlestadt (1988) have demonstrated that there are limits to this logic. Beliefs contain a substantial accuracy component, and as such, the degree to which they serve as mere justifications for attitudes is limited. Nevertheless, additional research is needed to more fully isolate the direction of causality when testing models within the TRA tradition.

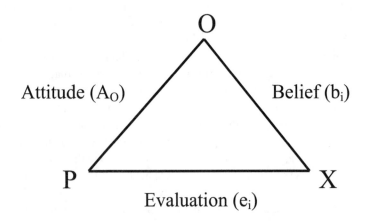

FIGURE 7–1.   Correspondence between elements of the Fishbein and Ajzen attitude model and the P–O–X triad.

CORRESPONDENCE (SPECIFICITY) OF MEASURES

Many of the chapters emphasize the critical role of *correspondence* within the TRA tradition (Ajzen & Albarracín; Capella; Jaccard & Blanton). The TRA approach correctly noted that the attitude-behavior correlation increases substantially when attitude and behavior are measured at corresponding levels of specificity. It is unreasonable to assume that an individual's global attitude toward an object (e.g., "I like my mother") will predict a specific behavior toward that object (e.g., "My buying my mother a ring"). Yet, early studies that investigated the attitude-behavior relation almost always committed this error, and more recent research often continues to do so. For example, Jaccard and Blanton correctly note that implicit attitude researchers commonly use an implicit measure of attitude toward an object (e.g., prejudice toward Blacks) when predicting a specific behavior (e.g., voting for a Black candidate).

The notion of correspondence constitutes an indispensable and extremely important addition to the attitude literature. Nevertheless, a descriptive model of human behavior might adopt a more flexible version of this principle. In some cases, individuals form an attitude toward a behavior that they are committed to under all circumstances. For example, some women are opposed to having an abortion under *any* circumstance. That is, they possess an extremely negative attitude toward this behavior that generalizes across all times and circumstances. When asked to report a multitude of specific abortion intentions (e.g., intention to have an abortion 6 weeks after conception, intention to have an abortion 8 weeks after conception, intention to have an abortion 10 weeks after conception), these individuals may not derive a specific attitude toward each behavior. For reasons of cognitive economy, these individuals may access their (more general) negative attitude toward the behavior, and use it as a basis for responding to the more specific behavior intention items. Individuals who are open to a behavioral possibility may be motivated to form more specific, correspondent attitudes. For example, a person who is seriously considering an abortion might form a more positive attitude toward an early term abortion than a late term abortion. It may be useful to adopt a flexible conceptualization of correspondence that accommodates this possibility.

IMPLICIT AND AUTOMATICALLY ACTIVATED ATTITUDES

Jaccard and Blanton identify numerous shortcomings associated with implicit attitude research that relies on the Implicit Association Test (IAT) measure. They suggest it is unlikely that implicit attitudes directly determine intentions or behavior. To the contrary, implicit attitudes may function primarily as *distal* variables. From this perspective, the effect of implicit attitudes on behavior is mediated by more proximal determinants of behavior already identified within the reasoned action tradition (e.g., behavioral beliefs, outcome evaluations). Jaccard and Blanton, however, do leave room for the possibility that implicit attitudes may exert a more direct influence on intentions or behavior. This might be demonstrated if implicit attitudes and behavior are measured at corresponding levels of specificity.

Implicit attitude researchers commonly assess global attitudes toward an object. This is not surprising. Implicit attitudes toward a specific behavior (e.g., "attending the Chicago Symphony on October 12th") are probably impossible to assess. Nonetheless, it is still possible to examine the implicit attitude-behavior relation without violating the principle of correspondence. Specifically, implicit attitudes toward an object can be used to predict a corresponding, global behavioral criterion (i.e., a behavioral index that summarizes the evaluative tone of *all* behaviors performed toward the object). Because implicit attitude researchers have failed to use a corresponding global behavioral criterion, it is not surprising that they have failed to obtain strong correlations between implicit attitudes and behavior (see Jaccard and Blanton).

It is also possible that a different kind of *correspondence* is relevant within this domain. Specifically, attitudes and behaviors that correspond in terms of automaticity may exhibit higher correlations than attitudes and behaviors that differ along this dimension. Whereas automatically activated attitudes may predict automatic behavioral reactions, more conscious and controlled attitudinal reports may predict more deliberative behavioral reactions. Consistent with this conceptualization, automatic evaluation of African Americans predicts a White person's non-verbal reactions to an African American person (Fazio, Jackson, Dunton, & Williams, 1995). Presumably, this occurs because non-verbal behavior is difficult to consciously control. On the other hand, more consciously controlled and explicit attitudinal reports may predict more deliberate and controlled behavior (e.g., hiring an African American). A proper test of this possibility should employ measures that correspond in terms of specificity—that is, researchers should assess automatic attitude toward the object, explicit attitude toward the object, a general index of automatic behavioral reactions to the object, and a general index of deliberative behavioral reactions to the object. If correspondence in terms of automaticity matters, the correlation between attitudes and behavior should be relatively strong when using the *matching* measures and relatively weak when using the *mismatching* measures. Previous attempts to uncover this pattern have failed to use measures that correspond in terms of specificity.

CONCLUSION

The theory of reasoned action continues to inspire research of the highest caliber. To increase our understanding of attitudes and behavior, future research might benefit by exploring creative extensions of this model. These might include expanding the concept of behavioral outcome to incorporate the notion of an emotional outcome, incorporating measures of beliefs at encoding when predicting attitudes, and adopting a more flexible and extended conceptualization of correspondence. We look forward to future research that explores these and other possibilities.

REFERENCES

Abelson, R. P., Kinder, D. R., Peters, M. D., & Fiske, S. T. (1982). Affective and semantic components in political person perception. *Journal of Personality and Social Psychology, 42*(4), 619–630.

Fazio, R. H., Jackson, J. R., Dunton, B. C., & Williams, C. J. (1995). Variability in automatic activation as an unobtrusive measure of racial attitudes: A bona fide pipeline? *Journal of Personality and Social Psychology, 69*(6), 1013–1027.

Fishbein, M., Ajzen, I. (1975). *Belief, attitude,intention, and behavior: An introduction to theory and research*. Reading: Addison-Wesley.

Hastie, R., & Park, B. (1986). The relationship between memory and judgment depends on whether the judgment task is memory-based or on-line. *Psychological Review, 93*(3), 258–268.

Ottati, V. (1996). When the survey question directs retrieval: Implications for assessing the cognitive and affective predictors of global evaluation. *European Journal of Social Psychology, 26*, 1–21.

Ottati, V., Fishbein, M., & Middlestadt, S. E. (1988). Determinants of voters' beliefs about the candidates' stands on the issues: The role of evaluative bias heuristics and the candidates' expressed message. *Journal of Personality and Social Psychology, 55*, 517–529.

Trafimow, D., & Sheeran, P. (1998). Some tests of the distinction between cognitive and affective beliefs. *Journal of Experimental Social Psychology, 34*(4), 378–397.

Triandis, H. C. (1980). Values, attitudes, and interpersonal behavior. In H. E. Howe, Jr. & M. M. Page (Eds.), *Nebraska Symposium on Motivation* (Vol. 27, pp. 195–259). Lincoln: University of Nebraska Press.

PART 2

Health Promotion

Does Perceived Control Moderate Attitudinal and Normative Effects on Intention? A Review of Conceptual and Methodological Issues

Marco Yzer

University of Minnesota

In the 35 years since the inception of reasoned action theory, thousands of studies have been conducted that used a reasoned action framework (Ajzen & Fishbein, 2005). With this vast volume in mind, it is remarkable that only a few studies have been published that sought to examine the moderating role of perceived control in intention formation. This chapter discusses why from a conceptual perspective perceived control should be expected to moderate attitudinal and normative effects on behavioral intention, and yet also why empirically these effects are often unlikely to be demonstrated. To this end, the first sections of this chapter review the role of perceived control in reasoned action frameworks, the rationale for perceived control interaction effects, and past research on these interactions. The next sections explain the paucity of published studies in terms of the method-ological difficulty of detecting interactions, and report perceived control by atti-tude and perceived control by subjective norm interactions in case studies of con-dom use, marijuana use, and smoking cessation. The last section considers why and how we should return to research on the moderating role of perceived control.

REASONED ACTION FRAMEWORKS AND PERCEIVED CONTROL

According to the theory of reasoned action, the intention to engage in a behavior is the most proximal determinant of behavior. Intention itself is a function of atti-tude, that is, one's evaluation of performing the behavior, and subjective norm, that is, the pressure one expects from relevant social networks when one would perform the behavior. Intention has been described as a decision to perform a behavior (Fishbein, 1980), which should make clear that if one is not in total command of a behavior, intention will not strongly predict behavior (Ajzen, 1991; Fishbein & Jaccard, 1973).

With respect to the prediction of intention, Ajzen (1991) argued that when behavioral performance is not a decision because of a lack of control over the behavior, attitude and subjective norm are not sufficient. Prediction of intention would be improved, it was proposed, by including perceptions of control as an additional determinant. The theory of planned behavior thus is a modification of the reasoned action framework, and differs from the theory of reasoned action in the inclusion of a perceived control construct. Control perceptions reflect expected capability of performing the behavior, and are defined as the extent to which we believe that a behavior is under our control.[1]

Causal Links of Perceived Control with Intention and Behavior

Perceived control should directly predict behavior (Ajzen, 1991). The logic here is that people who believe that they can perform a behavior should be more perseverant in their efforts than people who are less confident, even when intention is the same in both groups. Also, and following from the derivation of perceived control from actual control, the more accurate perceptions of control reflect actual control, the better it should predict behavior.

Control, or more specifically, actual control, also should moderate the relation between intention and behavior (Ajzen, 1991; Ajzen & Fishbein, 2005; Fishbein, 2000; Fishbein & Jaccard, 1973). In plain terms, I can act on my intention if I have the capability of acting, but not if I do not possess those capabilities. To the extent that perceptions of control are accurate, *perceived* control also should moderate intention effects on behavior.[2]

A third hypothesis is that perceived control will affect intentions. The role of perceived control as a predictor of intention has been much more extensively

---

[1]Although the general idea of perceptions of control is accepted, there remains controversy concerning the exact conceptual definition. For example, perceived control has been measured with items tapping into the degree to which behavioral performance is perceived to be under one's control, the degree to which behavioral performance is perceived to be difficult or easy, and the degree to which one feels capable of behavioral performance under increasingly challenging circumstances (i.e., self-efficacy; Bandura, 1977, 1997). A complete discussion of the conceptual differences between these measures is beyond the scope of this chapter. For the purposes of the present discussion, control perceptions are defined as expected capability, or "how sure I am that I can do it."

[2]Bandura (1977) also accepts a moderating role for control in explaining behavior. Instead of a control–intention interaction, however, he expects control to interact with attitude. Specifically, when explaining the conceptual difference between outcome expectations (conceptually equivalent to attitudinal beliefs) and efficacy expectations, he observes that "...individuals can believe that a particular course of action will produce certain outcomes, but if they entertain serious doubts about whether they can perform the necessary activities such information does not influence their behavior" (Bandura, 1977, p. 193; for empirical support of this perspective see Schultz & Oskamp, 1996).

studied than perceived control's direct effect on behavior. The arguments for a direct relationship between perceived control and intention actually have not been extensively discussed, however, as it seems self-evident that the intention to engage in a particular behavior is at least in part informed by expected capability. The influence of perceived control on intention has been proposed as additive to attitudinal and normative effects, following the general rule that the more favorable attitude and the subjective norm and the greater perceived control, the stronger the intention (Ajzen, 1991).

The fourth hypothesis is that perceived control moderates attitudinal and normative effects on intention. However, although this possibility has been recognized, it is not a formal theoretical proposition. Nonetheless, investigating such interactions would allow exploration of psychological processes that might advance our understanding of intention formation. We take the position here that because of its conceptual importance the moderating role of perceived control requires further review—it is the focus of this chapter.

Explaining Intention: A Moderating Role of Perceived Control

The current interpretation of the theory of planned behavior argues for additive effects of attitude, subjective norm, and perceived control on intention. One could also argue, however, that the theory of planned behavior suggests interactions of perceived control with attitude and subjective norm. Take, for example, the description of the theory of reasoned action as a special case of the theory of planned behavior. The theory of reasoned action can account for behaviors that are under complete volitional control (and thus, a measure of perceived control is irrelevant), whereas the theory of planned behavior is designed to account for behaviors that are not under complete control (and thus, a measure of perceived control is relevant). With respect to behaviors that are under volitional control, all should feel capable of performing the behavior and thus there should be no variance in perceived control. In terms of structural models, the theory of reasoned action therefore is the theory of planned behavior with the path from perceived control to intention empirically fixed to zero. This implies that for behaviors that are under volitional control, for example, choosing healthy food at a breakfast buffet, attitudinal and normative effects reflect effects under the condition of high perceived control. Conversely, one could argue that for behaviors that are not under volitional control, for example, ensuring male condom use for women, attitudinal and normative effects reflect effects under the condition of low perceived control. This suggests that attitudinal and normative effects are moderated by perceived control.

From a conceptual perspective, the argument for interpreting perceived control as a moderator seems more compelling than the argument for perceived control as an additive determinant. To be sure, control perceptions are considered when intentions are formed, but this does not necessarily mean that strong intentions are always formed when perceived control is high (Eagly & Chaiken, 1993). This is not yet a sufficient argument for conceptualizing perceived control to have interactive instead of additive effects. For example, Ajzen (1991) argued that perceived control is only one source of influence, and strong perceived control likely improves intention in conjunction with a positive attitude and subjective norm. But even when attitude and subjective norm are highly favorable, why would we even consider the particular behavior if we are sure that we cannot perform it? Accordingly, perceived control over behavioral performance might function as a precondition for attitude and subjective norm to predict intention. We should expect to see that the relationship of attitude and subjective norm with intention is stronger when perceived control is high than when it is low.

The idea of perceived control by attitude and perceived control by subjective norm interactions is by no means new. Indeed, the plausibility of these interactions has been acknowledged consistently albeit not discussed extensively. For example, Ajzen (2002) submits that "...logically, perceived behavioral control, rather than having a direct effect, is expected to interact with attitudes and with subjective norms in determining intentions... ." These interactions, however, have not become a central proposition in the theory. In an initial series of tests of the theory of planned behavior, Ajzen and colleagues tested for interactions of perceived control with attitude and intention, but typically found no support for these interactions (e.g., Ajzen & Driver, 1992; Ajzen & Madden, 1986. The lack of empirical support in fact led to the adoption of the simpler, additive model that does not explicitly assume perceived control interactions (Ajzen, 2002).

In a narrative review of the theory of planned behavior, Eagly and Chaiken (1993) attempted to renew interest in perceived control interactions. Their argument was that a main effect of perceived control on intention does not always make much sense. Eagly and Chaiken use shouting in a library as an example of a behavior that most people will perceive as under their control, but also as a negative thing to do. The logic of this example yields the hypothesis that perceived control predicts intention when attitude towards the behavior is positive but not when it is negative. As such interactions promise identification of explanatory psychological processes, Eagly and Chaiken advocate research on interactions between reasoned action and planned behavior constructs.

Despite compelling arguments for perceived control by attitude and perceived control by subjective norm interactions, and despite a call for more research attention, only a handful of studies have been published that specifically seek to demonstrate perceived control interactions. The studies that have been published roughly group together in two series. First, as noted earlier, Ajzen and his colleagues tested perceived control interactions in a series of initial tests of the theory of planned behavior. A second series is more recent and seems at least in part motivated by Eagly and Chaiken's (1993) suggestion that perceived control and attitude interact to predict intention.

The latter series of research on intention as a function of perceived control interactions includes six studies (Bansal & Taylor, 2002; Conner & McMillan, 1999; Kidwell & Jewell, 2003; McMillan & Conner, 2003; Povey, Conner,

Sparks, James & Shepherd, 2000; Umeh & Patel, 2004).[3] In contrast to Ajzen's earlier work, these studies detected statistically significant interactions of perceived control with attitude and/or subjective norm. It is therefore useful to review this work.

Past Research on Perceived Control Interactions

Table 8–1 summarizes a number of relevant features of the six studies that demonstrated interaction effects of perceived control on intention. Ten behaviors were examined between the six studies, and all but one of these 10 behaviors were health behaviors. Without exception the data were observed in survey research. Sample size ranged between 139 and 461. Of the two possible perceived control interaction effects on intention, the perceived control by attitude effect has been examined more often than the perceived control by subjective norm effect.

One can argue that the rather small sample sizes might have hurt the robustness of the demonstrated effects. On a positive note, however, the results summarized in Table 8–1 suggest consistent support for a perceived control by attitude interaction. Of the 12 tests that have been performed across the six studies, 11 reach statistical significance. Unfortunately, only one of these studies (Conner & McMillan, 1999) reports partial correlations for each of the effects in the regression models, which makes it difficult to univocally interpret the effect sizes of each of the reported interactions. The often reported change in squared multiple correlation as a result of entering the combined set of interactions to the equation, however, is uniformly small, which suggests that perceived control interactions are small in size. (An analysis of intention to use ecstasy is an exception to this pattern; see McMillan & Conner, 2003.)

A useful synopsis of past research on perceived control interactions focuses on three observations. First, there are very few published studies that report perceived control by attitude or perceived control by subjective norm effects on intention. Second, all of these studies use observational data. Third, the demonstrated interactions generally are small. To put these considerations in perspective we next discuss methodological points that are at issue when examining perceived control interactions.

---

[3]The search strategy aimed to identify peer-reviewed studies whose specific focus was on interaction effects on intention within reasoned action or planned behavior frameworks. It is likely that more research on perceived control interactions has been conducted than suggested here. For example, Albarracín, Johnson, Fishbein and Muellerleile (2001) performed a meta-analysis of reasoned action research on condom use. Although the original studies did not specifically test perceived control interactions, Albarracín and colleagues tested and found support for perceived control by attitude interaction effects on intended condom use.

TABLE 8–1.
Review of studies that examined effects of perceived control interactions on intention

Source (in chronological order)	Data type	Sample size	Target behavior	Number of tested interactions	Interaction effects on intention	
					PC x Att	PC x SN
Conner & McMillan, 1999	Observational	249	Cannabis use	5	Sign.	n.t.
Povey et al., 2000	Observational	235	Healthy eating	10	ns	ns [a]
Bansal & Taylor, 2002	Observational	371	Switching mortgage providers	3	Sign.	n.t.
Kidwell & Jewell, 2003 Study 1 [d]	Observational	139	Sunscreen use	5	Sign.[b]	Sign.
			Blood donation	5	Sign.[b]	Sign.
			Drinking and driving	5	Sign.[c]	ns
			Fast food consumption	5	Sign.[c]	ns
McMillan & Conner, 2003	Observational	461	LSD use	3	Sign.	n.t.
			Amphetamine use	3	Sign.	n.t.
			Cannabis use	3	Sign.	n.t.
			Ecstasy use	3	Sign.	n.t.
Umeh & Patel, 2004	Observational	200	Ecstasy use	5	Sign.	ns

Note: PC = perceived control, Att = attitude, SN = subjective norm. Sign. = statistically significant, ns = not statistically significant, n.t. = not tested. [a] But note that PC significantly interacted with perceived social support, which in turn correlated with SN, r = .47. [b] These effects concern attitude as measured with cognitive evaluation items only, and were replicated in a second study for fat and chocolate consumption when positive outcomes were used to describe the behaviors. [c] These effects concern positive (drinking and driving) and negative affect (fast food use) constructs. They are included in this review as indicative of PC x Att interactions, because the affect constructs likely correlate with affective attitude. Kidwell and Jewell's second study replicated a perceived control x negative affect effect for fat consumption when negative outcomes were used to describe the behavior.

METHODOLOGICAL CONSIDERATIONS

Conceptually one would expect perceived control to interact with attitude and subjective norm in determining intentions, but empirically it is hard to demonstrate such interactions (Ajzen, 2002). To fully appreciate this contention we must realize that the quintessential test for perceived control interactions is moderated regression analysis of observational data. In fact, as we touched upon in the previous section, the single most important explanation for the paucity of published research on perceived control interactions is that these tests have inadequate statistical power (Aiken & West, 1991; Cohen, Cohen, West, & Aiken, 2003; Jaccard & Turrisi, 2003; McClelland & Judd, 1993). It is therefore useful to discuss the factors that lead to inadequate power in moderated regression analysis of observational data.

It is of course not true that interaction effects are always difficult to detect. Indeed, the experimental literature reports little else than interactions. Interestingly, McClelland and Judd (1993) note that experimental studies outperform observational studies considerably in detecting the same hypothesized interactions. This difference is explained by experimental studies' far greater statistical power for detecting interactions. This is an important observation for the discussion of perceived control interactions within the context of reasoned action frameworks. Standard practice for reasoned action research is the collection of observational data in survey studies (Ajzen & Fishbein, 1980; von Haeften, Fishbein, Kasprzyk & Montano, 2001). Typically, an observational study is conducted that measures all theoretical constructs, and once data gathering has been completed, the data are used to explore theoretical issues. The point is that if one of those issues involves demonstration of perceived control interactions, we must realize that by using observational data we sacrifice a significant amount of statistical power relative to an experimental design (McClelland & Judd, 1993).

Several factors can reduce statistical power for interaction tests, but two issues are particularly relevant here. The first concerns the theoretical expectations of the scope of the interaction: Is it more reasonable to expect an interaction where within the range of possible values the simple slopes have the same sign, or a reversed interaction where the simple slopes have opposite signs? The literature on a possible moderating role of perceived control suggests interactions which produce slopes with the same signs. It is hypothesized that attitude can have a strong positive effect on intention if perceived control is high, and an attenuated effect if perceived control is low. Moreover, there does not seem to be a reason to expect that when perceived control is low, a negative attitude yields a stronger intention than a positive attitude. (For a different view see Conner & McMillan, 1999.) Because they are smaller in size, same sign interactions are more difficult to demonstrate than opposite sign interactions. Because we theorize same sign slopes and, hence, relatively small perceived control interaction effects, difficulty of detecting interactions should not come as a surprise. Indeed, successfully demonstrated perceived control interactions typically account for just a few percentage points of the variance once the main effects have been accounted for.

A second, and arguably more important threat to statistical power for interaction tests in moderated regression analysis, concerns the distribution of the predictor and moderator variables (McClelland & Judd, 1993). As a general rule, the smaller the variance of a variable, the more difficult it is to detect the variable's effect on another variable. This possibility has been recognized in the literature on perceived control interactions. For example, Ajzen (2002) recently argued that "... interactions of this kind can be expected only if values of the predictor variables cover the full range of possible scores, such that the product term is fully expressed in the prediction."

The conditions that yield optimal power for detecting interactions are in fact even more extreme. Optimal power requires maximum variance in the interaction term, or more specifically, the variance in the interaction term controlled for variance in the main effects. It is this residual variance that determines the statistical power for interaction tests (McClelland & Judd, 1993). The crucial point is that the residual variance of the interaction term is primarily determined by the joint distribution of the predictor and moderator variables. In effect, interaction variance is maximal when all observations jointly lie at the extreme points of the predictor and moderator scales (i.e., low-low, low-high, high-low, or high-high; McClelland & Judd, 1993). Observational data, however, typically suggest moderate to strong positive correlations of perceived control with attitude and subjective norm, which implies that off-diagonal cells (i.e., low-high and high-low) have only few observations.

Other factors that reduce variance are restricted range of observations and clustering of observations. When this occurs, reduced variances of the predictor and moderator variables are magnified in the variance of the interaction, thereby decreasing statistical power for the interaction test exponentially. This further explains why so little empirical evidence supports perceived control interactions with attitude and subjective norm. Probably true for most behaviors that have been subjected to reasoned action research, and very likely true for health behaviors in particular, the distributions of attitude, subjective norm, perceived control and intention are skewed and cluster around one of the scale end points. Thus, although demonstration of perceived control interactions is easier when many observations jointly reside at both ends of the predictor and the moderator scales, many if not most observational data sets simply do not have enough observations at both end points of the scales to detect the interaction.

For example, if all respondents in a sample report strong (e.g., a score of 4 on a 5-point scale) or very strong perceived control (a score of 5), it will be unlikely that an analysis can demonstrate an interaction of perceived control with another variable. The example distribution is tantamount to having only one level of the moderator variable. One could therefore argue that in many cases the use of observational datasets to demonstrate interactions corresponds to the wish to use a four-cell design when in fact only two cells contain observations. Many published attitudinal and normative main effects therefore might indicate simple effects at either high or low levels of perceived control.

Example Analyses

With these methodological considerations in mind, it is useful to discuss case studies to analyze perceived control by attitude and perceived control by subjective norm interactions in observational data. For this purpose we use two adult datasets and one youth dataset to describe attitude, subjective norm, perceived control, and intention with respect to condom use with new sexual partners (for detailed information see Yzer, Siero & Buunk, 2000), adolescent marijuana use (Yzer, Cappella, Fishbein, Hornik & Ahern, 2003), and smoking cessation (van den Putte, Yzer & Brunsting, 2005).

The three data sets are quite large, with $N_{\text{condom use}} = 1,502$, $N_{\text{marijuana use}} = 1,461$ and $N_{\text{smoking cessation}} = 3,456$. The samples were fairly equally distributed by gender, with female respondents providing 49% of the condom use data, 54% of the marijuana use data, and 57% of the smoking cessation data. Mean age in the condom use ($M = 34$ years) and smoking cessation studies ($M = 39$ years) is higher than in the marijuana use study ($M = 15$ years).

Correlations between attitude, subjective norm and perceived control are moderate to strong across all three behaviors (see Table 8–2). For condom use and smoking cessation, correlations of attitude and perceived control with intention are stronger than correlations of subjective norm with intention. This is in line with generally observed lower explanatory power for subjective norms (Albarracín, Johnson, Fishbein & Muellerleile, 2001; van den Putte, 1991). However, as predicted by the theory of reasoned action, the exact strength of these relationships is a function of the behavior under study. At the bivariate level subjective norm relates more strongly to condom use intention and marijuana use intention than to intention to quit smoking.

Importantly, Table 8–2 also shows that for condom use and marijuana use the mean levels of attitude, subjective norm, perceived control and intention are close to the scale end. The condom use and marijuana use data are highly skewed and cluster considerably, and as a result variances in these data are not very large. The situation is less dramatic in the smoking cessation data. Potentially promising for the detection of interaction effects is the negative kurtosis for perceived control, which suggests that perceived control observations do not cluster very much and have short tails. Overall, the dispersion and distribution results suggest that if perceived control interactions really exist, we will be better able to detect them in the smoking cessation data than in the condom use and marijuana use data.

In research seeking to demonstrate interaction effects, these descriptive results serve diagnostic purposes. Correlations and measures of dispersion (but less so measures of distribution) are routinely reported in empirical articles, but these results are usually not used to speculate either before or after the analysis about potential restrictions to effect size. Before taking the step of actually creating interaction terms and analyzing them in moderated regression, information that points at restricted range, clustering of observations, and reduced variance can already forewarn the analyst that detection of interaction effects will be difficult. We have performed such a diagnosis, and with the results in hand we can now proceed to the analysis.

TABLE 8-2.

Descriptive statistics: Correlations, variances, dispersion, and distribution of key variables.

Data set	Correlations and variances[a]				Scale range	dispersion		distribution	
	Att	SN	PC	BI		M	SD	Skew (SE)	Kurtosis (SE)
Condom use	Att	.47				1 to 5	4.76	.68	-3.54 (.06)	13.71 (.13)
N = 1,502	SN	.37	.92			1 to 5	4.48	.96	-2.25 (.06)	4.93 (.13)
	PC	.45	.32	.76		1 to 5	4.31	.87	-1.49 (.06)	2.56 (.13)
	BI	.51	.35	.56	.96	1 to 5	4.40	.98	-1.91 (.06)	3.40 (.13)
Marijuana use	Att	1.57				-3 to 3	-2.14	1.25	1.54 (.06)	1.67 (.13)
N = 1,461	SN	.48	.59			-2 to 2	-1.62	.77	2.37 (.06)	5.88 (.13)
	PC[b]	-.28	-.18	1.23		-2 to 2	1.28	1.11	-1.70 (.06)	1.91 (.13)
	BI	.67	.38	-.33	.90	1 to 4	1.53	.95	1.63 (.06)	1.29 (.13)
Smoking cessation	Att	.89				-2 to 2	.84	.94	-.63 (.04)	.02 (.08)
N = 3,456	SN	.42	.69			-2 to 2	1.17	.83	-.69 (.04)	.01 (.08)
	PC	.29	.10	1.19		-2 to 2	-.13	1.09	.16 (.04)	-.54 (.08)
	BI	.42	.28	.42	1.57	-2 to 2	-.52	1.25	.43 (.04)	-.77 (.08)

Note: [a] Values on the diagonal are variances. Att = attitude, SN = subjective norm, PC = perceived control, and BI = behavioral intention. [b] Measured as confidence in ability to <u>not</u> use marijuana.

The analysis is moderated regression, where in a first step main effects are entered as mean-centered independent variables, and in a second step the interaction effect is entered as the product of the mean-centered independent variables (Aiken & West, 1991). Specifically, the mean-centered attitude, subjective norm and perceived control variables were used to create perceived control by attitude and perceived control by subjective norm interaction terms. An important advantage of mean-centering is the reduction in nonessential multicollinearity between independent variables and the interaction term (Aiken & West, 1991; Cohen et al., 2003). One implication of this method is that for appropriate interpretation of the results unstandardized b-coefficients and not standardized β-coefficients should be reported (Aiken & West, 1991).

Table 8–3 has the results. The b-coefficients and the partial correlations strongly suggest that perceived control moderates attitudinal and normative effects on the intention to quit smoking. The samples were large enough, however, to also detect much smaller moderator effects on condom use and marijuana use.

To interpret the interaction effects, results from Tables 8–2 (standard deviations) and 8–3 (constants and b-coefficients) were used to compute and test simple regression equations for attitude and subjective norm at low (one SD below the mean) and high (one SD above the mean) values of perceived control (Aiken & West, 1991; Cohen et al., 2003).

The simple slopes confirm that the interaction effects on condom use intention and marijuana use intention are not very large. Attitude predicts condom use intention more strongly when perceived control is high ($b = .49, p < .001$) than when it is low ($b = .43, p < .001$). There is a small effect of subjective norm on condom use intention under low perceived control ($b = .04, p < .001$), but no effect when perceived control is high ($b = .00, ns$).

Recall that in the marijuana use data attitude, subjective norm and intention referred to using marijuana, whereas perceived control referred to *not* using marijuana. This correspondence problem calls for care in interpreting the interactions. As expected, attitude towards using marijuana predicts marijuana use intention more strongly when lower control over *not* using marijuana is perceived ($b = .47, p < .001$) than when higher control is perceived ($b = .43, p < .001$). In contrast to expectations, subjective norm concerning marijuana use predicts marijuana use intention more strongly under high perceived control over *not* using marijuana ($b = .17, p < .001$) than under low perceived control ($b = .05, p < .10$).

The clearest moderator pictures emerge in the smoking cessation data. As hypothesized, attitude predicts quit intention more strongly when perceived control is high ($b = .56, p < .001$) than when it is low ($b = .22, p < .001$). Similarly, subjective norm predicts quit intention more strongly under high perceived control ($b = .32, p < .001$) than under low perceived control ($b = .10, p < .001$).

GENERAL CONCLUSION

This chapter discussed why conceptually perceived control should be expected to moderate attitudinal and normative effects on intention, and why conventional approaches should not be expected to provide overwhelming empirical support for

TABLE 8–3.

Intention regressed on attitude, subjective norm, perceived control (step 1), and the interactions of perceived control with attitude and subjective norm (step 2)

Behavior	Condom use			Marijuana use			Smoking cessation		
	b	$R^2\Delta$	pr	b	$R^2\Delta$	Pr	b	$R^2\Delta$	pr
Model after step 1									
Constant	4.35			1.53			-.52		
Attitude	.44		.35	.46		.58	.35		.26
Subjective norm	.02		.04	.09		.08	.20		.14
Perceived control	.48	.41	.42	-.12	.48	-.18	.39	.29	.35
Model after step 2									
Constant[a]	4.34			1.53			-.58		
Attitude	.46		.31	.45		.55	.39		.29
Subjective norm	.02		.04	.11		.10	.21		.15
Perceived control	.48		.42	-.12		-.18	.41		.38
Perceived control x attitude	.03		.03	-.02		-.05	.16		.15
Perceived control x subj. norm	-.02	.01	-.03	.05	.01	.06	.10	.04	.09

Note: pr = partial correlation coefficient. All coefficients are statistically significant. [a] Scale range for condom use intention is 1 to 5, for marijuana use intention 1 to 4, and for quit intention −2 to +2.

these interactions. This closing section reflects on the implications of some conceptual and methodological points for research on the moderating role of perceived control in reasoned action frameworks.

Conceptual Issues

Theoretical versus empirical sufficiency. The conceptual discussion of the role of perceived control raises an important point. Perceived control has been proposed as an additional behavioral determinant because of a concern that attitude and subjective norm are not sufficient to account for behaviors that are not under volitional control. Empirical support for this argument was subsequently sought and found. This approach to sufficiency questions first builds a theoretically compelling argument for inclusion of a construct, and then finds empirical support for the argument. Very often, however, research on the sufficiency of the reasoned action framework follows a different order. If a particular construct is found to explain a sizeable portion of variance in intention, it is concluded that it must be an important predictor and some argument is needed to justify inclusion. This approach reflects an explained variance or empirical sufficiency criterion, which potentially invites overly inductive reasoning. As such, it will not advance reasoned action theory much.

The explained variance criterion in relation to the sufficiency of the reasoned action framework also bears on the moderating role of perceived control. Interaction effects in observational data are small. Hence, if we deem large proportions of explained variance as a necessary condition for further consideration of a construct, then perceived control interactions with attitude and subjective norm should not be accepted as useful. This underscores the problem of failing to interpret the sufficiency issue as referring to theoretical sufficiency. If we accept theoretical arguments for perceived control interactions, then frameworks without those interactions are theoretically insufficient.

Perspectives on perceived control as a moderator. Interestingly, two different conceptual perspectives on interaction effects of perceived control can be discerned. A first approach follows the logic that no matter how positively people feel about performing a behavior, they will not even consider performing it if at the same time they are convinced that they cannot perform the behavior. Hence, perceived control is a precondition for attitudinal and normative influence. According to this reasoning attitude and subjective norm should particularly predict intention when people feel in control over behavioral performance (cf. Ajzen, 2002). A second perspective sees a positive attitude and a positive subjective norm as preconditions for perceived control to influence intention. The rationale for this idea is that many behaviors that are under people's control, for example, socially inappropriate behaviors, are not performed because people hold negative attitudinal and normative beliefs with respect to these behaviors (cf. Eagly & Chaiken, 1993).

These hypotheses reflect an interesting difference in perspective. Empirically, however, interactions demonstrated by moderated regression analysis of observational data cannot prove the superiority of one perspective over the other.

For example, Umeh and Patel (2004) report on a perceived control by attitude interaction and plot simple slopes for attitude with perceived control on the x-axis. The resulting graph shows that perceived control predicts intention to use ecstasy when attitude is positive (at low control $M \approx 9$ and at high control $M \approx 11$), but not when attitude is negative (at low control $M \approx 6$ and at high control $M \approx 6$). These same results can also be plotted with attitude on the x-axis. Now the graph suggests that attitude particularly predicts intention when perceived control is high (at negative attitude $M \approx 6$ and at positive attitude $M \approx 11$), and less so when perceived control is low (at negative attitude $M \approx 6$ and at positive attitude $M \approx 9$). This example illustrates that the same perceived control by attitude interaction can be interpreted as suggesting that either perceived control or attitude is the moderator, but as these interpretations are based on the same interaction result they offer no proof that one perspective is better than the other.

Methodological Issues

The danger of inadequate statistical power for tests of perceived control interactions lurks when observational data are used. It is possible, however, to improve statistical power for interaction tests in moderated regression analysis of observational data (McClelland & Judd, 1993), but these options are not without problems.

A first possible strategy is to increase overall sample size. There are, however, two reasons why a sufficiently large sample might not be attainable. To start, variables in observational research are not measured with perfect reliability, and even a small degree of unreliability is exacerbated when these variables are used to create interaction terms (Aiken & West, 1991). Cohen et al. (2003) illustrate that if both predictor and moderator are measured with quite acceptable reliabilities of .80, a sample of over 1,000 cases would be required for .80 power to detect an interaction of small size. Such large samples often are beyond the researcher's resources.

What is more, predictor and moderator variables typically are skewed with the great majority of observations clustering at one end of the scale. Thus, randomly sampling more cases will add mostly to already clustered observations, and it would require huge sampling efforts to yield the necessary cases that reside at the joint extremes of the scales.

Selective oversampling has been proposed as an alternative to random additional sampling (McClelland & Judd, 1993). This strategy selectively samples cases with joint extreme values for the predictor and moderator variables. This strategy can greatly improve statistical power for detecting an interaction effect of small size. A serious practical problem, however, is that oversampling requires prior knowledge about where to find those cases, and as such it is not a very useful strategy for the field researcher who typically does not have this knowledge.

A strategy that is closely related to oversampling uses a random sample and then selects only those cases that have observations of the predictor and moderator variables at the joint extreme ends of the scales. This seems a reasonable strategy, as it increases residual variance of the interaction term. For several reasons, however, this strategy should not be used to demonstrate interaction effects in observational data. First, the benefits of increased residual variance can be offset by the resulting reduced sample size (McClelland & Judd, 1993). Second, although selecting only extreme cases should not necessarily affect unstandardized effect estimates, it will reduce standard errors of those effects and thus inflate standardized effect estimates such as the squared multiple correlation. Selecting extreme cases, and then relying on the squared multiple correlation to indicate the effect size of the interaction, thus will suggest a larger effect than really exists in the population.

Does the Moderating Role of Perceived Control Have a Future?

Inadequate power for interaction tests in observational data explains why it is so difficult to demonstrate perceived control interactions. At the same time, methodological difficulties of detecting interactions leave the theoretical argument for perceived control interactions intact. If our goal is to further our understanding of psychological processes in intention formation, the moderating role of perceived control should return to the research agenda.

One could argue that such research is not very meaningful if most people in the population have either highly positive or highly negative attitudes, subjective norms, and perceived control concerning a particular behavior. Small effect sizes for perceived control interactions may therefore accurately reflect the true size of the effect. This cannot imply, however, that such effects are unimportant. Suppose, for example, that most members of a particular population perceive strong control and have a positive attitude concerning condom use. Suppose further that the relatively few who have a positive attitude but low perceived control concerning condom use also are at greatest risk of HIV infection. If a positive attitude translates in condom use intention when perceived control is high but not when it is low, it clearly is very important to improve perceived control for this relatively small part of the population. In this example the possibility of a perceived control by attitude interaction is of great practical significance, even though statistically the interaction effect may be small.

The potential theoretical and practical importance of perceived control interactions should of course not lead researchers to relax standards and accept very small effects as sufficiently indicative of meaningful population effects. If the available data are observational, then dispersion and distribution of the data should at least be screened and findings should be interpreted in the context of weak power. The design of observational studies that explicitly seek to test perceived control interactions should include a power analysis for the specific interaction tests (Maxwell, 2004).

Most promising for theoretical advancement is experimental research. For example, experiments can be designed to maximally affect perceived control and attitude. As a result experimental data can be equally distributed over the four extreme ends of the perceived control and attitude continua, thereby optimizing statistical power for the interaction test. Such experimental results may not generalize well, but they can greatly advance our understanding of the processes that theoretically make so much sense (Mook, 1983). This includes the possibility of separately manipulating perceived control and attitude to test whether perceived control or attitude is the moderator in the interaction.

Further research on the moderating role of perceived control in reasoned action frameworks can greatly advance our understanding of intention formation. It is possible to overcome methodological difficulties by improving statistical power in observational studies, and particularly by designing experimental research. A first step is to add empirical support for the role of perceived control as a moderator. This chapter contributes to this goal. A next step is to theorize and examine the boundaries of the moderator hypothesis; when is perceived control particularly likely to moderate attitudinal and normative effects on intention? In addition, we need to know more about the shape of the interaction. The analyses presented here assume multiplicative linear relationships, but non-linear relationships also seem possible. For example, when there is no perceived control at all, attitudes likely will not affect intentions, but even with small increments of perceived control, attitudes might become rapidly important. The future promises exciting new research programs.

ACKNOWLEDGMENTS

I thank Doloris Albarracín, Bob Hornik, Brian Southwell and Jim Jaccard for their valuable comments on an earlier version of this chapter.

REFERENCES

Aiken, L. S., & West, S. G. (1991). *Multiple regression: Testing and interpreting interactions*. Newbury Park, CA: Sage.

Ajzen, I. (1991). The theory of planned behavior. *Organizational Behavior and Human Decision Processes, 50*, 179–211.

Ajzen, I. (2002). Perceived behavioral control, self-efficacy, locus of control, and the theory of planned behavior. *Journal of Applied Social Psychology, 32*, 665–683.

Ajzen, I., & Driver, B. L. (1992). Application of the theory of planned behavior to leisure choice. *Journal of Leisure Research, 24*, 207–224.

Ajzen, I., & Fishbein, M. (1980). *Understanding attitudes and predicting social behavior*. Englewood Cliffs, NJ: Prentice Hall.

Ajzen, I., & Fishbein, M. (2005). The influence of attitudes on behavior. In D. Albarracín, B. T. Johnson, & M. P. Zanna (Eds.), *The handbook of attitudes* (pp. 173–221). Mahwah, NJ: Lawrence Erlbaum Associates.

Albarracín, D., Johnson, B. T., Fishbein, M., & Muellerleile, P. (2001). Theories of reasoned action and planned behavior as models of condom use: A meta-analysis. *Psychological Bulletin, 127*, 142–161.

Bandura, A. (1977). Self-efficacy: Toward a unifying theory of behavioral change. *Psychological Review, 84*, 191–215.

Bandura, A. (1997). *Self-efficacy: The exercise of control*. New York: Freeman & Co.

Bansal, H. S., & Taylor, S. F. (2002). Investigating interactive effects in the theory of planned behavior in a service-provider switching context. *Psychology & Marketing, 19*, 407–425.

Cohen, J., Cohen, P., West, S. G., & Aiken, L. S. (2003). *Applied multiple regression/correlation analysis for the behavioral sciences* (3rd ed.). Mahwah, NJ: Lawrence Erlbaum Associates.

Conner, M., & McMillan, B. (1999). Interaction effects in the theory of planned behaviour: Studying cannabis use. *British Journal of Social Psychology, 38*, 195–222.

Eagly, A. H., & Chaiken, S. (1993). *The psychology of attitudes*. Forth Worth, TX: Harcourt Brace Jovanovich.

Fishbein, M. (1980). A theory of reasoned action: Some applications and implications. In H. Howe & M. Page (Eds.), *1979 Nebraska Symposium on Motivation* (pp. 65–116). Lincoln, NE: University of Nebraska Press.

Fishbein, M. (2000). The role of theory in HIV prevention. *AIDS Care, 12*, 273–278.

Fishbein, M., & Jaccard, J. J. (1973). Theoretical and methodological considerations in the prediction of family planning intentions and behavior. *Representative Research in Social Psychology, 4*, 37–51.

Jaccard, J., & Turrisi, R. (2003). *Interaction effects in multiple regression*. Thousand Oaks, CA: Sage.

Kidwell, B., & Jewell, R.D. (2003). The moderated influence of internal control: An examination across health related behaviors. *Journal of Consumer Psychology, 13*, 377–386.

Maxwell, S. E. (2004). The persistence of underpowered studies in psychological research: Causes, consequences, and remedies. *Psychological Methods, 9*, 147–163.

McClelland, G. H., & Judd, C. M. (1993).Statistical difficulties of detecting interactions and moderator effects. *Psychological Bulletin, 114*, 376–390.

McMillan, B., & Conner, M. (2003). Applying an extended version of the theory of planned behavior to illicit drug use amongst students. *Journal of Applied Social Psychology, 33*, 1662–1683.

Mook, D. G. (1983). In defense of external invalidity. *American Psychologist, 38*, 379–387.

Povey, R., Conner, M., Sparks, P., James, R., & Shepherd, R. (2000). The theory of planned behaviour and healthy eating: Examining additive and moderating effects of social influence variables. *Psychology & Health, 14*, 991–1006.

Schultz, P. W., & Oskamp, S. (1996). Effort as a moderator of the attitude-behavior relationship: General environmental concern and recycling. *Social Psychology Quarterly, 59*, 375–383.

Umeh, K., & Patel, R. (2004). Theory of planned behaviour and ecstasy use: An analysis of moderator-interactions. *British Journal of Health Psychology, 9*, 25–38.

van den Putte, B. (1991). *20 years of the theory of reasoned action of Fishbein and Ajzen: A meta-analysis*. Unpublished manuscript, University of Amsterdam.

van den Putte, B. , Yzer, M. C., & Brunsting, S. (2005). Social influences on smoking cessation: A comparison of the effects of six social influence variables. *Preventive Medicine, 41*, 186–193.

von Haeften, I., Fishbein, M., Kasprzyk, D., & Montano, D. (2001). Analyzing data to obtain information to design targeted interventions. *Psychology, Health and Medicine, 6*, 151–164.

Yzer, M. C., Cappella, J. N., Fishbein, M., Hornik, R., & Ahern, R. K. (2003). The effectiveness of gateway communications in anti-marijuana campaigns. *Journal of Health Communication, 8*, 1–15.

Yzer, M. C., Siero, F. W., & Buunk, B. P. (2000). Can public campaigns effectively change psychological determinants of safer sex? An evaluation of three Dutch safer sex campaigns. *Health Education Research, 15*, 339–352.

CHAPTER 9

What Is the Behavior? Strategies for Selecting the Behavior to be Addressed by Health Promotion Interventions

Susan E. Middlestadt

Indiana University

The purpose of this chapter is to discuss a critical task in the development of health promotion interventions, the selection of the behavior. While there are many approaches to intervention design which call for applying theories of behavior to improve the effectiveness of health promotion interventions, less attention has been paid to the process of selecting the behavior to use in the application of the theory. This chapter will present questions to ask and steps to take when selecting which behavior to target with a health promotion intervention. An approach to primary research to help select and identify the behavior will be outlined. Throughout, illustrations will be drawn from the behaviors underlying obesity and overweight.

BACKGROUND

Developing Theory-Based and Empirically Grounded Health Promotions

A number of theories of behavior and behavior change are used to inform the development of health promotion interventions (Ajzen, 1991; Ajzen & Fishbein, 1980; Bandura, 1977, 1986; Fishbein & Ajzen, 1975; Janz & Becker, 1984; Kirscht, 1974; Prochaska, 1994; Prochaska & DiClemente, 1983; Rosenstock, 1974; Rosenstock, Strecher & Becker, 1988). In most cases, once the behavior has been selected, application of the theories is relatively straightforward. Briefly, given a behavior, these theories specify a set of determinants of the behavior which, if addressed, will result in an improved behavior. While there are differences in the determinants identified by each theory, there is considerable overlap

(Fishbein, et al. 2001). For example, many of the theories identify a construct that captures advantages and disadvantages of performing the behavior in an expectancy-value formulation. In the Theories of Reasoned Action and Planned Behavior, this appears as behavioral beliefs about the consequences of the behavior and the evaluations of these outcomes; in the Health Belief Model, benefits and barriers; in Social Cognitive Theory, outcome expectations; and in the Transtheoretical Model, pros and cons.

To develop a theory-based and empirically-driven health promotion intervention, the practitioner reviews or conducts formative behavioral research with members of the priority segment of the population of interest to identify behavioral determinants. Often preliminary research is needed to provide specific instantiations of general determinants. For example, qualitative salient belief elicitation research (Ajzen & Fishbein, 1980; Middlestadt, Bhattacharyya, Rosenbaum, Fishbein, & Shepherd. 1996) can help identify salient outcomes that members of the priority group believe will occur if the behavior is performed. Given the specific instantiations of the determinants, quantitative formative research can determine which of the possible determinants are more strongly associated with the behavior in the priority group. Then the practitioner can proceed to develop intervention activities and components to address these key determinants.

Fundamental to this logic of using theory and data to inform intervention design is the assumption that interventions need to be different if the determinants are different and if determinants are different if the behavior is different. Thus, a crucial task in developing health promotions is the selection and complete identification of the behavior of interest.

Previous Discussions of the Selection of the Behavior

Within the social marketing literature, factors to consider in segmenting the population and in selecting which segments to address with a health promotion intervention are discussed (Academy for Educational Development, 2001; Andreasen, 1995; Donovan & Henley, 2003; Siegel & Doner, 1998). Social marketers recommend that factors such as segment size, incidence of the behavior in the segment, ease of reaching the segment, the willingness or responsiveness of the segment to change, the cost of reaching and moving the segment, and the mission or capacity of the sponsoring agency to reach the segment be taken into account. Basically, these factors are balanced to achieve a marketing plan that optimizes health improvement within the financial and human resources available. Less attention has been paid to factors to consider in selecting and identifying the behavior to be targeted by the intervention. Although many descriptions point to the behavioral focus as a key defining characteristic of the social marketing approach (Academy for Educational Development, 2001; Andreasen, 1995) and recommend the analysis of competitive as well as target behaviors, few provide details on the task of selecting the behavior.

Within the attitude and behavior literature, there has been discussion of the definition of the behavior (Ajzen & Fishbein, 1980; Fishbein & Middlestadt,

1989; Fishbein, Middlestadt & Hitchcock, 1991; Jaccard & Blanton, 2005). First, according to these discussions, it is important to distinguish a behavior from the health status or outcome resulting from the practice of a behavior. Theories of behavior work best when used with behaviors rather than outcomes. Presumably, improving outcomes is likely to involve factors other than behavioral determinants and may involve improving many behaviors. Second, it is important to distinguish a single, specific, observable action from a category of behaviors, comprised of several single performed actions. Third, the full identification of the behavior requires specifying four components: the observable action; the target at which the action is directed; the context in which it occurs; and the time at which it is performed. Fourth is the issue of quantification. A behavior can be a matter of yes/no (i.e., did the action occur?) or a matter of amount or frequency of the action (i.e., how much or how often was the action).

These types of differentiations in the definition of the behavior (i.e., action vs. outcome; single act vs. category of behavior; elements of action, target, context, and time; and different quantifications of amount and frequency) are important for two reasons. They matter for measuring behavior, examining how well intention predicts behavior, and assessing how well the behavior improves health outcomes. In addition, and the focus of this chapter, these differentiations are important for understanding the determinants of the behavior with the goal of designing interventions to improve the behaviors. More specifically, the behavior, the determinants of the behavior, and thus interventions effective at changing the determinants may need to be different if any of these parameters change. In the literature on behaviors relevant to the prevention of HIV and other sexually transmitted infections, there is ample evidence that changing any of these parameters changes the specific determinants that are more strongly associated with the behavior and thus the specific determinants to be addressed by a change attempt. For example, the behavioral belief about the effect of using a condom on the trust between partners is a more critical determinant for condom use with a steady partner than for condom use with a new or occasional partner (Middlestadt et al., 1996). With new domains, it is critical to learn how to define behavior and to identify the parameters that most impact the underlying cognitive structure.

Overweight and Obesity

Overweight and obesity is a major problem in the U.S. (Koplan & Dietz, 1999; USDHHS, 2001) and it is fast becoming the number one preventable health issue. The proportion of adults who are overweight or obese has been increasing rapidly since the Centers for Disease Control and Prevention (CDC) began measuring Body Mass Index; overweight among children and teenagers has more than tripled in the past three decades (Institute of Medicine, 2004). Overweight and obesity result in diabetes, elevated blood pressure, high blood cholesterol, coronary artery disease, gallbladder disease, and osteoarthritis. Thus, the problem takes an immense emotional and economic toll (Koplan & Dietz, 1999; Institute of Medicine, 2004; USDHHS, 2001) and requires effective health promotion interventions. On the one hand, controlling the obesity epidemic is a simple matter of balancing calories in with calories out. On the other hand, it is a more complex one of addressing two sets of behaviors, eating and physical activity behaviors, both of which consist of many different specific behaviors. As individual and environmental health interventions are being developed, there is a clear need for systematic input on the task of selecting the behavior(s) to be changed.

SELECTING THE BEHAVIOR TO CHANGE

This chapter argues that a health promotion intervention is more likely to successfully improve health if explicit attention is paid to the task of selecting the behavior. More specifically, the task of selecting the behavior should be a multidisciplinary effort that involves input from several perspectives and that balances considerations from these different perspectives. An explicit behavioral selection process can be identified in terms of questions to ask and steps to take.

Questions to Ask

Table 9–1 presents a list of questions that can be asked when selecting and identifying a behavior to be changed by a health promotion intervention to improve a health status or outcome. The questions are grouped into four categories that represent different perspectives: (1) the perspective of the health scientist or epidemiologist who understands the hard science underlying morbidity and mortality; (2) the consumer perspective which captures the views of the community and the members of the priority group; (3) the perspective of the program planner who is designing the intervention; and (4) the views of the behavioral scientist who understands what a behavior is and the theories that can be used to explain and change behavior. The questions from each of these perspectives will be discussed with examples from eating and physical activity behaviors underlying the obesity epidemic.

Health Scientist and Epidemiologist.   The perspective of the health scientist or epidemiologist ensures that the selection of the behavior takes into consideration what is known about the relationship between the behavior and morbidity and mortality. These scientists know the literature connecting behavior to health outcomes. They have identified categories of actions that are important and ways to measure behavior. With respect to obesity, the health sciences of nutrition, kinesiology, and exercise physiology need to be represented.

Behavioral surveillance data and epidemiological studies can be examined to ensure that there is evidence that the behavior, if practiced, will reduce morbidity and mortality. The CDC's Behavioral Risk Factor Surveillance System (BRFSS) monitors behaviors that have been identified as responsible for adult health risks. Similarly, the Youth Risk Behavior System (YRBS) assesses the behaviors known to influence the health of the nation's youth.

The practitioner can use guidelines developed by agencies whose role is to define public health standards. The U.S. Department of Agriculture (USDA) recently released dietary guidelines for Americans with recommendations for the general population as well as special populations on what to eat and what to do for

TABLE 9–1
Factors to Consider in Selecting a Behavior

Perspective	Question
Health Scientist or Epidemiologist	• Is there evidence that a positive health status outcome will result if the action is performed? • Is the action consistent with (or moving in the direction of) established guidelines? • How does the action fit with the categories used by scientists who study the health topic?
Priority Group	• Is the action feasible given the current level of the behavior of the priority group? • Is the action phrased in language that is meaningful to priority group? • Is it possible for the action to be performed in the current environment? • To what extent is the action under the voluntary control of members of the priority group?
Program Planner	• Is the action of interest to and within the mandate of institutions and organizations interested in supporting and implementing interventions and programs? • Can the action be addressed with the types of intervention activities available to those interested in improving health? • Is the action relevant to the segments of the target population of interest to the program planner?
Behavioral Scientist	• Is the behavior an observable action rather than a health status outcome that results from the performance of the action? • Is the behavior a single, specific action that can be observed rather than a behavioral category of actions? • Is it useful to identify the target, context, and time frame of the behavior as well as the action? • Should the quantity of the behavior be specified in terms of yes/no, frequency, or amount? • Is there a way to phrase the action as doing a healthy action (walking) rather than stopping an unhealthy one (decrease TV watching)?

physical activity and fitness to maintain or lose weight, achieve fitness, and reduce risk of chronic disease (USDA, 2005). The guidelines for the general population consist of: general recommendations (e.g., consume a variety of nutrient-dense foods and beverages within and among the basic food groups while choosing foods that limit saturated and trans fats, cholesterol, added sugars, salt, and alcohol); specific recommendations about the food groups to encourage (e.g., consume sufficient fruits and vegetables while staying within the energy limits; choose a variety of fruits and vegetables; consume whole-grain products; consume fat-free or low-fat milk or milk products); and specific recommendations about fats (e.g., consume less than 10% of calories from saturated and trans fats), carbohydrates (e.g., choose and prepare foods with little added sugars and caloric sweeteners), sodium/potassium (e.g., choose and prepare foods with little added salt), and alcohol (e.g., limit to one drink per day for women and two for men).

The CDC, the American College of Sports Medicine (ACSM), and the U.S. Surgeon General develop guidelines for physical activity (USDHHS, 1996). The current recommendation for adults is to "accumulate 30 minutes or more of moderate-intensity physical activity on most or, preferably all, days" (Pate, et al. 1995). For youth, the CDC monitors the percent who participate in vigorous activity and sets indicators based on the percent who engage in at least 20 minutes of vigorous physical activity 3 or more days a week (USDHHS, 2000).

In defining physical activity, exercise scientists specify the intensity of the activity, the duration of the activity, and the frequency per week. The respondents on the CDC's Behavioral Risk Factor Surveillance System (BRFSS) are asked about moderate-intensity activity—"activities for at least 10 minutes at a time, such as brisk walking, bicycling, vacuuming, gardening, or anything else that causes small increases in breathing or heart rate" and vigorous-intensity activity— "activities for at least 10 minutes, such as running, aerobics, heavy yard work, or anything else that causes large increases in breathing or heart rate."

Exercise scientists also differentiate physical activity in terms of how the activity fits into a person's life. As described on the CDC Web site, physical activity is any bodily movement produced by skeletal muscles that result in an expenditure of energy. Exercise is physical activity that is planned or structured and that involves repetitive bodily movements done to improve or maintain one or more of the components of physical fitness, including cardio-respiratory endurance, muscular strength, flexibility, and bodily composition. Blair, Kohl, and Gordon (1992) outlined three theoretical patterns: the sedentary pattern in which the person expends little energy throughout the day; the leisure-time exercise pattern in which the individual is primarily sedentary except for a 20- to 30-minute bout of vigorous activity that is planned for as part of their leisure activity; and the lifestyle exercise pattern in which the person integrates activity into their daily routine and expends energy in short bouts throughout the day.

Among health scientists, there can be controversy about guidelines. Different researchers and organizations often come up with different recommendations; and recommendations change over time. Both the standards and the phrasing of the standards can be different. For example, in the eating domain, earlier guidelines, under the 5-a-day program, recommended at least 5 servings of fruits and vegetables a day. The more recent 2005 guidelines discuss cups (i.e., 2 cups of fruits and 2.5) cups of vegetables). In terms of physical activity, earlier recommendations specified participation in vigorous-intensity activity at least 20 minutes at least 3 times a week. Based on updated studies of moderate-intensity activity, the current guidelines recommend the accumulation of moderate-intensity activity at least 30 minutes at least 5 days a week. Additional research provided support for the value of 10-minute bouts (Andersen, 1999). And, the approach of counting steps relaxes even this 10-minute minimum of continuous exercise. Nevertheless, guidelines established by national organizations should be considered in selecting the behavior. And, in fact, the areas of controversy are issues that are likely to be ripe for input from other perspectives.

Priority Group and the Community. It is vital to define behaviors that make sense and are feasible to the members of the priority group and that fit into the priorities as defined by the communities that are the beneficiaries of the health promotion interventions. Priority groups may use language, words, and categories different from scientists. Communities may have more urgent priorities than those of the program planners designing interventions. There are a variety of research techniques that can be used to get the consumer and community perspective on the selection of the behavior. Input can be obtained through research with members of the priority group (Donovan & Henley, 2003; Siegel & Doner, 1998) and through the engagement of community stakeholders and leaders on community advisory boards and using participatory planning and evaluation models (e.g., Fetterman, Kaftarian & Wandersman, 1996; Green & Kreuter, 1999).

For a behavioral intervention to successfully change behavior, the behavior must be phrased so that it is understandable to the participants being addressed rather than being in the technical language of the scientists. Further, it can be argued that if the level of the behavior being recommended is feasible to the segment of the priority group given their current level of the behavior and the environment, the intervention is more likely to be successful.

As an example, consider designing an intervention to increase the fruit and vegetable consumption of adolescents. The CDC YRBS data can be used to identify the current level of the behavior among youth, overall, by gender, race, and state. In 2003, 20.3% of female students in grades 9 to 12 and 23.6% of male students reported eating fruits and vegetables 5 or more times a day during the preceding 7 days (Grunbaum, et al. 2004). As described previously, the phrasing of the recommendation for fruits and vegetables has shifted from at least 5 a day to 2 cups of fruit and 2.5 cups of vegetables, which comes to 9 servings. While this is the level recommended by the USDA, the practitioner designing a program will want to ask how this new level is perceived by the community. To illustrate, when the new recommendations came out, 26 young adults were asked what came to their mind when they thought of eating at least 9 servings of fruits and vegetables every day. In response to this question, 16 participants replied that this amount was too much, overwhelming, unlikely to be done, or hard to do, and an additional 4 participants mentioned the cost and time barriers to the behavior—that is, fully 67% expressed some reservations as the first thing that came to their mind when asked about this behavior. The current level of intake in this segment of the population was about 3.5 servings per day. The practitioner might want to consider a lower initial level when defining the behavior to be targeted by a health promotion intervention directed at this segment of the population.

Program Planner and Sponsoring Agency. Considering the perspective of the program planner and their institutional context when defining the behavior may help ensure that the interventions planned can be fully implemented by the agencies funding and sponsoring the program. There are many different kinds of activities, ranging from communication and education components through policy and environmental change, which can be implemented to improve behavioral determinants and thus improve behavior and health. Agencies and collaborations of agencies often have limitations on the type and content of activities that are feasible for them to implement. Furthermore, sponsoring agencies often have missions defined in terms of communities or priority groups. Organizations with national mandates may need to select general behaviors; local organizations serving specific segments of a priority group and with more information about current levels may be able to be more specific. For example, while the Food and Nutrition Service (FNS) of the USDA is concerned with healthy weight, it places a primary emphasis on nutrition education and eating behaviors. The FNS has a national mandate and accesses its constituents through state and local programs making educational interventions in a workshop format easy to implement.

Behavioral Scientist.   The perspective of the behavioral scientist helps ensure that what is selected is truly a behavior and is specified in a way that leads to the optimal identification of determinants. Table 9–1 summarizes the four differentiations outlined in the first section of this chapter (i.e., action vs. outcome; single act vs. category of behavior; the elements of action, target, context, and time; and different quantifications of amount and frequency). Most importantly, it is essential that the target of the intervention actually be an action rather than a resulting health status or outcome. Achieving a healthy weight and reaching an optimal level of fitness are both health statuses rather than health actions. Theories of health behavior are designed to address health behaviors, not health statuses. When using a theory of behavior to develop a health promotion intervention to help a priority group achieve or maintain a healthy weight, it is essential to identify the actions or behaviors that lead to improved weight and increased fitness. While the main impetus for a behavioral emphasis comes from the behavioral scientist, there is increasing recognition within the fields of nutrition education (Contento et al., 1995) and exercise physiology (Hardman, 2001) that designing interventions that promote behavior rather the accumulation of nutrients or energy expenditure might lead to interventions more effective at changing behavior.

Steps to Take

Given these perspectives and questions to consider, a number of recommendations can be made about steps to take in the selection process. Throughout the process, input from key informants and stakeholders representing the multiple perspectives is helpful. Meetings and other collaborative mechanisms can facilitate dialogue between the representatives of these perspectives. As described previously, the practitioner should look for guideline documents that can serve as rapid summaries of what the hard scientists know about the behavior, its categories, and definitions. Various literatures should be consulted, including formative research on the psychosocial and environmental determinants of the behavior, intervention research evaluating the effectiveness of interventions, literature recommending measures, and epidemiological studies. These literatures may show how the behavior is defined and illuminate critical definitional issues. Finally, primary research with members of the priority group may be beneficial.

Although a review of the literature on eating and physical activity is beyond the scope of this chapter, two prior reviews make clear suggestions. A review of interventions for older adults (Middlestadt et al., 2004) focused on the period between 1996 and 2002, looked for intervention studies on two specific behaviors among older adults, eating fruits and vegetables and walking, and included studies which used some form of comparison group. Eight of the nine nutrition intervention studies identified tried to increase consumption of fruits and vegetables; only two of the nine physical activity intervention studies specifically considered walking. Instead, the physical activity interventions tried to increase participation in various types of exercise classes and programs.

A review in progress of theory-based studies of the determinants of specific physical activity behaviors, like walking, and of eating fruits and vegetables, yielded a similar conclusion. Most of the studies of physical activity examined general exercise or physical activity (e.g., adhere to a program of physical activity; participate in regular exercise; exercise regularly, that is 3 or more times per week for at least 20 minutes; participate in physical activity during free time; exercise during the next month; exercise 3 days per week; intend to be active so that the heart beats fast) rather than specific actions like walking 30 minutes almost every day. In contrast, in the nutrition behavior literature, it was easy to locate studies of the specific behavior of eating fruits and vegetables.

AN APPROACH TO FORMATIVE RESEARCH TO IDENTIFY THE ACTION

As argued herein, primary formative research to define the behavior might be a useful step. Open-ended qualitative formative research to elicit actions in the words of the priority group might help the practitioner choose among various options for behaviors to be targeted by a health promotion. The approach taken here is to ask members of the priority group what actions they could take to improve a health issue. The elicitation is followed by: a content analysis; a frequency analysis to identify the salient responses; a comparison of behaviors elicited from the participants with the recommendations by the relevant health scientists and epidemiologists and the differentiations important to the behavioral scientists; and a summary description of the structure of the behavior space.

Tables 9–2 and 9–3 present results from 92 undergraduate and graduate students of a Midwestern university who were asked open-ended questions about what they could do to eat better and move more. While many of the participants were young adults, about one third were older adults returning for an MPH degree. The participants were asked, "List the actions that you can take to maintain or achieve a healthy weight. Name two that involve eating better and two that involve moving more." Each table lists the behavior, some examples of specific responses, and the percent and frequency who mentioned each. Since participants could mention more than one action, the percents sum to more than 100%. These data were collected when the guidelines for fruits and vegetables were 5 a day.

TABLE 9–2
Behaviors Elicited to Help Achieve or Maintain Healthy Weight: Eating Better

Percent	Behavior	Examples
43 (40)	Eat more fruits and/or vegetables	• Eat fruits and vegetables every day • Eat lots of fruits and vegetables • Eat veggies
21 (19)	Eat a balanced diet	• Eat a balanced diet • Eat according to the food pyramid • Balance your diet • Eat 3 to 4 well-balanced meals a day
10 (9)	Eat healthy	• Eat healthy • Eat health snacks
12 (11)	Eat smaller portions	• Eat smaller portions • Eat small portions • Limit portion sizes
14 (13)	Eat less junk and fast food	• Eat less junk food • Stay away from junk food • No fast food
11 (10)	Snack less	• Less snacking • No snacking between meals
15 (14)	Drink water instead of soda	• Drink lots of water • Drink water instead of soda • Replace soda with water • Stop drinking soda
9 (8)	Stop eating when full	• Stop eating when you are full • Stop when you are full • Don't eat unless you are hungry • Eat only when you are hungry, not for emotional/social reasons
3 (3)	Eat slowly	• Eat slowly • Eat slowly, chew longer
9 (8)	Eat at correct time	• Don't eat in the evening • Eat small meals throughout the day • Not eating a lot of food before bed
13 (12)	Watch or count calories	• Count calories (4) • Watch calories (3) • Control total calories to 3,000 a day • Eat less than you expend (3) • Eat less high calorie foods (3)
5 (5)	Eat high fiber foods	• Eat a lot of fiber • Eat higher fiber foods

(continued)

TABLE 9–2 *(continued)*

Percent	Behavior	Examples
7 (6)	Eat sugar-free products (3) and/or avoid sugary foods (3)	• Eat sugar-free products • Minimize sugar intake • Stop eating sugary foods • No cookies
23 (21)	Eat low-fat food or avoid high-fat food	• Eat low-fat food • Cook low-fat food • Lower fat • Limit high-fat food • Avoid oily and fatty foods • Minimize fat intake
11 (10)	Eat other specific foods	• Eat protein (1) • Eat meat (1) • Eat carbohydrates (3) • Eat grains (1) • Limit caffeine (1) • Limit chocolate (3) • Less salty foods (1)
9 (8)	Facilitating Behaviors - shop differently	• Shop daily • Plan meals • Buy healthy foods instead of convenience foods
8 (7)	Facilitating Behaviors - eat at home more often	• Cook more • Eat at home • Eat out less • Bring lunch from home (3)

Eating Better

The behaviors that involve eating better described in Table 9–2 can be analyzed in terms of the four behavioral science differentiations (i.e., action vs. outcome; single act vs. category; elements of action, target, context, and time; and quantification). The participants were asked about the behaviors to achieve a status or outcome of healthy weight and had no problem coming up with behaviors to achieve this outcome. By far, most of the participants identified some form of eating as the action. Some participants mentioned facilitating behaviors or ways to achieving the recommendations on how much and what to eat, in particular shopping differently and cooking differently.

Many of the participants were specific about the behavior by selecting a target of the action. The most frequently mentioned target was fruits and vegetables. Almost half (43%) of the participants mentioned this target. The next most frequently mentioned target was food lower in fat. In addition to fruits and vegetables and fats, participants also mentioned fiber, sugar, carbohydrates, meat, and protein as foods or food groups to eat or to avoid eating. About one third of respondents did not mention specific foods or food groups as a target, but instead listed eating better generally (i.e., eat a balanced diet).

Some participants mentioned time when giving an action they could take to achieve a healthy weight. While the day seemed to be the implicit time frame for most respondents, only nine explicitly mentioned daily or each day. A few participants mentioned timing as a strategy (e.g., eat throughout the day).

Considering the amount of the behavior, about one third (34%) of participants gave an action that involved eating more and about one fourth (27%) mentioned eating less or smaller amounts. Only five participants mentioned specific amounts (e.g., eat 3 to 4 balanced meals a day; eat 3 servings of vegetables and 1 to 2 of fruit; eat much more fruit, at least 1 serving a day).

Overall, there is some correspondence between the USDA guidelines and the responses of these participants. Both include the idea of balance. For both, fruits and vegetables is the first mentioned food group. Both also mention fats, fiber, and sugar as other food groups. Both mention what to eat and what to avoid or limit. For both, the behavior can be either general (i.e., eating nutrient-dense in the language of the USDA or eating healthy foods from the food pyramid in the language of the participants) or specific (i.e., eating specific foods of which fruits and vegetables is clearest). Both the USDA (not mentioned in the summary recommendations but discussed in other documents) and the participants discuss facilitating behaviors like shopping and cooking differently that may help individuals eat specific healthy foods.

Unlike the USDA guidelines, few of these participants mentioned amounts. In addition, the USDA is more specific when describing some of the foods. That is, the USDA talks about saturated and trans fats, added sugar, and whole grains. Within the guidance, USDA discusses dark green and orange vegetables. Participants referred to fats, sugars, grains, and fruits and vegetables.

Moving More

Table 9–3 shows the behaviors elicited when the participants were asked for actions that involved moving more. Once again, the participants were explicitly asked for behaviors to achieve the health outcome and had no difficulty coming up with behaviors to achieve a healthy weight. In contrast to eating better in which eating was by far the most frequently mentioned action, participants had many different actions when asked about moving more. Walking was the most frequently mentioned action: 28% explicitly listed walking instead of driving or taking the bus; 22% just listed walking. While both these behaviors have the same action (walking), these were coded differently since their context is different. The first implies using walking instead of driving as a way of incorporating physical activity into everyday life; the second implies that walking is an activity planned to be done for its own sake. In terms of specific actions, running, biking, jogging, swimming, and dancing were the vigorous actions mentioned. Yoga and stretching were mentioned as specific actions in the area of flexibility fitness. Lifting weights was mentioned as actions in strength fitness (see Table 9–3).

TABLE 9–3
Behaviors Elicited to Help Achieve or Maintain Healthy Weight: Moving More

Percent	Behavior	Examples
28 (26)	Walk (as transportation)	• Walk instead of drive • Walk instead of bus • Walk to class, store, work
2 (2)	Bike (as transportation)	• Bike to class • Use bike to run errands
22 (20)	Walk (as exercise)	• Go for a walk • Take walks • Walk every day • Walk after dinner • Take walks for 30 minutes a day
26 (24)	Take stairs	• Take stairs instead of elevator • Use stairs at work • Climb stairs 3 times a week
30 (28)	Exercise	• Exercise regularly • Exercise for 30 minutes 3 times a week • Exercise at least 5 times a week • Increase exercise activity
10 (9)	Work out	• Work out • Working out more • Work out every few days
5 (5)	Do aerobic or cardio activity	• Get 30 minutes of cardio • Do more aerobic
3 (3)	Do physical activity	• Get 30 minutes of physical activity • Do physical activity every day • Maintain a physical activity routine
3 (3)	Just start moving	• Just start moving • Be active - play sports • Expend more than you eat
22 (20)	Do specific physical activities for cardio-respiratory fitness	• Running (9) • Jogging (3) • Biking (8) • Swimming (2) • Dance for 30 minutes every day
11 (10)	Lift weights	• Start lifting weights every day • Weight train twice a week • Lift weights
7 (6)	Do specific flexibility activities	• Yoga (4) • Stretching (2)
5 (5)	Decrease sedentary activity	• Reduce lazy days • Turn off TV and go outside • Get up from your computer
13 (12)	Facilitating behaviors	• Train for an event (3) • Go to the gym (2) • Ask a friend to exercise with me (4) • Make a contract with rewards (2) • Break into 10 minute sessions (1)

Fully 30% of the participants used the word *exercise*. It is unclear from these data whether these participants follow the CDC's definition (i.e., structured or planned physical activity done to improve or maintain a component of fitness). An additional 10% listed *working out* and 5% doing *aerobic or cardio activity*. Interestingly, only 3% used the words *physical activity*. As with the eating behaviors, some respondents (13%) mentioned facilitating behaviors, such as asking a friend to exercise or training for an event that might help them accumulate the necessary minutes of activity.

In comparison to eating better, more of the participants listed a specific amount or frequency. Specifically, 13% mentioned 30 minutes of activity, most of these 30 minutes a day. Overall, 22% mentioned every day; 16% mentioned 3 to 5 days a week, every other day, or almost every day. Only 7% described an action of increasing or doing more, and 5% discussed doing less of sedentary activities.

Again there is some overlap between the perspectives of the exercise scientists and of the participants. Both mention moderate (e.g., walking) as well as vigorous (e.g., running and swimming) activities. Both are open to counting the number of minutes and the times per week. For both, there are two types of physical activity behaviors: there are the physical activity behaviors that the scientists describe as exercise that is structured and planned; and there are behaviors that provide ways to incorporate physical activity into daily life such as by walking instead of driving and taking the stairs instead of the elevator. The main difference between the perspectives of the exercise scientists and the participants is in the use of the term *physical activity*. Physical activity is a generally used by the exercise scientists to describe the recommendations they make for expending energy and to summarize the many types of actions people can take to accumulate minutes of activity. Few participants used the term *physical activity* and instead mentioned specific actions like walking.

Map of the Behavior Space

Table 4 summarizes this analysis of the behavioral domain of eating and physical activity behaviors underlying overweight and obesity with a map of the behavior space. While it is based on a review of the guidelines and findings of a small preliminary study, this table is not meant to show definitive guidelines, to recommend specific behaviors to select, to be comprehensive, or to capture the different recommendations for different types of individuals. Instead the table proposes a conceptual framework for describing the behavior space in the domain of eating better and moving and illustrates an approach that might be relevant to any domain. Implicit in this framework is a flow from upstream facilitating behaviors (Column 5) through specific behaviors (Column 4) to furthest downstream, the health status outcomes (Column 1) (see Table 9–4).

At the far right is the health status or outcome. This is defined in terms of morbidity and mortality and is clearly an outcome and not a behavior. Here it is phrased for someone with a healthy weight to maintain. It lists healthy weight, but could also include reduced risk of chronic disease and other health status outcomes. Immediately upstream from the health outcome is a column that reflects

TABLE 9–4

Conceptual Framework Outlining Types of Behaviors in the Overweight and Obesity Domain

Health Status Outcome (1)	Balance of Eating & Physical Activity (2)	Behavior Accumulations (3)	Specific Behaviors (4)	Facilitating Behaviors (5)
• Maintain healthy weight • Reduce morbidity & mortality	• Balance calories in with energy expended	• Consume variety of nutrient-dense foods and beverages among basic food groups while choosing foods that limit saturated and trans fats, cholesterol, added sugars, and alcohol • Meet recommended intakes by adopting balanced eating plan	• Consume 2 cups of fruit and 2.5 cups of vegetables per day • Consume a variety of fruits and vegetables every day • Consume 3 or more oz equivalents of whole grains every day • Consume 3 cups per day of fat-free or low-fat milk or milk products	• Shop and buy differently • Ask preparer to serve fruits and vegetables • Prepare differently • Count calories • Eat breakfast • Eat smaller portions
		• Engage in vigorous-intensity activity for at least 20 minutes 3 days a week • Engage in moderate-intensity activity for at least 30 minutes on most days of the week • Take at least 6000 steps per day	• Run 20 minutes 3 days a week • Jog 20 minutes 3 days a week • Swim 20 minutes 3 days a week • Walk briskly 30 minutes a day mostly every day • Park some distance from work/school/store and walk • Take elevator instead stairs	• Go to the fitness facility • Train for an event • Walk with a companion • Wear pedometer to count steps

the fact that individuals must balance calories in with calories out, a complicating factor when it comes to overweight and obesity. In the table it is phrased as "maintaining the balance." This would be phrased as "making small decreases in calories in and small increases in physical activity" if the individual needs to achieve a healthy weight or to prevent weight gain with age.

From the middle column to the left, the top rows of the table outline eating behaviors; the bottom rows focus on physical activity behaviors. The middle column is labeled accumulation. Both nutritionists and exercise physiologists use language that calls for the individual to ultimately achieve an accumulation of either nutrients or minutes (or other measures) of physical activity. This column is on the border between the clear outcome (e.g., achieve healthy weight) and the specific actions (e.g., eat fruits and vegetables or walk). Specific behaviors are upstream from these accumulations. In terms of eating, these behaviors include eating food from the several foods groups. In terms of physical activity, these behaviors include specific actions like walking and running.

At the most upstream in this table are the facilitating behaviors. Theoretically, these behaviors if practiced will lead to the practice of the specific behaviors which ideally will lead to the accumulation of nutrients and minutes that will balance calories in with calories out and ultimately achieve or maintain a healthy weight. With obesity, as with other health issues, it is clear that, for long-term and wide-ranging success, environmental as well as individual factors need to be addressed in health promotion interventions (Koplan & Dietz, 1999). Viewed from the perspective of the program planner, these facilitating behaviors could represent a way for individuals to shape and choose their environment. In addition, they might provide a way to influence several specific downstream behaviors. The program planner faces a challenge when trying to change many specific behaviors and often resorts to phrasing the behavior generally, such as, eating healthy foods. Addressing facilitating behaviors represents an alternative solution to the dilemma of multiple behaviors. The table could be extended with facilitating behaviors that are even further upstream.

There are a number of limitations to this table. The table does not capture the different outcomes and behaviors for different segments of the priority group defined on the basis of initial level of obesity and overweight or other factors, such as race/ethnicity, age, gender, or other demographic or psychographic characteristics. It is set up for a person whose goal is to maintain a healthy weight, not an overweight, or obese individual whose goal is to achieve one. At this stage of the work on the behaviors underlying achieving a healthy weight, it is unclear which behavior or class of behaviors to select for an intervention. However, it is hoped that this map of the behavior space underlying the eating better and moving more behaviors that contribute to a healthy weight helps the practitioner articulate some of the possibilities from which to choose. And it is hoped that the map illustrates an approach that can be applied to other health domains.

CONCLUSION

This chapter has tried to make three points relevant to designing effective theory-based and data-grounded health promotion interventions. First, the issue of the selection and identification of the behavior to be improved by a health promotion intervention deserves increased attention. Second, this chapter has outlined some of the issues that make the selection of behavior complex. In terms of overweight and obesity, there are many options the practitioner could select and considerable diversity of terminology used. The decision about which behavior to target lies at the interface of the behavioral scientist who examines the behavior and its relationship to its determinants, the health scientist or epidemiologist who focuses on the behavior and its relationship to health status, and the consumer and their community.

Third, the chapter suggests a number of questions to ask and steps to take in this critical task of intervention design. The main recommendation is to involve multiple perspectives and to use input from a number of literatures in making the decision. As with the issue of selecting the priority group to be addressed by an intervention, it is unlikely that there is just one right answer when it comes to selecting the behavior to target by an intervention. It is more likely that practitioners will need to balance the multiple perspectives to select the behavior that makes the most sense for their setting and circumstances.

This analysis of the task of the selection of the behavior provides three clear suggestions for next research steps. First, documents describing interventions and summarizing behavioral and intervention research could be more explicit about the reasoning used and factors considered in selecting the behavior to be changed or studied. Intervention research articles generally provide support for their final choice of behavior, but less often discuss options rejected. Behavioral research is less restricted in terms of space for detail on the selection of the behavior. If progress is to be made on a systematic approach to the selection of the behavior, information is needed on options, process, and rationale.

Second, it might be fruitful to review the literature in fields like HIV and AIDS with many successful interventions from the perspective of analyzing the specific behavior that was selected. Was it general or specific? Which specific parameters of action, target, context, and time had the most impact on determinants or on the effectiveness of the intervention? Was the magnitude or frequency of the behavior specified? How was this selected? There are likely to be lessons specific to HIV, as well as lessons relevant to other domains.

Third, research is needed on the patterns of the specific behaviors. The eating and physical activity behaviors of interest are those that occur on a daily basis and can change over time of year and stage in the life of an individual. It is likely that different actions are more feasible among people with different histories. How many adults have never been active? Do the sedentary begin with moderate-intensity activity and then progress to more vigorous activity? Have moderately active individuals been active all of their lives or have they had periods of inactivity? While national surveillance data can provide summaries of overall levels, there is a limit to the detail that is possible. The selection task would be improved if there were more solid data on patterns.

REFERENCES

Academy for Educational Development. (2001). *Social marketing lite*. Washington, DC: AED.

Ajzen, I. (1991). The Theory of Planned Behavior. *Organizational Behavior and Human Decision Processes, 50*, 179–211.

Ajzen, I. & Fishbein, M. (1980). *Understanding attitudes and predicting behavior*. Englewood Cliffs, NJ: Prentice Hall.

Andersen, R.A. (1999). Exercise, an active lifestyle, and obesity. *The Physician and Sportsmedicine, 27*, 10.

Andreasen, A. (1995). *Marketing social change: Changing behavior to promote health, social development, and the environment*. San Francisco, CA: Jossey-Bass Publishers.

Bandura, A. (1977). *Self-efficacy: Toward a unifying theory of behavior change. Psychological Review, 84*, 191–215.

Bandura, A. (1986). *Social foundations of thought and action*. Englewood Cliffs, NJ: Prentice Hall.

Blair, S. N., Kohl, H. W. & Gordon, N. F. (1992). Physical activity and health: A lifestyle approach. *Med Ex Nutrition and Health, 1*, 54–57.

Contento, I., Balch, G. I., Bronner, Y. L., Lytle, L. A., Maloney, S. K., Olson, C. M., et al. (1995). The effectiveness of nutrition education and implications for nutrition education policy, programs, and research: A review of research—Executive summary. *Journal of Nutrition Education, 27*, 227–283.

Donovan, R and Henley, N. (2003). *Social marketing: Principles and practice*. Victoria, Australia: IP Communications.

Fetterman, D., Kaftarian, S., & Wandersman, A. (Eds.). (1996). *Empowerment evaluation*. Thousand Oaks, CA: Sage.

Fishbein, M., & Ajzen, I. (1975). *Belief, attitude, intention, and behavior: An introduction to theory and research*. Reading, MA: Addison Wesley.

Fishbein, M., & Middlestadt, S. E. (1989). Using the Theory of Reasoned Action as a framework for understanding and changing AIDS related behaviors. In V. M. Mays, G. W. Albee, & S. F. Schneider (Eds.), *Primary prevention of AIDS: Psychological approaches* (pp. 93–110). Newbury Park, CA: Sage.

Fishbein, M., Middlestadt, S. E., & Hitchcock, P. J. (1991). Using information to change STD related behaviors: An analysis based on the Theory of Reasoned Action. In J. Wasserheit, S. Aral & K. Holmes (Eds.), *Research issues in human behavior and sexually transmitted diseases in the AIDS era*. Washington, DC: American Society for Microbiology.

Fishbein, M., Triandis, H. C., Kanfer, F. H., Becker, M., Middlestadt, S. E., & Eichler, A. (2001). Factors influencing behavior and behavior change. In A. Baum, T. A. Revenson, & J. E. Singer (Eds.), *Handbook of Health Psychology* (pp. 1–7). Mahwah, NJ: Lawrence Erlbaum Associates.

Green, L. W., & Kreuter, M. W. (1999). *Health education planning: A diagnostic approach*. Mountain View, CA: Mayfield.

Grunbaum, J. A., Kann, L., Kinchen, S., Ross, J., Hawkins, J., Lowry, R., et al. (2004). Youth Risk Behavioral Surveillance–United States, 2003. In *Surveillance Summaries*, May 21, 2004. *MMWR: Morbidity and Mortality Weekly Report, 53* (No. SS–2), 1–95.

Hardman, A.E. (2001). Physical activity and health: Current issues and research needs. *International Journal of Epidemiology, 30*, 1193–1197.

Institute of Medicine. (2004). *Preventing childhood obesity: Health in the balance*. Washington, DC: National Academies Press.

Jaccard, J. & Blanton, H. (2005). The origins and structure of behavior: Conceptualizing behavior in attitude research. In D. Albarracín, B. T. Johnson, & M. P. Zanna (Eds.). (2005). *Handbook of attitudes* (pp. 125–171). Mahwah, NJ: Lawrence Erlbaum Associates.

Janz, N. K. & Becker, M. H. (1984). The health belief model: A decade later. *Health Education Quarterly, 11*, 1–47.

Kirscht, J. P. (1974). The health belief model and illness behavior. *Health Education Monographs, 2*, 2387–2408.

Koplan, J. P. & Dietz, W. H. (1999). Caloric imbalance and public health policy. *Journal of the American Medical Association, 282*, 1579–1582.

Middlestadt, S. E., Bhattacharyya, K., Rosenbaum, J. E., Fishbein, M., & Shepherd, M. (1996). The use of theory-based semi-structured elicitation questionnaires: Formative research for CDC's Prevention Marketing Initiative. *Public Health Reports, III, Supplement I*, 18–27.

Middlestadt, S. E., Jimerson, A., Lehman, T. C., Tensuan, L., Lane, A., & Bates, K. (2004). *Improving the eating and physical activity behaviors of the low-income elderly: Promising practices report*. Washington, DC: Academy for Educational Development. Report prepared for U. S. Department of Agriculture, Food and Nutrition Service.

Pate, R. R., Pratt, M., Blair, S. N., Haskell, W. L., Macera, C. A., Bouchard, C., et al. (1995). Physical activity and public health: A recommendation from the Centers for Disease Control and Prevention and the American College of Sports Medicine. *Journal of the American Medication Association, 273*, 402–407.

Prochaska, J. O. (1994). Strong and weak principles for progressing from precontemplation to action based on twelve health behaviors. *Health Psychology, 13*, 47–51.

Prochaska, J. O., Velicer, W. F., Rossi, J. S., Goldstein, M. G., Marcus, B. H., Rakowski, W., et al., (1994). Stages of change and decisional balance for twelve health behaviors. *Health Psychology, 13*, 39–46.

Prochaska, J. O. & DiClemente, C. C. (1983). Stages and processes of self-change of smoking: Toward an integrated model of change. *Journal of Clinical and Consulting Psychology, 51*, 390–395.

Rosenstock, I. (1974). The historical origins of the health belief model. *Health Education Monographs, 2*, 328–335.

Rosenstock, I. M., Strecher, V. J., & Becker, M. H. (1988). Social Learning Theory and the Health Belief Model. *Health Education Quarterly, 15*, 2, 175–183.

Siegel, M., & Doner, L. (1998). *Marketing public health: Strategies to promote social change*. Gaithersburg, MD: Aspen Publishers.

USDA. (2005). *Dietary Guidelines for Americans 2005*. U.S. Department of Agriculture.

USDHHS. (1996). *Physical Activity and Health: A Report of the Surgeon General*. Atlanta, GA: U.S. Department of Health and Human Services, Centers for Disease Control and Prevention.

USDHHS. (2000). *Healthy People 2010: Understanding and improving health*. 2nd ed. Washington, DC: U.S. Printing Office.

USDHHS. (2001). *The Surgeon General's Call to Action to Prevent and Decrease Overweight and Obesity: 2001*. Rockwell, MD: U.S. Department of Health and Human Services, Public Health Service, Office of the Surgeon General.

CHAPTER 10

Application of an Integrated Behavioral Model to Understand HIV Prevention Behavior of High-Risk Men in Rural Zimbabwe

Danuta Kasprzyk and Daniel E. Montaño

Battelle Centers for Public Health Research and Evaluation, Seattle

The work we describe in this chapter was conducted to determine the utility of the integrated behavioral model (IBM; Kasprzyk, Montaño, & Fishbein, 1998) using components of the theory of reasoned action (TRA) and the theory of planned behavior (TPB) to explain safe sex behavioral intentions in Zimbabwe. This work was carried out within the context of an applied HIV/STD prevention research trial. This international HIV/STD Prevention Trial to implement and evaluate the Community Popular Opinion Leader (CPOL) model intervention to increase safe sex behavior in Zimbabwe is part of a broader study currently being conducted in five countries as a randomized community-based trial. It is important to first describe this larger research program. Within this context we describe the formative research on which the behavioral model was based, how we selected final constructs to measure, and how we measured those constructs. Based on the model analyses, we also provide recommendations to better tailor prevention messages among high-risk men in Zimbabwe.

BACKGROUND

Zimbabwe, situated in southeastern Africa, has been especially devastated by the HIV epidemic. With one of the highest HIV prevalence rates (34%) among adults in the world at the end of 2001 (UNAIDS/WHO, 2002), Zimbabwe continues to be one of the highest prevalence countries today. Antenatal clinic (ANC) sentinel surveys conducted to monitor the epidemic show the prevalence among pregnant women in Zimbabwe climbed from 25% in 1997 to 35% in 1999, with rates in 2000 and 2001 declining to 33% and 27%, respectively (Kububa, Dube, Midzi, Nesara, & St. Louis, 2002). The Young Adult Survey (YAS), conducted among a nationally representative sample in 2001–2002, showed population prevalence rates of 22% among 15- to 29-year-old women and 10% among 15- to 29-year-old men (Ministry of Health and Child Welfare [MOHCW], 2004). New modeling based on ANC and other data in Zimbabwe currently estimates that overall prevalence in the population of 15 to 49 year olds is about 20.1% (MOHCW, 2005; UNAIDS, 2005; UNAIDS/WHO, 2004). Zimbabwe is experiencing a generalized HIV epidemic, with women having about twice the prevalence as men. Urban (25%), as compared to rural areas (17%), have higher HIV rates, but areas considered neither urban nor rural, such as commercial farming areas and growth points, have the highest estimated current prevalence (27%) (MOHCW, 2005). Mortality is high (Blacker, 2004), with an estimated 3,252 men, women, and children dying each week from AIDS in Zimbabwe (MOHCW, 2005). As a result of Zimbabwean National AIDS Council and Ministry of Health and Child Welfare (MOHCW) priorities, we chose to implement a comprehensive HIV/STD prevention program in growth points in Zimbabwe. Growth points are designated sites in rural areas in Zimbabwe slated for economic and infrastructure development by the government, surrounded by many traditional villages. To encourage individuals in Zimbabwe to increase safer sexual behavior, in the context of such high AIDS rates, we are implementing the CPOL model, based on Diffusion of Innovation (Rogers, 1985), among residents of 30 growth points. This intervention involves popular opinion leaders talking to their peers about safe sex behavior.

Since the early 1990s, research has demonstrated that this intervention has resulted in declines in risky sexual behavior among gay men and heterosexual minority women (Kelly, St. Lawrence, & Diaz, 1991; St. Lawrence, Brasfield, Diaz, & Jefferson, 1994; Kelly et al., 1997; Sikkema et al., 2000). This community-level intervention is hypothesized to encourage normative change in behavior (Kelly, 1999). While these studies showed behavior change attributable to the CPOL intervention, research in the United Kingdom did not replicate these results (Elford, Bolding, & Sherr, 2001; Elford, Hart, Sherr, Williamson, & Bolding, 2002a, Flowers, Hart, Williamson, Frankis, & Der, 2002). A number of explanations have been attributed to this finding (Kelly, 2004; Elford, Sherr, Bolding, Serle, & Macguire, 2002b), but one possibility is that the CPOL model intervention did not shift mediators (e.g., attitudes, self-efficacy, intentions, norms) we know are linked to HIV risk-reduction behaviors. Such mediators are constructs that come directly from social-cognitive theories such as the TPB and Social Cognitive Theory (SCT). These have extensive research support showing they affect behavior (Albarracín et al., 2003; Armitage & Conner, 2001; Bandura, 1994; CDC AIDS Community Demonstration Project Research Group, 1999; Fishbein & Ajzen, 1975; Fisher & Fisher, 2000; Jaccard, Dodge, Dittus, & Feldman, 2002; Jemmott & Jemmott, 2000).

While the assumption underlying the CPOL model is that normative change in behavior occurs, only two studies have assessed norms, and they show conflicting results. Amirkhanian, Kelly, Kabakchieva, McAuliffe, and Vassileva (2003) showed AIDS knowledge, attitudes, normative perceptions, self-efficacy, intentions, and condom use changed from baseline to a 4-month post-assessment while Miller and colleagues (1998) showed condom use behavior increased, but community and individual norms did not change. To date there has been no research conducted by Kelly, using established behavioral models, such as the TPB or the IBM, to determine which mediators actually change in the CPOL conversational process. Kelly has never assessed longitudinally among a cohort of CPOLs, or community members, the very constructs (attitudes, norms, intentions, and self-efficacy) that he recommends need to be targeted in interventions (Kelly, 2002, 2004). These constructs have not been assessed to determine which of them change, and how. Thus, the conversational process Kelly motivates in CPOLs essentially remains a "black box." We have no explanation of what mediators change. Thus, within the context of the CPOL intervention for the HIV/STD Prevention Trial in Zimbabwe, we wanted to determine which of these mediators are most strongly associated with behavioral intention for the targeted safe sex behaviors. These mediators then should be the focus of CPOL conversations. Ultimately the evaluation should determine whether these mediators change as a result of the intervention, and whether this leads to change in those behaviors.

As part of preparation for the intervention Trial, a formative phase was conducted that included an epidemiologic study to assess behavioral risk and HIV prevalence in Zimbabwe growth points (Woelk, Kasprzyk, & Montaño, 2002a; Montaño, Kasprzyk, & Woelk, 2002; Kasprzyk, Woelk, Montaño, Bittner, & Richard, 2004). The epidemiologic study collected survey and biologic data from a household-based sample of 1,600 people ages 16 to 30 in 32 rural growth points. Overall HIV prevalence was 25% (15% for male, 34% for females), while prevalence among sexually active individuals was 33%. The prevalence of most other sexually transmitted infections (STIs) was relatively low, probably due to an effective STD control program launched in the 1990s by the Ministry of Health and Child Welfare (MOHCW). Gonorrhea, chlamydia, and chancroid, previously relatively common infections, had prevalence rates of less than 5%, and syphilis less than 1% (Woelk et al. 2002a). Of the total sample, 82% had ever had sex (75% males and 87% females). Men reported a lifetime mean number of 6.8 partners (Median = 3), while women reported a mean of 2.6 partners (Median = 1). Overall, 27% had more than one partner in the past year (49% men, 12% women); 15% had more than one regular partner in the past year (27% men, 6% women); 24% had a casual partner in the past year (45% men, 11% women); and 15% exchanged money or goods for sex (24% men, 9% women). In the context of the generalized HIV epidemic in Zimbabwe, even a small number of sexual contacts with multiple partners will result in a high probability of encountering an infected partner. Over half (55%) of men, but only 13% of women, drink at least monthly, 78% of the men who drink reported getting drunk at least monthly (Montaño et al., 2002), and about 60% of those who report getting drunk had multiple partners.

HIV prevalence among males and females was associated with number of partners, alcohol use, and intoxication. HIV prevalence among males was also associated with condom use and transactional sex. Female HIV risk appears to be determined more by their partners' behavior rather than their own (Mbizvo et al., 2005). Men do not use condoms at a high enough frequency to control the spread of HIV in Zimbabwe. Men, who are older on average in a sexual relationship, are more likely to be infected (HIV prevalence > 40% among men ages 27–30), and to in turn infect their younger wife or steady partner.

These results point to a focus on men for HIV prevention programs, especially men who engage in multiple risk behaviors. Women are much lower risk through their own behavior, but not through their partner's behavior. Interventions in Zimbabwe may be most effective using a *multi-message* approach (AVERT, 2005) including messages about remaining monogamous, using condoms with all partners if one is not able to commit to monogamy, discouraging drinking before having sex (Fritz et. al., 2002), and avoiding commercial sex workers (Cowan et. al., 2005) or using condoms with them. Thus, although the CPOL intervention Trial and development of our IBM survey instrument included men and women, the analyses presented in this chapter focused on higher-risk men. Our rationale for studying these men was to identify behavioral model constructs that might be the focus of prevention intervention messages to such men, thereby also potentially having a large impact on their partners' risk of HIV acquisition.

There has been criticism about applying *Western* cognitive models such as the TRA, TPB, and IBM to understand or explain HIV and AIDS health-related behaviors in developing countries (Joffe, 1996; Airhihenbuwa & Obregon, 2000). The commonly put forth argument is that such models do not apply to non-Western cultures and cannot be used to explain behavior or to inform the design of interventions to change behavior because they are based on the *rational man* approach. Thus, in other cultures which are more group or community oriented, these models would not explain behavior. We would argue that these models *are* applicable cross-culturally. The expectancy-value nature of cognitive models has led to the misperception that these are models of *rational behavior*. This is far from correct. The underlying assumption of the cognitive models is only that individuals are *rational actors*—that is, all individuals process information within their cultural context, and act based on their perceptions, beliefs and values. The models assume that there are underlying reasons that determine an individual's motivation to perform a behavior. These reasons, made up of a person's values and beliefs (affective, behavioral, normative, control, self-efficacy), determine motivation, regardless of whether those beliefs are rational, logical, or correct by some objective standard. These models also assume that we can identify and measure those beliefs, to understand and explain intention and behavior. The strength of these cognitive models is that they provide a framework for identifying the beliefs underlying behavior, and this can inform interventions to encourage behavior change (Abraham, Sheeran, & Orbell, 1998).

Thus, the work presented here had four main goals:

1. To assess through qualitative interviews whether cognitive-behavioral factors specific to unsafe sex could be elicited among a group of Zimbabwean men and women;

2. To determine whether measures of the cognitive-behavioral model constructs with respect to safe sex behaviors are understandable, and to develop *best measurement* strategies for the model constructs in Zimbabwe—a developing world, non-Western country;

3. To assess how well the model explains behavioral intentions related to multiple safe-sex behaviors among higher-risk men in Zimbabwe; and

4. To analyze the measures in order to identify specific target messages for tailored behavior change interventions for higher-risk men.

We will describe how qualitative data were collected and analyzed to design the IBM survey, followed by the IBM survey data collection. We then present analyses showing the association of behavioral model constructs with behavioral intention for six safer-sex behaviors among selected high-risk men.

METHODS

The IBM is a behavioral model that posits six main constructs as determinants of behavior. These constructs include affect, attitude, subjective norm, and self-efficacy with regard to the behavior. For some behaviors affect, consisting of a person's emotional response to the idea of the behavior, is distinct from attitude which comprises a cognitive response. The model also includes a construct to measure community and individual level facilitators and barriers, and perceived behavioral control over a behavior (Kasprzyk, et. al. 1998). Our previous research found that these constructs are measurable, and the measures were reliable and valid in Zimbabwe (Kasprzyk & Montaño, 2001; Kasprzyk & Montaño, 1994; Montaño, Kasprzyk, & Wilson, 1993). However, it was necessary to develop an IBM questionnaire specific to the target population (residents of rural growth points) and the safe-sex behaviors being targeted by the CPOL intervention. The IBM questionnaire was thus developed using qualitative data collected as part of a comprehensive formative phase of the HIV/STD Prevention Trial. This phase also allowed us to pilot test and finalize the IBM construct measures as described herein.

Qualitative Study

Qualitative data collection.   The formative research was conducted in 32 growth points throughout Zimbabwe. Ethnographers carried letters of introduction and approval from the Ministry of Health and the Department of Community Medicine, University of Zimbabwe Medical School, when they met with key informants and stakeholders in each selected community. Ethnographers randomly selected 15 households in the village closest to each growth point in order to conduct open-ended in-depth elicitation interviews with 16–30 year olds. They also compiled lists of stakeholders and key informants in each community. In addition, ethnographers compiled lists of 16–30 year olds for recruitment for four focus group discussions with 6–10 participants each.

The ethnography team approached each of the selected households, and randomly selected a person between ages 16 and 30. The interviewer explained the project and administered informed consent before proceeding with the interview. Open-ended interviews lasted between 45 minutes and 1.5 hours. Stakeholders and key informants were identified purposively, and were recruited to be interviewed individually. Stakeholder and key informant interviews lasted from 1 to 2 hours. Individual interviews were primarily conducted outside, sitting under trees. When participants were willing, interviews were conducted in the home. If there was no appropriate private place available, the interview was conducted in the project vehicle. All individuals recruited to participate in focus group discussions gathered in a central location in the village. Focus groups were held in rooms, in school rooms, outside under trees, or in the kraal (village) head's home. Focus group discussions lasted 1.5 to 2 hours.

For both interviews and focus groups, the interviewer followed an interview guide that asked a variety of questions intended to help design the CPOL intervention, including knowledge and opinions about HIV, causes of HIV/AIDS, and sexual behavior. The interview guide also included questions designed to elicit information relevant to each of the IBM model constructs. Participants were asked to describe their feelings, beliefs, sources of normative influence, barriers and facilitators with respect to several safe-sex behaviors. These behaviors included condom use with various partners (spouse, steady partner, casual partner, commercial sex worker), monogamy (sticking to one partner), avoiding alcohol before sex, avoiding commercial sex workers (CSWs), and talking about safe sex with partners. All open-ended interviews and focus groups were audio tape-recorded.

Qualitative Data Analysis.   Qualitative audio-recorded interviews and focus groups were transcribed verbatim, translated, and typed. All typists followed layout instructions to facilitate easy conversion to text files for NUD*IST. All typed interviews were then read into a qualitative database created in NUD*IST version N5. Data were coded by a team of four study coders. Summaries were conducted on the coded transcripts to provide ethnographic data required to tailor the CPOL intervention (Armstrong, et. al., 2002), and to determine all issues related to IBM constructs (affect, attitude, subjective norm, perceived control, self-efficacy, and barriers and facilitators). These summary results were used in the development of the IBM questionnaire.

Qualitative Study Results.   Participants were able to name many advantages and disadvantages, normative influences, and barriers and facilitators regarding condom use with different partners, monogamy, drinking and sex, avoiding commercial sex workers, and talking about safer-sex issues with partners (Armstrong et al. 2002; Woelk, Armstrong, Kasprzyk, & Montaño, 2002b; Kasprzyk, Terera, Montaño, & Woelk, 2003). Specific beliefs regarding these behaviors are presented in more detail following in the IBM results section.

Development of the IBM Survey Instrument

Coding of the qualitative interviews yielded lists of beliefs related to all IBM behavioral model constructs, coded into listings of affect, attitude, subjective norm, and barriers and facilitators in regards to condom use, monogamy, and avoiding CSWs. Coding schemes also allowed us to capture specific beliefs regarding the use of alcohol, and talking about sexual risk issues with partners. In addition, coding schemes allowed us to capture more general beliefs or stereotypes related to condom use and alcohol use. These lists were compared to previous beliefs generated in research in Zimbabwe (Kasprzyk & Montaño, 2001; Kasprzyk & Montaño, 1994; Montaño et. al., 1993) to validate issues raised. Once lists specific to model constructs for each targeted behavior were generated, questionnaire items were constructed. We used 5-point *strongly agree-strongly disagree* scales for general attitudes towards condoms, behavioral beliefs, and normative beliefs (see tables later in this chapter for specific content of these beliefs). Direct measures of attitude were assessed on 5-point semantic differential scales with the end points of "extremely good-bad," "extremely difficult-easy," and "extremely safe-unsafe." Pilot study interviews assessing affect and direct attitude using these three items did not factor into subscales, thus we did not include affect as a separate construct measure. We piloted scales to measure perceived control and self-efficacy by asking questions concerning barriers or facilitators in two ways. For example, "If you have been drinking before sex, it makes it 'very easy-very difficult' to use a condom" on a 5-point scale; and "If you have been drinking before sex, how certain are you that you could always use condoms" scaled from "Extremely certain I could not" to "Extremely certain I could" on a 5-point scale.

We conducted pilot studies to test all measures including beliefs, outcome evaluations, motivation to comply with referents, and especially to compare measures of perceived control (control beliefs and perceived power) and self-efficacy with respect to the same set of barriers. We found that the perceived control questions (easy-difficult scale) did not generate varied responses among individuals; essentially everyone agreed with the perceived ease or difficulty. By contrast, the self-efficacy measure (certain I could vs. could not) generated more varied responses. Thus, in the final version of the survey, we decided to measure self-efficacy instead of perceived control. In regards to subjective norm, we found essentially no variance on the direct (single item) measure for various safe-sex behaviors (i.e., most people important to me think I should...). By contrast there was variance in participants' normative beliefs with respect to specific referents. Thus, we decided to exclude the direct measure of subjective norm and rely only on the indirect measure, by measuring normative beliefs with respect to various referent individuals and groups. When asked to provide belief evaluations and motivation to comply with referents, study participants had trouble rating these questions—they seemed obvious to study participants. There seemed to be overall general agreement about the valence of behavioral outcome evaluations and motivation to comply with social referents. As a result, we found little variance in the outcome evaluation and motivation to comply with various referents. Our previous research in HIV prevention behavior has also shown that the value aspect of behavioral and normative beliefs does not impact intention as much as the beliefs themselves (von Haeften, Fishbein, Kasprzyk, & Montaño, 2001a; von Haeften & Kenski, 2001b; Fishbein, von Haeften, & Appleyard, 2001). Because of these pilot results and the length of the questionnaire to measure model components with respect to multiple behaviors, we decided to exclude these measures. Thus, our indirect attitude measures consisted only of behavioral beliefs, without the corresponding outcome evaluation. Similarly, our subjective norm measure consisted only of normative beliefs, without weighting them by motivation to comply. In addition we created a *Condom Stereotypes Scale*, which allowed us to explore further the nature of attitudes in regards to condoms (Ajzen, 2001). This scale consisted of two subscales of myth and moral statements made in relation to condoms, such as "only promiscuous people use condoms," and allowed us to test whether these moral and myth attitudes had separate and independent effects on condom use intentions.

The format of the final instrument was a paper-and-pencil questionnaire, delivered as a face-to-face interview that measured model constructs with respect to six behaviors: condom use with spouse, steady, casual, and commercial sex partners; avoiding CSWs; and monogamy (sticking to one partner). The survey measured recent behavior, behavioral intention, attitude, behavioral beliefs, self-efficacy (direct), self-efficacy beliefs, and normative beliefs with respect to each behavior.

IBM Survey Data Collection Methods

The IBM survey data were collected within the context of the larger baseline data collection effort for the CPOL Intervention Trial. Study participants for the Trial were 185 individuals in each of 30 rural growth points, approximately equally distributed between males and females. Participants were recruited by nurse interviewers between November 2003 and December 2004. All individuals entering selected study venues of bottle stores, general dealers, and markets during the course of a seven-day period were intercepted, screened for eligibility, and if eligible, recruited. People were eligible if they were between the ages of 18 and 30, had lived in the growth point for at least 1 year, expected to stay in the growth point area for the next 2 years, and came to the growth point shops at least twice a week. After recruitment, participants were scheduled for interviews in private rooms rented by the project.

All participants were provided with informed consent and reimbursement for their time. Interviews took place in Shona or Ndebele, Zimbabwe's majority languages, with survey instruments that had been translated from English and back-translated using a decentering process to translate for meaning. After obtaining informed consent, the nurse conducted a behavioral risk assessment using a standardized computer assisted personal interview (CAPI) developed for the five-country Trial. This instrument was designed to collect data on participants' demographics, residential stability, health status including a history of STDs, drug and alcohol use, overall sexual risks, condom use, injection or medical exposures, and body-piercing experiences. The CAPI interview took 15–20 minutes to complete, depending on the skip sections for each participant.

Nurses next conducted a syndromic assessment for STD symptoms, carried out pre-test counseling, and collected biological samples to screen participants for HIV and other STDs. Study participants received syndromic treatment for curable STDs based on the Zimbabwe MOHCW protocol for symptomatic participants (MOHCW, 2001). This phase of the interview took from 40 to 60 minutes. This was followed by the IBM interview, which took from 20 to 40 minutes to complete (Mode = 20 minutes), depending on the types of partners participants reported.

Biological Outcomes.   Participants provided blood, urine, and cervical specimens that were tested in the University of Zimbabwe project laboratory following standardized laboratory protocols. Twenty percent of specimens were sent to Johns Hopkins University School of Medicine for quality control. HIV testing was performed using three ELISA tests, two initially, and a third as a tie breaker for discordant results. HSV–2 testing was performed using Herpeselect 2 EIA (MRL, Focus Technologies, Los Angeles, CA, USA). Syphilis testing was performed by Rapid Plasma Reagin (RPR) and confirmed using the *Treponema pallidum* Particle Agglutination test. Vaginal swabs were cultured for *Trichomonas vaginalis* using the InPouch TV 20 test kit (Biomed, San Jose, CA, USA). Urine from males and vaginal swabs from females were tested for chlamydia and gonorrhea DNA using Amplicor CT/NG PCR (Roche, Branchburg, NJ, USA).

At the time of the post-test counseling appointment, treatment for curable STDs was provided to individuals diagnosed via lab results, about 4 weeks after their interview. During post-test counseling, participants could choose whether or not they wanted to learn their STD results and HIV status separately.

Data Processing and Data Entry.   All quantitative study data were entered into data management systems. Biological test results were entered into a laboratory management system that was used to determine results. Reports were then generated for the nursing team to take back to each community to notify study participants of their STD or HIV test results. All biological sample test results were double-checked by the laboratory manager and supervisor, who signed off on the results before they were given to the nurse's team to provide results to study participants.

RESULTS OF IBM SURVEY

At the time that this chapter was written, data had been processed and cleaned for 1,998 male participants who reported that they had ever had sex. Of these, 458 (23%) were identified to be higher-risk men based on their report of either having a casual partner in the past year or having ever had sex with a CSW. Results are presented for these 458 higher-risk men.

Study Participant Characteristics

Table 10–1 presents demographic and other characteristics of the 458 high-risk men surveyed. These men were on average nearly 24 years of age and over one fourth (26%) were married. Nearly three fourths were of Shona and one fourth of Ndebele ethnicity. Nearly all men reported that they know how to use a male condom (96%) and had ever used a condom (94%). They reported an average age at first intercourse of nearly 18 years, and they reported a median of 8 lifetime sex partners, with 3 partners in the previous 12 months.

Table 10–2 lists the various sample subgroups based on risky behavior, and their respective HIV prevalence. The HIV prevalence of the entire sample of higher-risk men was 26%, while the overall study HIV prevalence was 20%. Over 70% of the men reported ever having sex with a CSW, with over 50% having had sex with a CSW within the previous year. Of the men reporting ever having had sex with a CSW, 74% reported having sex with one in the past 12-months (not tabled). The HIV prevalence of men who reported sex with a CSW was 29%. Half of the men reported having sex with a casual partner in the past year. These men reported an average of 2.4 casual partners in the last 12 months, and their HIV prevalence was almost 25%.

Due to their sexual behavior with CSWs and casual partners, this study sample of higher-risk men may also be at risk for transmitting HIV to their spouses or steady partners. Over one fourth (26%) of the study sample reported having sex with a spouse in the previous year. The HIV prevalence of this subgroup was 37%. Sixty percent of study participants reported having had sex with a steady partner in the previous year, and their HIV prevalence was 26%. Since HIV prevalence is positively associated with age in Zimbabwe, the higher HIV prevalence of the subgroup of men who had sex with a spouse may be partially attributed to being on average slightly older than the other subgroups as shown in Table 10–2.

TABLE 10–1
Characteristics of Survey Participants

Characteristics	Mean/%
Age (mean)	23.8
Married (%)	25.8%
Ethnicity:	
Shona	73.4%
Ndebele	26.6%
Know how to use a condom (%)	96.3%
Ever used a condom (%)	94.3%
Age at first intercourse (mean)	17.7
Number of sex partners:	
lifetime (median)	8.0
past 12 months (median)	3.0
Ever exchanged money/goods for sex (%)	43.4%

TABLE 10–2
Survey Participant Risk Behaviors and HIV Prevalence

Sample Group	N (%)	HIV Prevalence	Age (mean)
Total	458 (100%)	26.1%	23.8
Ever had sex with CSW	323 (70.5%)	28.7%	24.2
Sex with CSW in past year	239 (52.2%)	28.6%	23.7
Sex with casual partner past year	228 (49.8%)	24.7%	23.4
Partner risk subgroups:			
Sex with spouse	117 (25.5%)	37.4%	25.3
Sex with steady partner	275 (60.0%)	25.7%	23.8

Correlation and Regression of Model Constructs to Explain Behavioral Intention

Prior to carrying out correlation and regression analyses to test the theoretical model, the various model component scores were calculated. Appropriate attitude and belief item scores were first reflected so that a higher score was associated with a positive opinion about each behavior. Internal consistency analyses with computation of Cronbach's alpha were then carried out for the items making up each model construct for each of the six behaviors investigated (see Table 10–3). The direct measure of attitude consisted of 3 items, resulting in adequate Cronbach's α between .46 and .76 for the six behaviors. Between 9 and 14 behavioral belief items were used to obtain an indirect measure of attitude toward each behavior. Internal consistency of behavioral beliefs was high resulting in Cronbach's α between .73 and .92 for the six behaviors. Between 4 and 6 normative beliefs were used to measure subjective norm, resulting in very adequate internal consistency, with Cronbach's α between .63 and .82 for the six behaviors. In addition to a single direct measure of self-efficacy, indirect self-efficacy measures were obtained by measuring 11 self-efficacy beliefs for each condom use behavior and 6 self-efficacy beliefs for monogamy. The self-efficacy beliefs resulted in high internal consistency with Cronbach's α between .91 and .95 for the six behaviors.

Model component scores were next computed by taking the mean of the appropriate items underlying them. A direct measure of attitude toward each behavior was computed as the mean of the three semantic differential items measured. Indirect attitude scores were obtained by computing the mean of the behavioral beliefs measured with respect to each behavior. Subjective norm scores were obtained by computing the mean of the normative beliefs measured with respect to each behavior. Indirect self-efficacy scores were obtained by computing the mean of the self-efficacy beliefs concerning each behavior.

In addition to the model component computation, two general condom attitude scores were computed from the general condom belief measures. One score was computed as the mean of six beliefs concerned with myths about condoms. The second score was computed as the mean of five beliefs concerned with morals associated with condom use. Items comprising both scores had adequate internal consistency (Cronbach's α = .65 for condom myths and .63 for condom morals).

TABLE 10–3
Reliabilities of Model Construct Scales (Cronbach's alpha)

	Condom Use Spouse (n = 111)	Condom Use Steady (n = 270)	Condom Use Casual (n = 224)	Condom Use CSW (n = 239)	Avoid CSW (n = 323)	Mono-gamy (n = 438)
Attitude (direct)	.67	.64	.64	.76	.53	.46
Behavioral Beliefs	.92	.92	.82	.73	.73	.84
Normative Beliefs	.82	.66	.63	.66	.74	.61
Self-Efficacy Beliefs	.93	.95	.94	.93	.94	.91

Multiple regression analyses were next conducted to explain behavioral intention for each of the six behaviors. These analyses were carried out in three steps. On the first step the direct measure of attitude and subjective norm were entered to test how well the TRA explains each behavioral intention. On the second step the direct measure of self-efficacy was entered (in place of perceived control) to test the TPB. On the third step, stepwise regression was used, including the indirect measure of attitude (mean of belief items), and the indirect measure of self-efficacy (mean of self-efficacy beliefs). Condom moral attitude and condom myth attitude were also included in the four condom intention analyses. This third step was used to determine whether any of these measures, especially moral attitude (Ajzen, 2001), improve the TPB in explaining behavioral intentions.

Table 10–4 lists the correlations between the model components and behavioral intention. All correlations were significant with $p < 0.01$. Table 10–4 also presents the multiple regression results of applying the TPB to explain each behavioral intention. The regression analysis results for each behavior are described below.

Condom Use Intention with Spouse (N = 111).   Attitude and subjective norm each obtained significant beta weights in explaining men's intentions to use condoms with their spouses, obtaining a multiple $R = 0.47$. Attitude had a larger beta weight than subjective norm. When self-efficacy was added to test the TPB, a multiple $R = 0.53$ was obtained. Both self-efficacy and attitude had significant beta weights, but subjective norm was no longer significant in this model. No other variables were significant on the last regression step.

Condom Use Intention with Steady Partners (N = 270).   Attitude and subjective norm had significant beta weights, with subjective norm having the larger weight. This test of the TRA resulted in a multiple $R = 0.50$. The addition of self-efficacy to test the TPB resulted in a multiple $R = 0.73$. Self-efficacy and subjective norm had significant beta weights while attitude was no longer significant in this model. Stepwise regression resulted in the mean behavioral belief score being added to the equation with a multiple $R = 0.74$. Although this is

TABLE 10–4
Correlation and Regression to Explain Intention

	Condom Use Spouse (n = 111) r (beta)	Condom Use Steady (n = 270) r (beta)	Condom Use Casual (n = 224) r (beta)	Condom Use CSW (n = 239) r (beta)	Avoid CSW (n = 323) r (beta)	Monog-amy (n = 438) r (beta)
Attitude	.44 (.31**)	.38 (.04 ns)	.41 (.23**)	.28 (.17**)	.36 (.18**)	.43 (.25**)
Subj. Norm	.31 (.10 ns)	.44 (.16**)	.36 (.13*)	.36 (.20**)	.15 (.07 ns)	.20 (.00 ns)
Self Efficacy	.44 (.27**)	.71 (.63**)	.61 (.49**)	.49 (.42**)	.51 (.42**)	.59 (.49**)
Multiple R	.53	.73	.67	.57	.53	.63

All correlations and multiple R in table significant with p < 0.01;
* beta weight significant with p < 0.05;
** beta weight significant with p < 0.01

a small increase in variance accounted for, this finding suggests that the direct attitude measure may not have adequately assessed attitude toward using condoms with steady partners. Alternatively, the direct attitude measure and the mean belief measure may have assessed different dimensions of attitude, such as affective and cognitive dimensions.

Condom Use Intention with Casual Partners (N = 224). Attitude and subjective norm each had significant beta weights, with attitude having the larger weight, resulting in a multiple $R = 0.49$ for the TRA. The multiple R increased to $R = 0.67$ when self-efficacy was added, and all three model components had significant beta weights for the TPB. The stepwise regression resulted in the addition of the mean self-efficacy beliefs, with a multiple $R = 0.72$. This finding suggests that the direct measure of self-efficacy may not have been adequately assessed, or that the direct and indirect measures assessed different constructs.

Condom Use Intention with CSWs (N = 239). Attitude and subjective norm each had significant beta weights, with subjective norm having the larger weight. This test of the TRA resulted in a multiple $R = 0.40$. The addition of self-efficacy to test the TPB resulted in all three constructs having significant beta weights, and a multiple $R = 0.57$. The stepwise regression resulted in no other variables entering the equation.

Intention to Avoid CSWs (N = 323). The test of the TRA resulted in both attitude and subjective norm having significant beta weights, with attitude having the larger weight, and a multiple $R = 0.37$. The addition of self-efficacy resulted in multiple $R = 0.53$ for the TPB. Both attitude and self-efficacy had significant beta weights, while subjective norm was no longer significant. The stepwise regression resulted in the addition of the mean self-efficacy belief score, with multiple $R = 0.57$. This finding suggests that the direct measure of self-efficacy may not have been adequately assessed, or that the direct and indirect measures assessed different constructs.

Intention to Stick to One Partner (Monogamy; N = 438). Both attitude and subjective norm obtained significant beta weights, with attitude having the larger weight. This test of the TRA resulted in a multiple $R = 0.44$. The addition of self-efficacy to test the TPB resulted in a multiple $R = 0.63$, with both self-efficacy and attitude having significant beta weights. Subjective norm was no longer significant. The stepwise regression resulted in the addition of both the mean self-efficacy score and the mean behavioral belief score, with multiple $R = 0.66$. This suggests that the direct measures of attitude and self-efficacy may not have been adequately assessed for this intention, or that the direct and indirect measures captured slightly different constructs.

Individual Indicator Analysis to Identify Key Beliefs

The previous regression analyses identified the most important model constructs to target by interventions to change behavioral intention and behavior for each of the six behaviors. In order to change attitude toward the behavior it is necessary to change the underlying behavioral beliefs. Similarly, to change subjective norm one must change the underlying normative beliefs, and underlying self-efficacy beliefs must be changed in order to change self-efficacy. Rather than target all of these underlying beliefs for each behavior, it is important to identify a smaller number of key beliefs that will have the most impact in changing each model construct.

Therefore, the next step in our analysis was to identify the belief items underlying attitude, subjective norm, and self-efficacy that best explain each behavioral intention. We began with a correlation analysis to identify the beliefs within each construct that were significantly associated with each behavioral intention. Next, the significant beliefs underlying each model construct were entered in a stepwise multiple regression to identify those beliefs that make an independent contribution to explaining each behavioral intention. Thus, separate stepwise regressions were carried out for: (1) behavioral beliefs, (2) normative beliefs, and (3) self-efficacy beliefs.

Table 10–5 presents the correlations between each of the four condom use behavioral intentions and the beliefs underlying each model construct. Table 10–6 presents these correlations for intentions to avoid CSWs and stick to one partner (monogamy). These tables also show the results of the stepwise multiple regression analyses to identify the key beliefs within each construct that independently contribute to explaining each behavioral intention. It is important to note that in our earlier analyses to test the overall models (Table 10–4), subjective norm did not obtain a significant beta weight for three behaviors (condom use with a spouse, avoid CSWs, monogamy), and attitude did not obtain a significant beta weight for one behavior (condom use with a steady partner). However, these constructs were included in the current regression analyses for two reasons: (1) they had significant correlations with behavioral intentions yet their non-significant beta weights may have been due to collinearity with other construct measures, (2) the effect of a few important underlying beliefs may have been suppressed in the computation of construct scores. The results of these analyses for each behavioral intention are described below.

Condom Use Intention with Spouse.   Twelve of the 14 behavioral beliefs were significantly correlated with behavioral intention. When these 12 beliefs were entered in a stepwise regression, only 2 beliefs obtained significant beta weights: (1) show that you are diseased or unclean, and (2) encourage promiscuity in her. Among the 5 normative beliefs, only the normative belief about whether the spouse wants him to use a condom was significantly correlated with behavioral intention. All of the 11 self-efficacy beliefs were significantly correlated with intention. The stepwise regression resulted in only 2 self-efficacy beliefs obtaining significant beta weights: (1) when carried away and cannot wait to have sex, and (2) having a condom with you. These results suggest that interventions to increase intention to use condoms with a spouse could target 2 behavioral beliefs to impact attitude, partner norm to impact subjective norm, and 2 self-efficacy beliefs to impact self-efficacy.

TABLE 10–5
Correlation and Regression to Identify Key Item Predictors of Condom Use Intentions

	Condom Use Spouse r (beta)	Condom Use Steady r (beta)	Condom Use Casual r (beta)	Condom Use CSW r (beta)
Behavioral Beliefs				
Make her angry	−.39	−.37	−.24 (−.17)	−.13
Show lack of respect for her	−.35	−.42 (−.17)	−.15	−.12 NS
Show you think she is unclean/diseased	−.32	−.37	−.12 NS	−.04 NS
Show that you are unclean/diseased	−.40 (−.29)	−.32	−.18	−.15
Be embarrassing	−.24	−.28	−.22	−.24 (−.17)
Make her think you don't love her	−.33	−.38	—	—
Protect you from HIV	.07 NS	.21 (.14)	.12 NS	.16 (−.15)
Spoil the relationship	−.35	−.41 (−.17)	−.26 (−.21)	—
Show you don't trust her	−.36	−.38	—	—
You would get less pleasure	−.22	−.13	−.12 NS	−.06 NS
Make her think you have other partners	−.42	−.39 (−.21)	—	—
Unnecessary—she has no other partners	−.24	−.33	—	—
You will not have sexual release	−.14 NS	−.27	−.19	−.09 NS
Encourage promiscuity in her	−.39 (−.22)	−.24	—	—
Not get what you paid for	—	—	—	.03 NS
Expensive	—	—	—	−.23 (−.17)
Multiple R	**.45**	**.51**	**.31**	**.33**
Normative Influence				
Your family	.15 NS	.31 (.18)	.12 NS	.27
Her family	.17 NS	—	—	—
Your closest friends	.17 NS	.22	.30 (.23)	.35 (.35)
Radio shows or dramas	.18 NS	.08 NS	.19	.23
Your partner	.49 (.49)	.55 (.50)	.40 (.36)	.19 (.16)
Multiple R	**.49**	**.58**	**.46**	**.39**
Self-Efficacy				
Carried away and can't wait to have sex	.45 (.32)	.56 (.19)	.39	.23
You drink before sex	.39	.47	.41	.16
She drinks before sex	.37	.40	.47	.28
Use another method of birth control	.31	.61 (.30)	.49 (.25)	—
She doesn't want to use condom	.32	.53	.42	.31
Believe AIDS will affect you	.23	.37	.45	.38 (.14)
Having condom with you	.39 (.22)	.52	.45	.35
Know how to use a condom	.35	.51	.50	.23
Condom availability in community	.37	.59	.53	.26
Had to talk about it with her	.31	.57 (.27)	.54	.46 (.97)
You think she had other partners	.20	.41	.57 (.43)	.24 (−.68)
Multiple R	**.49**	**.66**	**.61**	**.59**

NS = correlation not significant
— = not measured for the behavior

Condom Use Intention with Steady Partners.   All 14 of the behavioral beliefs were significantly correlated with intention. The stepwise regression resulted in 4 of these beliefs obtaining significant beta weights: (1) show lack of respect for her, (2) protect you from HIV, (3) spoil the relationship, and (4) make her think you have other partners. Three of the normative beliefs were significantly correlated with intention, and the stepwise regression resulted in the normative beliefs about the steady partner and family obtaining significant beta weights. All of the self-efficacy beliefs were significantly correlated with intention. When these were entered into the stepwise regression, 3 self-efficacy beliefs obtained significant beta weights: (1) when carried away and cannot wait to have sex, (2) using another method of birth control, and (3) having to talk about it with her. These results suggest that interventions to increase intention to use condoms with a steady partner could best target 4 behavioral beliefs to impact attitude, 2 normative beliefs to impact subjective norm, and 3 self-efficacy beliefs to impact self-efficacy.

Condom Use Intention with Casual Partner.   Six of the 9 behavioral beliefs were significantly correlated with intention to use condoms with casual partners. These 6 behavioral beliefs were entered into a stepwise regression, and 2 beliefs obtained significant beta weights: (1) make her angry, and (2) spoil the relationship. Three normative beliefs were significantly correlated with intention. The stepwise regression resulted in 2 of these normative beliefs obtaining significant beta weights: (1) normative belief about the casual partner, and (2) normative belief about closest friends. All of the self-efficacy beliefs were significantly correlated with intention, and the stepwise regression resulted in 2 self-efficacy beliefs obtaining significant beta weights: (1) using another method of birth control, and (2) you think she has had other partners. In summary, interventions to increase intention to use condoms with a casual partner could best target 2 behavioral beliefs to impact attitude, 2 normative beliefs to impact subjective norm, and 2 self-efficacy beliefs to impact self-efficacy.

Condom Use Intention with CSWs.   Five of the 10 behavioral beliefs were significantly correlated with intention to use condoms with CSWs. When these 5 behavioral beliefs were entered into a stepwise regression, 3 beliefs obtained significant beta weights: (1) would be embarrassing, (2) protect you from HIV, and (3) would be expensive. All 4 normative beliefs were significantly correlated with intention, and the stepwise regression resulted in 2 normative beliefs obtaining significant beta weights: (1) normative belief about closest friends, and (2) normative belief about the CSWs. All 10 self-efficacy beliefs were significantly correlated with intention. The stepwise regression resulted in 3 of these self-efficacy beliefs obtaining significant beta weights: (1) believing AIDS will affect you, (2) having to talk about it with her, and (3) thinking she has other partners. These findings indicate that interventions to increase intention to use condoms with a CSW could target 2 behavioral beliefs to impact attitude, 2 normative beliefs to impact subjective norm, and 3 self-efficacy beliefs to impact self-efficacy.

Intention to Avoid CSWs.   Three of the 7 behavioral beliefs were significantly correlated with intention to avoid CSWs, and only 1 of these beliefs was significant in the stepwise regression analysis: difficult when wife/steady is

TABLE 10–6
Correlation and Regression to Identify Key Item Predictors of Avoiding CSWs and
Monogamy Intentions

	Avoid CSW r (beta)	Monogamy r (beta)
Behavioral Beliefs		
Not get type sex wife/girlfriend does not provide	−.12	—
Not get sexual release when want it	−.09 NS	—
Goes against our culture	.02 NS	—
Not have something to occupy time	−.22	—
Difficult when wife/steady not available	−.31 (−.30)	—
Friends won't go drinking with you at beer hall	−.07 NS	—
Not have sex anytime when want it	−.08 NS	—
Not get variety in sex partners you need	—	−.11 (.13)
Not be sexually satisfied	—	−.33 (−.26)
Does not fit into our culture	—	−.09 NS
Difficult because you have high sex drive	—	−.37 (−.20)
Difficult since traditional for multiple partners	—	−.32 (−.13)
Makes men less manly	—	−.15 (.13)
You will not get HIV	—	.17 (.15)
Something you cannot commit to	—	−.32 (−.20)
Would get sick	—	−.19
Would lose prestige or standing in community	—	−.16
Multiple *R*	**.30**	**.50**
Normative Influence		
Your family	.14 (.12)	.12
Your closest friends	.18 (.14)	.17 (.13)
Friends at beer hall	.11	—
Your church	.03 NS	.02 NS
Your culture	.12	.19 (.14)
Radio shows or dramas	.07 NS	.11
Multiple *R*	**.21**	**.22**
Self–Efficacy		
Drinking with friends at beer hall	.39 (.23)	—
You have money	.39	—
You need sexual release when wife/steady gone	.37	—
In mood for things wife/steady does not do	.36	—
CSW is attractive	.41 (.27)	—
Have regular CSW you see	.40	—
Talking about it with partner	—	.54 (.32)
Trust partner is also monogamous	—	.44
You and partner being apart a lot	—	.45 (.18)
Partner did not want sex as often as you	—	.40
You spot a beautiful girl	—	.43
CSWs entice you	—	.42
Wife or steady partner being pregnant	—	.48 (.17)
Multiple *R*	**.44**	**.57**

NS = correlation not significant
— = not measured for the behavior

not available. Four of the 6 normative beliefs were significantly correlated with intention. Two of these were significant in the stepwise regression: (1) normative belief about your family, and (2) normative belief about closest friends. All 6 self-efficacy beliefs were significantly correlated with intention, and the stepwise regression resulted in 2 of these obtaining significant beta weights: (1) drinking with friends at the beer hall, and (2) CSW is attractive. Thus, interventions to increase intention to avoid CSWs could best target 1 behavioral belief to impact attitude, 2 normative beliefs to impact subjective norm, and 2 self-efficacy beliefs to impact self-efficacy.

Intention to Stick to One Partner (Monogamy).   Nine of the 10 behavioral beliefs were significantly correlated with intention to stick to one partner. When these were entered into the stepwise regression, 7 behavioral beliefs were significant: (1) would not get variety in sex partners you need, (2) would not be sexually satisfied, (3) difficult because have high sex drive, (4) difficult since it is traditional for men to have multiple partners, (5) makes men less manly, (6) means you will not get HIV, and (7) is something you cannot commit to. Four normative beliefs were significantly correlated with intention, and 2 of these obtained significant beta weights in the stepwise regression: (1) normative belief about closest friends, and (2) normative belief about your culture. All 7 self-efficacy beliefs were significantly correlated with intention, and the stepwise regression resulted in 3 self-efficacy beliefs obtaining significant beta weights: (1) talking about it with partner, (2) you and partner being apart a lot, and (3) wife or steady partner being pregnant. These results indicate that interventions to increase intention to stick to one partner could target 7 behavioral beliefs to impact attitude, 2 normative beliefs to impact subjective norm, and 3 self-efficacy beliefs to impact self-efficacy.

CONCLUSION

Our qualitative study phase was very successful in eliciting from rural Zimbabweans relevant behavioral outcomes, social referents, and barriers and facilitators for each of the safe-sex behaviors investigated. Qualitative study participants understood the concepts behind each of the model constructs and were able to provide excellent information. This served as the basis for designing an initial draft of the survey instrument to measure the various model constructs. Pre-testing of this instrument and discussions with participants resulted in the development of appropriate wording for each question and response scales that were understandable. This also led to exclusion of some measures. For example, we chose to use measures of self-efficacy instead of control beliefs and perceived power. We also excluded measures of behavioral outcome evaluations and motivation to comply.

The TRA and TPB constructs were good at explaining safe-sex behavioral intentions among this rural Zimbabwe population. Multiple correlations ranged between 0.53 and 0.73 for explaining the six safe-sex behavioral intentions. Only for condom use intention with spouse did attitude have the largest beta weight. For all five other behavioral intentions, self-efficacy had the largest beta weight. It is important to note that the two general condom attitude measures (condom moral attitude and condom myth attitude) had low correlations with condom use behavioral intentions, and never entered the regression equations. This finding shows that even with attitudes that have clear and measurable moral underpinnings (Ajzen, 2001), the specific attitude towards the behavior is a better indicator of behavioral intention. This finding clearly supports the importance of measuring attitudes that are specific to the behavior.

All three model constructs had significant correlations with all six behavioral intentions. In the multiple regression analyses to explain condom use intentions, all three model constructs had significant beta weights only for intention to use condoms with casual partners and with CSWs. Subjective norm was not significant in the multiple regression to explain condom use with a spouse, and attitude was not significant in the regression to explain condom use with steady partners. Despite these constructs being non-significant (likely due to collinearity with the other two constructs), we included them in the individual indictor analysis because they were moderately correlated with intention and they include belief items that appear to be important determinants of intention.

The individual indicator analysis identified key beliefs within all three model constructs for interventions to target. Partner norm is particularly important for intention to use condoms with spouse, steady partner, and casual partner. This coincides with other research showing the partner is a particularly important referent in regards to condom use behavior (von Haeften et. al., 2001a). Normative belief about closest friends is more important for condom use with CSWs, and is also important for condom use with casual partners. The significant behavioral beliefs varied considerably by behavioral intention, though "spoil the relationship" was significant for condom use with steady and casual partners and was also correlated with intention to use condoms with a spouse. Similarly, the significant self-efficacy beliefs varied by behavioral intention, though several beliefs were significant for two behaviors (getting carried away and can't wait to have sex; using another birth control method; having to talk about it with her; thinking she has other partners).

Our analyses identified the beliefs within each construct that were most highly correlated with, and that provide independent contributions to explaining, each behavioral intention. Thus, in most of the analyses only two or three beliefs were significant. The significant beliefs may be the most important ones to consider for targeting by intervention programs through large audience modes, such as public health media campaigns. However, it is important to note that interventions should not be limited to these beliefs. Other important beliefs may be related to those identified and were not significant simply due to collinearity. These beliefs therefore might also be targeted by the intervention. For example, the regression analysis of behavioral beliefs correlated with intention to use condoms with a spouse resulted in only two significant beliefs. There are at least five other beliefs that are nearly as highly correlated as the significant beliefs, and that could be considered for intervention targets.

With respect to the multiple regression analyses to explain intention to avoid CSWs and intention to stick to one partner, subjective norm did not have a significant beta weight. Although subjective norm was significantly correlated with intention for both behaviors, these correlations were low compared with the other model constructs. The individual indicator analysis of subjective norm items found two items to be significant for each behavior, but their beta weights were fairly low. Thus, interventions to change these two behavioral intentions may be more effective if they focus on attitude and self-efficacy rather than subjective norm. The individual indicator analysis identified only one key behavioral belief to target to impact attitude toward avoiding CSWs. By contrast this analysis identified seven behavioral beliefs to target attitude toward sticking to one partner. Clearly interventions to promote these two behaviors will require different message strategies.

Implications for CPOL Intervention

Many interventions either implicitly or indirectly target IBM, TRA, or TPB constructs in order to change behavior. However, it is rare that these constructs are explicitly targeted and that the issues (beliefs) to target are systematically identified in behavior change interventions (Hardeman et. al., 2002). For example, we have implemented the CPOL model intervention, to increase safe-sex behavior among residents in half of 30 rural areas in Zimbabwe. Following the HIV/STD Intervention Trial CPOL protocol, we recruited popular opinion leaders and taught them to have conversations with their peers about safe-sex behavior. The assumption underlying the training is that over time these conversations will result in changes in beliefs, attitudes, and ultimately in the perception that the safe-sex behavior is normative. However, the CPOL model does not specify a mechanism for CPOLs to systematically identify and target behavioral constructs in their conversations. Conversations take place and it is assumed that appropriate cognitive-behavioral issues are addressed in the conversations, and through modeling of behavior. It is believed that a gradual shift in the perception of norms related to safer sexual behavior occurs. However, we do not really know whether CPOLs are identifying and addressing the most important issues with their friends and peers. We also do not know whether the CPOL conversations result in change in the important issues, and whether such changes are then associated with behavior change. The current CPOL study only looks at behavioral and biological outcomes, and does not assess the important underlying beliefs to see if and how they are affected by the intervention.

Therefore we have begun to address these limitations. In our roll-out to control sites we are working with our intervention team to train CPOLs to carry out more targeted conversations. First, they will elicit information from people they talk to using the IBM as a conversation guide. Then, they will specifically target the issues identified in the conversation, using persuasive arguments identified from analysis of the data just presented. Next, we would propose an outcome evaluation to assess whether in fact the intervention results in changes in the critical beliefs we identified previously. Thus, it can be established empirically whether beliefs targeted through more specific conversations do in fact change, leading to a change in the behaviors of interest.

ACKNOWLEDGMENTS

This work was carried out in conjunction with three research projects funded by CDC (S-Z1150-01-M-575), NIMH (U10 MH061544), and NIAAA (RZI AA014802).

We would like to acknowledge our ZiCHIRe team in Zimbabwe, led by Dr. Godfrey Woelk, project director, Ms. Sherla Greenland, office manager; our teams: Ethnography, led by Ms. Norma Tshuma and Ms. Priscilla Maphosa; nurses led by Ms. Reggie Mutsindiri, and field supervisors Ms. Margaret Moyo, and Eva-Clothilda Moyo; Intervention team led by Mr. Walter Chikanya; Process Evaluation team led by Mr. Pesenai Chatikobo; Laboratory, Mr. Patrick Mateta, manager, Ms Luanne Rodgers, supervisor; Data Entry, Ms. Patricia Chikuse-Gundidza; Transcription, led by Ms. Rachel Gatsi; Administrative, Ms. Gay Hendrikse, head secretary; IT, Mr. Adam Greenland; Drivers, led by Mr. Gift Mutepfe; and all other ZiCHIRe employees who made this research possible. We would also like to acknowledge all the Zimbabweans who have participated in all phases of our research studies with grace, freely giving up their time to talk to our multiple teams. In addition, for her help in carrying out the analyses, we would like to acknowledge Dr. Melanie Gallant.

REFERENCES

Abraham, C., Sheeran, P., & Orbell, S. (1998). Can social cognitive models contribute to the effectiveness of HIV-preventive behavioral interventions? A brief review of the literature and a reply to Joffe (1996; 1997) and Fife-Schaw (1997). *British Journal of Medical Psychology, 71*, 297–310.

Airhihenbuwa, C. O., & Obregon, R. (2000). A critical assessment of theories/models used in health communication for HIV/AIDS. *Journal of Health Communication, 5*(Suppl.), 5–15.

Ajzen, I. (2001). Nature and operation of attitudes. *Annual Review of Psychology, 52*, 27–58.

Albarracín, D., McNatt, P. S., Findley-Klein, C., Ho, R., Mitchell, A., & Kumkale, G. T. (2003). Persuasive communications to change actions: An analysis of behavioral and cognitive impact in HIV prevention. *Health Psychology, 22*, 166–177.

Amirkhanian, Y. A., Kelly, J. A., Kabakchieva, E., McAuliffe, T. L., & Vassileva, S. (2003). Evaluation of a social network HIV prevention intervention program for young men who have sex with men in Russia and Bulgaria. *AIDS Education & Prevention, 15*, 205–220.

Armitage, C. J., & Conner, M. (2001). Efficacy of the theory of planned behaviour: A meta-analytic review. *British Journal of Social Psychology, 40*, 471–499.

Armstrong, K., Kasprzyk, D., Woelk, G., Ndimande, G., Nhira, S., Terera, G., & Nyamutsaka, G. (2002). Zimbabwe Ethnographic Rapid Assessment Summary Report. (2002). Presented to NIMH, March 2002, Battelle, Seattle, WA and ZiCHIRe, Harare, Zimbabwe.

AVERT (2005). HIV & AIDS in Uganda: Why is Uganda Interesting? Retrieved December 19, 2005, from http://www.avert.org/aidsuganda.htm

Bandura, A. (1994). Social cognitive theory and control over HIV infection. In R. J. DiClemente & J. L. Peterson (Eds.). *Preventing AIDS: Theories and methods of behavioral interventions* (pp. 25–59). New York: Plenum Press.

Blacker, J. (2004). The impact of AIDS on adult mortality: Evidence from national and regional statistics. *AIDS, Jun.18, Suppl 2*:S19–S26.

CDC AIDS Community Demonstration Project (ACDP) Research Group. (1999). Community-level HIV intervention in 5 cities: Final outcome data for the CDC AIDS Community Demonstration Projects. *American Journal of Public Health, 89*, 336–345.

Cowan, F. M., Langhaug, L. F., Hargrove, J. W., Jaffar, S., Mhuriyengwe, L., Swarthout, T. D., et al. (2005). Is sexual contact with sex workers important in driving the HIV epidemic among men in rural Zimbabwe? *Journal of Acquired Immune Deficiency Syndrome, 40*, 371–6.

Elford, J., Bolding, G. & Sherr, L. (2001). Peer education has no significant impact on HIV risk behaviours among gay men in London (letter). *AIDS, 15*, 535–537.

Elford, J., Hart, G., Sherr, L., Williamson, L. & Bolding, G. (2002a). Peer led HIV prevention among homosexual men in Britain (Editorial). *Sexually Transmitted Infections, 78*, 158–159.

Elford, J., Sherr, L. Bolding, G., Serle, F. & Macguire, M. (2002b). Peer-led HIV prevention among gay men in London: Process evaluation. *AIDS Care, 14*, 351–360.

Fishbein, M., & Ajzen, I. (1975). *Belief, attitude, intention, and behaviour: An introduction to theory and research*. Reading, MA: Addison-Wiley.

Fishbein, M., von Haeften, I., & Appleyard, J. (2001). The role of theory in developing effective interventions: Implications from Project SAFER. *Psychology, Health and Medicine, 6*, 223–238.

Fisher, J. D., & Fisher, W. A. (2000). Theoretical approaches to individual-level change in HIV risk behavior. In J. L. Peterson & R. J. DiClemente (Eds.), *Handbook of HIV prevention AIDS prevention and mental health* (pp. 3–55). New York: Kluwer Academic/Plenum.

Flowers, P., Hart, G. J., Williamson, L. M., Frankis, J. S., & Der, G. J. (2002). Does bar-based, peer-led health promotion have a community-level effect amongst gay men in Scotland? *International Journal of STD and AIDS, 13*, 102–108.

Fritz, K. E., Woelk, G. B., Bassett, M. T., McFarland, W. C., Routh, J. A., Tobaiwa, O., & Stall, R. D. (2002). The Association between Alcohol Use, Sexual Risk Behavior, and HIV Infection among Men Attending Beerhalls in Harare, Zimbabwe. *AIDS and Behavior, 6*, 221–228.

Hardeman, W., Johnston, M., Johnston, D. W., Bonett, D., Wareham, N. J., & Kinmonth, A. L. (2002). Application of the Theory of Planned Behaviour in behaviour change interventions: A systematic review. *Psychology and Health, 17*, 123–158.

Jaccard, J., Dodge, T. Dittus, P., & Feldman, S. (2002). Parent-adolescent communication about sex and birth control: A conceptual framework. In E. D. Shirley & D. A. Rosenthal (Eds.). *Talking sexuality: Parent-adolescent communication. New directions for child and adolescent development* (No. 97, pp. 9–41). San Francisco: Jossey-Bass.

Jemmott, J. B. 3rd, & Jemmott, L. S. (2000). HIV risk reduction behavioral interventions with heterosexual adolescents. *AIDS, 14*(Suppl. 2), 540–552.

Joffe, H. (1996). AIDS research and prevention: A social representational approach. *British Journal of Medical Psychology, 70*, 75–83.

Kasprzyk, D, Montaño, D. E, & Fishbein, M. (1998). Application of an Integrated Behavioral Model to Predict Condom Use: A Prospective Study Among High HIV Risk Groups. *Journal of Applied Social Psychology, 28*, 1557–1583.

Kasprzyk, D. & Montaño, D. E. 1994, February 16–20). *The process of developing culturally relevant survey instruments measuring HIV prevention behavior in Zimbabwe and Seattle*. Paper presented at the Society for Cross Cultural Research Meeting, Santa Fe, NM.

Kasprzyk, D., & Montaño, D. E. (2001) *Correlational analyses of Integrated Behavioral Model constructs and items with condom use intention and monogamy intention; Zimbabwe SAFER Project*. Report submitted to Zim-CDC, July, Battelle; Centers for Public Health Research and Evaluation, Seattle, WA.

Kasprzyk, D, Terera, G., Montaño, D. E.,& Woelk, G. (2003). Zimbabwe Phase One Results: Summary Report, May 2003. Battelle, Seattle, WA and ZiCHIRe, Harare, Zimbabwe.

Kasprzyk, D., Woelk, G. B., Montaño, D. E., Bittner, A. B., & Richard, C. (2004, July). *NIMH Collaborative HIV/STD Prevention Trial: Modeling risk factors associated with HIV prevalence in rural Zimbabwe: Demographic, medical, behavioural, and STD, including HSV2.* Paper presented at the 15th International AIDS Conference, Bangkok, Thailand.

Kelly, J. A. (1999) Community-level interventions are needed to prevent new HIV infections (editorial). *American Journal of Public Health, 89*, 299–300.

Kelly, J. A. (2002). Innovation in the Application of Social Cognitive Principles to Develop Prevention Interventions to Reduce Unsafe Sexual Behaviors Among Gay and Bisexual Men. In M. A. Chesney, & M. H. Antoni (Eds.), *Innovative Approaches to Health Psychology: Prevention and Treatment Lessons from AIDS.* American Psychological Association (APA).

Kelly, J. A. (2004) Popular opinion leaders and HIV prevention peer education: Resolving discrepant findings, and implications for the development of effective community programmes. *AIDS Care 16*(2), 139–150.

Kelly, J. A., Murphy, D. A., Sikkema, K. J., McAuliff, T. L., Roffman, R. A., Solomon, L. J., Winett, R. A., Kalichman, S. C. and the Community HIV Prevention Research Collaborative (1997). Randomised, controlled, community-level HIV-prevention intervention for sexual-risk behaviour among homosexual men in US cities. *Lancet*, 350, 1500–1505.

Kelly, J. A., St. Lawrence, J. S., & Diaz, Y. E. (1991). HIV risk behavior reduction following intervention with key opinion leaders of a population: An experimental community-level analysis. *American Journal of Public Health, 81*, 168–171.

Kububa, P., Dube, L. B., Midzi, S., Nesara, P., & St Louis, M. E. (2002, July). *First Suggestion of a Decline in ANC HIV Sero-Prevalence?* Paper presented at the 14th International AIDS Conference, Barcelona, Spain.

Mbizvo, E. M., Msuya, S., Hussain, A., Chirenje, M., Mbizvo, M., Sam, N., & Stray-Pedersen, B. (2005). HIV and sexually transmitted infections among women presenting at urban primary health care clinics in two cities of sub-Saharan Africa. *African Journal of Reproductive Health, 9*, 88–98.

Miller, R. L., Klotz, D., & Eckholdt, H. M. (1998). HIV prevention with male prostitutes and patrons of hustler bars: Replication of an HIV preventive intervention. *American Journal of Community Psychology, 26*, 97–132.

Ministry of Health and Child Welfare (MOHCW), Zimbabwe National Family Planning Council, National AIDS Council, and U.S Centers for Disease Control and Prevention, Zimbabwe-CDC AIDS Program. (2004). The Zimbabwe Young Adult Survey (YAS), 2001–2002: Final Report. Report prepared by H. M. B Dube, R. Kambarami, S. Laver, L. Gavin, A. D. McNaghten, M. E. St. Louis, & J. M. Herold.

Ministry of Health and Child Welfare (MOHCW), Health Information and Surveillance Unit, Department of Disease Prevention and Control, AIDS & TB Programme. (2005). Zimabwe National HIV/AIDS Estimates, 2005: Preliminary Report.

Ministry of Health and Child Health Welfare. Essential Drugs List for Zimbabwe. Causeway; Zimbabwe, Harare; Ministry of Health & Child Welfare. 2001.

Montaño, D. E., Kasprzyk, D., & Wilson, D. (1993, June 6–11). *Theory based correlates of condom use in Zimbabwe.* Poster presented at the 9th International Conference on AIDS, Berlin, Germany.

Montaño, D. E., Kasprzyk, D., & Woelk, G. B. (2002, July). *NIMH Collaborative HIV/STD Prevention Trial. National survey of behavioral risk for STDs and HIV among residents in rural growth point villages in Zimbabwe.* Paper presented at the 14th International AIDS Conference, Barcelona, Spain.

Rogers, E. M. (1985). *Diffusion of innovation.* New York: Free Press.

Sikkema, K. J., Kelly, J. A., Winett, R. A., Solomon, L. J., Cargill, V. A., Roffman, R. A., McAuliffe, T. L., Heckman, T. G., Anderson, E. A., Wagstaff, D. A., Norman, A. D., Perry, M. J., Crumble, D. A., & Mercer, M. B. (2000). Outcomes of a randomized community-level HIV prevention intervention for women living in 18 low-income housing developments. *American Journal of Public Health, 90*, 57–63.

St. Lawrence, J. S., Brasfield, T. L., Diaz, Y. E., Jefferson, K. W., Reynolds, M.T., & Leonard, M.D. (1994). Three-year follow-up of an HIV risk reduction intervention that used popular peers. *American Journal of Public Health, 84*, 2027–2028.

UNAIDS/WHO. (2002). Epidemiological Fact Sheets on HIV/AIDS and STIs: Zimbabwe.

UNAIDS/WHO. (2004). Epidemiological Fact Sheets on HIV/AIDS and STIs: Zimbabwe.

UNAIDS (2005). AIDS Epidemic Update, December 2005.

von Haeften, I., Fishbein M,, Kasprzyk D, & Montaño, D. E. (2001a). Analyzing data to obtain information to design targeted interventions. *Psychology, Health and Medicine, 6*, 151–164.

von Haeften, I., & Kenski, K. (2001b). Multi-partnered heterosexuals: Men's and women's condom use with their main partner as a function of attitude, subjective norm, partner norm, perceived behavioral control, and weighted control beliefs. *Psychology, Health and Medicine, 6*, 165–178.

Woelk, G. B., Kasprzyk, D., & Montaño, D. E. (2002a, July). *NIMH Collaborative HIV/STD Prevention Trial. National survey of STDs and HIV from residents in Rural Growth Point Villages in Zimbabwe.* Paper presented at the 14th International AIDS Conference, Barcelona, Spain.

Woelk, G. B., Armstrong, K., Kasprzyk ,D., & Montaño, D. E. (2002b, July). *NIMH Collaborative HIV/STD Prevention Trial: National beliefs and practices of alcohol use and risky sexual behavior among rural Zimbabweans.* Paper presented at the 14th International AIDS Conference, Barcelona, Spain.

CHAPTER 11

Understanding and Motivating Condom Use among At-Risk and HIV-Seropositive Persons: A Review and Demonstration of the Applicability of the Theories of Reasoned Action and Planned Behavior

Richard J. Wolitski and Jun Zhang

Centers for Disease Control and Prevention

Although it has been more than 25 years since the first cases of acquired immunodeficiency syndrome (AIDS) were diagnosed, the human immunodeficiency virus (HIV) continues to exact a devastating toll on the health of individuals, families, and entire countries. Worldwide, an estimated 38.6 million persons were living with HIV at the end of 2005 (United Nations Programme on HIV/AIDS [UNAIDS], 2006). In that year alone, an estimated 4.1 million persons, or more than 11,000 per day, were newly infected with HIV (UNAIDS, 2006). Approximately 2.8 million persons with AIDS were believed to have died in 2005. Many of these deaths were preventable, but the high cost of antiretroviral treatments that dramatically slow the progression of HIV disease makes them unavailable to many who need them most. In the United States, 1.0-1.2 million people are believed to be living with HIV, and roughly 40,000 new HIV infections are estimated to occur each year (Fleming et al., 2002; Glynn & Rhodes, 2005). Heterosexual intercourse is the primary route of HIV transmission in much of the world, but in the United States, and most other industrialized countries, sex between men who have sex with men (MSM) accounts for the largest proportion of new HIV infections (UNAIDS, 2006).

An effective vaccine that can prevent HIV infection remains elusive and may not be available for 10 or more years. Motivating individuals to modify behaviors that can transmit HIV infection remains the most effective strategy for stemming the tide of the epidemic. The only 100% effective strategies for preventing the sexual acquisition of HIV infection are abstinence from all sexual intercourse or having sex with only uninfected partners. Reliably choosing uninfected partners is difficult outside of a mutually monogamous relationship as some partners do not have accurate knowledge of their HIV status (Centers for Disease Control and Prevention [CDC], 2005a), may not disclose this information (Simoni & Pantalone, 2005), or may engage in risky sexual behaviors with other partners without their primary partner's knowledge (Buunk & Bakker, 1997). For many sexually active persons, avoiding sexual practices that are most likely to transmit HIV (i.e., anal and vaginal intercourse) or consistently using condoms represent the most acceptable strategies for preventing HIV infection. When used consistently, latex condoms are highly effective and have been shown to reduce the risk of HIV transmission by at least 80% to 94% (Warner, Stone, Macaluso, Buehler, & Austin, 2006).

Developing a better understanding of factors associated with risk behavior and how to motivate at-risk individuals to eliminate or reduce their risk is a priority for public health. This chapter reviews research examining the application of the Theory of Reasoned Action (TRA) and the Theory of Planned Behavior (TPB) to the prediction and promotion of condom use among persons who are at-risk of contracting HIV and those living with HIV whose behavior may transmit the virus to others. Results of a study that extends prior research on factors associated with condom use among persons living with HIV are described and implications of these findings for health behavior theory and future research are discussed.

Understanding HIV Risk Behavior within At-Risk Populations

Research on the determinants of HIV risk behaviors and the factors that affect the adoption and maintenance of risk reduction strategies has been reported in hundreds of studies that have been published since the mid-1980s (for selected reviews see Albarracín, Johnson, Fishbein, & Muellerleile, 2001; Bandura, 1994; Becker & Joseph, 1988; Fisher & Fisher, 2000; Hospers & Kok, 1995; Rosenstock, Strecher, & Becker, 1994). Given the breadth of the literature, it is not surprising that many different conceptual frameworks and theories have guided this research. The TRA is one theory that has been used in a large number of HIV-related studies and has received considerable empirical support.

The TRA is a general theory of human behavior that has been used to predict a wide range of health promoting and other behaviors (Ajzen & Fishbein, 1980; Fishbein, 1967; Fishbein & Ajzen, 1975; Fishbein, Middlestadt, & Hitchcock, 1991). In brief, TRA assumes that the most powerful predictor of future behavior is one's intention to perform a given behavior. Intention is determined by attitudinal and normative influences. Attitudes (one's assessment of the behavior in positive or negative terms) are in turn determined by one's underlying beliefs about the behavior and the expected outcomes of performing the behavior. Subjective norm represents one's overall perception of social pressure to perform (or not to perform) a given behavior. Subjective norm is determined by one's belief that specific individuals or groups think that he or she should (or should not) perform a given behavior and one's motivation to comply with the desires of various individuals or groups.

An assumption of TRA is that the individual has control over the target behavior. However, some behaviors are not entirely under an individual's control. The ability to act on an intention may be limited by factors that affect an individual's ability to exert control over the behavior such as one's own ability to use condoms or a partner's willingness to wear a condom. To improve the prediction of behaviors that are not entirely volitional, Ajzen (1985; 1991) added a new construct, perceived behavioral control, to the TRA. The resulting model was named the TPB. Perceived behavioral control accounts for an individual's belief that the behavior is under his or her control (e.g., that one can perform the behavior if one wants to) and is predicted to directly affect future behavior as well as to indirectly affect behavior through intention.

TRA and TPB have provided important insights into the adoption of condom use to prevent HIV transmission in a large number of studies conducted with diverse samples of at-risk persons. An extensive meta-analytical review of 96 datasets provides strong support for the ability of TRA and TPB variables to predict condom use (Albarracín et al., 2001). Consistent with TRA, the authors of this review found that across studies intention to use condoms was strongly associated with condom use (weighted mean $r = .45$), and that attitudes about condom use ($r = .58$) and subjective norms ($r = .39$) were associated with intention to use condoms. The meta-analysis also demonstrated the importance of perceived behavioral control in determining condom use. Consistent with TPB, perceived behavioral control was strongly associated with intention to use condoms ($r = .45$), but perceived behavioral control did not have a direct influence on condom use when intention was taken into account (i.e., the association between perceived behavioral control and condom use was fully mediated by condom use intention).

The conclusions of Albarracín and colleagues (2001) were consistent with those of an earlier independent review of the literature on the ability of TRA/TPB variables to predict condom use intentions (Sheeran & Taylor, 1999). This meta-analytic review of data from 67 study samples also concluded that attitude, subjective norm, and perceived behavioral control were associated with condom-use intentions as specified by TRA/TPB. Unlike the later review, these authors also examined the extent to which the addition of perceived behavioral control improved the prediction of condom use intentions over and above variance accounted for by TRA variables. Using data from 18 studies, Sheeran & Taylor found that studies based on TPB accounted on average for 5% more of the variance in condom use intentions compared to studies based only on TRA variables. In addition, they reported that perceived behavioral control was a significant independent predictor of condom use in 7 out of 10 studies that tested TPB variables. Thus, the authors concluded that accounting for an individual's perceived behavioral control was important for the prediction of condom use intentions.

Although there is strong support for the ability of TRA/TPB variables to predict condom use behavior, the importance of individual components of these models has been shown to vary across at-risk populations and with regard to the specific behavior being addressed (e.g., Corby, Jamner, & Wolitski, 1996; Jamner, Wolitski, Corby, & Fishbein, 1998). Whether one is the insertive or the receptive partner presumably affects an individual's control over condom use. The insertive partner is likely to have more control in most situations because he is the one who wears the condom. The receptive partner is likely to have less control because she or he (in the case of receptive anal sex for MSM) does not wear the condom. For receptive partners, the ability to have condom-protected sex depends upon their ability to ask their partner to use a condom, negotiate condom use if the insertive partner is resistant to using a condom, or to refuse sex if their partner is unwilling to wear a condom. Within heterosexual couples, differences in men's versus women's control over condom use may be compounded by power differentials that limit women's power in sexual decision making (Guinan & Leviton, 1995).

In addition to the specificity of the behavior, research has shown that it is important not only to be clear about the individual's role during a sexual act, but also with whom the behavior occurs. An individual's relationship with his or her partner is associated with differences in sexual behavior and beliefs about the behavior. In general, research conducted with samples from a variety of at-risk populations has found differences in sexual risk with primary or main partners compared to casual or non-main partners (Misovich, Fisher, & Fisher, 1997), and the correlates of condom use intentions and behavior can vary depending on the partner type (Corby et al.,1996; Jamner et al., 1998).

Not surprisingly, the known or assumed HIV status of one's sex partner also affects risk behavior, individuals' perceptions of the behavior, and whether one takes action to protect oneself from HIV. HIV-seronegative persons are much less likely to engage in unprotected sex with persons they know or believe are HIV-seropositive compared to persons they believe are uninfected (Hoff et al., 1997). Similarly, HIV-seropositive persons are less likely to engage in unprotected sex with persons they know are HIV-seronegative than they are to engage in this behavior with partners who are also HIV-seropositive (Parsons et al., 2005). When HIV serostatus is not discussed, sexual decision making may be affected by non-verbal and contextual cues that some persons use to infer HIV status (Gold & Skinner, 1992, 1996; O'Leary, 2005). Unfortunately, these cues may be processed in a biased manner that may lead some HIV-seronegative and HIV-seropositive persons to assume that they and their partners have the same HIV status, increasing the likelihood that unprotected sex will occur (Suarez & Miller, 2001).

Interventions to Prevent HIV Acquisition

TRA and TPB have informed development of interventions that have been shown to reduce HIV risk behavior. Two projects initiated by the CDC, Project RESPECT and the AIDS Community Demonstration Projects (ACDP), provide strong evidence of the efficacy of these interventions in motivating change at both the individual and community levels. Project RESPECT (Kamb et al., 1998) was

a randomized controlled trial of HIV interventions for at-risk heterosexual sexually transmitted disease (STD) clinic patients. The trial evaluated the efficacy of a
four-session enhanced individual counseling intervention, a two-session standard
individual counseling intervention, and didactic messages delivered by a health
care provider during two clinic visits. The enhanced counseling intervention was
based on TRA and incorporated the concept of self-efficacy from social cognitive
theory (Bandura, 1986, 1994). Perceived self-efficacy " ...is concerned with people's beliefs that they can exert control over their own motivation, thought
processes, emotional states, and patterns of behavior" (Bandura, 1994; p. 26) and
is similar to the concept of perceived behavioral control in TPB. The enhanced
counseling intervention included activities that focused specifically on changing
attitudes toward condom use, enhancing self efficacy, and changing perceived
norms and perceived community support for condom use (Fishbein et al., 2001).

Compared to participants who received the didactic messages, participants
assigned to the enhanced intervention were less likely to report unprotected vaginal sex and more likely to report any condom use at the 3-month and 6-month follow-up assessments (Kamb et al., 1998). Similar differences between the standard
counseling and didactic message arms were observed for unprotected sex, but not
for any condom use. Importantly, the enhanced and standard counseling interventions were also associated with a significantly decreased rate of new STDs at 6 and
12 months, relative to those who received the didactic messages.

Subsequent analyses of the Project RESPECT provide evidence linking inter-
vention-associated changes in the theoretical constructs targeted in the enhanced
counseling intervention with changes in condom use with main partners (Fishbein
et al., 2001). These analyses showed that changes in attitude, subjective norm, and
self-efficacy were associated with changes in condom-use intentions, and that
changes in intention were associated with the observed changes in condom use.
For men and women, receiving the enhanced intervention was associated with
changes in attitude and self-efficacy, but not subjective norms. These findings
raise questions about the efficacy of activities that were designed to change perceived norms, but, as a whole, Project RESPECT provides compelling evidence
of the ability of a theory-based intervention to motivate reductions in HIV risk
behavior at the level of the individual.

The ability of a theory-based intervention to effect change in entire communities of at-risk individuals was tested in the ACDP. The ACDP was based on an
integrative model that drew from TRA, social cognitive theory, the health belief
model, and the transtheoretical model (CDC ACDP Research Group, 1999). This
intervention sought to reduce the risk of entire communities of high-risk persons
using specially tailored role-model stories that were distributed (along with condoms and bleach for cleaning injection equipment) by networks of peer volunteers
from the target communities. Role model stories described the experiences of real
individuals from the target community who had made progress toward consistently using condoms or avoiding risks associated with drug injection (Corby,
Enguidanos, & Kay, 1996). These stories were elicited using an interview guide
that ensured that information about key theoretical variables (e.g., attitudes,
norms, self-efficacy, risk perceptions) was collected. The stories were then

written to emphasize certain theoretical variables that were most strongly associated with behavior change in cross-sectional surveys that were conducted as part of the outcome evaluation with the local target audience. Each story focused on a successive step toward achieving a sustained reduction in risk. The specific stage of change depicted by the role model stories (e.g., forming an intention to use condoms, asking a partner to use condoms for the first time, trying to use condoms after an initial failed attempt) was keyed to the stage of change in the target audience. In this way, the distribution of the stages of change depicted in the stories was intended to be about one stage ahead of the existing distribution in the community.

Over a 3-year period, more than 15,000 interviews were conducted during 10 cross-sectional waves in 10 intervention and community pairs (CDC ACDP Research Group, 1999). Exposure to the role model stories in the intervention communities peaked at 54% about 2 years into the study. Thus, about half of the target population had been reached in the intervention communities by the end of the study. At the community level, the presence of the intervention in a given community was associated with movement toward consistent condom use with main and non-main partners, as well an increase in observed condom carrying, regardless of whether or not a given individual had been personally exposed to the role model stories. Individual-level analyses clearly linked the community-level changes to exposure to the ACDP intervention. When data from persons who were exposed to the intervention were compared to those who were not, exposure to the intervention was associated with increased stage of change for consistent condom use with main and non-main partners, consistent use of bleach to clean injection equipment, and condom carrying.

The utility of TRA/TPB in the development of effective HIV-prevention interventions is further supported by the results of a meta-analytic review on the effects of HIV-intervention studies conducted during the past 17 years (Albarracín et al., 2005). The authors of this review reported that intervention strategies targeting attitudes, norms (for adolescents only), and perceived behavioral control were associated with significant changes in risk behavior. More importantly, they determined that there was sufficient evidence to conclude that intervention-related changes in attitudes, norms, and perceived behavioral control mediated behavior change. Taken as a whole, the published literature provides strong support for the ability of HIV-prevention interventions based on TRA/TPB constructs to motivate behavior change among persons who are at risk for contracting HIV.

Understanding and Preventing HIV Risk Behavior among Persons Living with HIV

Public health programs have placed greater emphasis on the development of interventions for persons living with HIV since the late 1990s (CDC, 2003; Janssen et al., 2001; Wolitski, Janssen, Onorato, Purcell, & Crepaz, 2005). Although many persons who learn that they are HIV-seropositive change their risk behavior (Weinhardt, Carey, Johnson, & Bickman, 1999), some continue to engage in sexual practices that place others at risk or resume risk behavior later in life

(Kalichman, 2000; Marks, Burris, & Peterman, 1999; Parsons et al., 2005). The increased attention on the risk behavior of persons living with HIV called attention to the relative lack of information about the determinants of condom use among HIV-seropositive persons.

Until the late-1990s, most HIV-prevention research had not differentiated between the behaviors of persons who were at risk for HIV infection from those who had been diagnosed with HIV. The majority of these studies exclusively focused on persons who were at risk for contracting HIV rather than those who were at risk for transmitting it. The lack of data regarding the behavior of persons living with HIV raised important questions about fundamental differences between the factors that motivate individuals to adopt self-protective behaviors (e.g., using condoms to protect oneself from HIV) versus behaviors that may be viewed by at least some person living with HIV as primarily protecting the health of others.

A growing number of studies have sought to better understand the factors that influence sexual practices among persons living with HIV (Crepaz & Marks, 2002; Kalichman, 2000; Kok, 1999; O'Leary et al., 2005; Ostrow, McKirnan, Klein, & DiFranceisco, 1999; Parsons, Halkitis, Wolitski, Gómez, & SUMS Team, 2003; Schiltz & Sandfort, 2000; Wolitski, Parsons, & Gómez, 2004). To the best of our knowledge, however, only one published study has specifically addressed the ability of the TRA/TPB to predict behaviors that reduce the risk of HIV transmission by persons living with HIV. This study examined the utility of the TPB in predicting condom use and avoidance of anal sex among 96 men who have sex with men (Godin, Savard, Kok, Fortin, & Boyer, 1996). The study used cross-sectional data to assess the association of attitude, subjective norm, and perceived behavioral control with behavioral intention and longitudinal data to assess the ability of these variables to predict behaviors that were measured 6 months later. The results provided only partial support for predictions based on TPB. Intention was not significantly associated with future behavior for either condom use during anal intercourse or abstaining from anal intercourse. Perceived behavioral control was the only variable associated with condom use intention, with higher perceived behavioral control scores being associated with stronger intention to use condoms during anal intercourse. With regard to abstaining from anal intercourse, subjective norm and perceived behavioral control, but not attitude, were significantly associated with intention.

Godin and colleagues' findings raised questions about the ability of TPB to provide a sufficient theoretical basis for the development of sexual behavior change interventions for persons living with HIV. The findings indicated that control beliefs are likely to be an important target for these intervention efforts. On the other hand, the evidence regarding the role of subjective norms was inconsistent, and attitudes were not significantly associated with condom use intention in any analyses. The lack of association between intention and behavior is even more troubling, as it suggests that risk behavior may be driven less by reasoned action and more by emotional, contextual, or other determinants that may be less amenable to change through standard behavioral interventions.

These results may reflect true differences in the determinants of sexual risk reduction among HIV-seronegative and HIV-seropositive persons, or they may be the result of known and unknown factors unique to Godin and colleagues' study. The relatively small number of participants and the reliance on a convenience sample from medical clinics limited the statistical power to detect meaningful effects and the generalizability of these findings to other samples. In addition, a number of measurement issues may affect the validity of their findings. The measures employed by Godin and colleagues asked about anal sex in general (i.e., were not specific to insertive versus receptive anal sex) and did not specify the respondent's relationship to the partner (i.e., whether this person was a primary/main partner or a non-main partner). As discussed previously, research with HIV-seronegative persons has shown this level of specificity in the behavioral target to be important. In addition, the measures did not address the HIV serostatus of the partner. HIV serostatus is an important determinant of unprotected sex and condom use among persons living with HIV, and HIV-seropositive persons perceive the benefits of condom use differently for HIV-seropositive, HIV-seronegative, and partners whose HIV serostatus they do not know (Halkitis, Gómez, & Wolitski, 2005; Suarez & Miller, 2001).

Findings from the study by Godin and colleagues raised difficult issues for the TPB view. The remaining sections of this chapter describe a study that addresses some of those issues. The study described next sought to better understand the influence of variables derived from the TRA/TPB on intentions and reported condom use in a larger sample of HIV-seropositive MSM. The study went beyond the work of Godin and colleagues by limiting the scope of the variables included in analyses to those pertaining to non-main partners and by measuring TRA/TPB variables and behavior separately for insertive versus receptive anal sex with HIV-seronegative, HIV-seropositive, and unknown HIV status partners.

Methods

Prior to implementation, all procedures were reviewed by institutional review boards at the CDC and Research Triangle Institute, Inc.

Participants

Convenience samples were recruited from 12 cities in the northeastern (Baltimore, Boston, New York, Philadelphia, Washington, DC), southern (Atlanta, Houston, Fort Lauderdale, Miami), mid-western (Chicago), and western (Los Angeles, San Diego) regions of the United States. Participants were recruited from June to September of 2004 as part of a larger study evaluating HIV-prevention messages for MSM. Recruitment methods included advertisements in gay-oriented publications, flyers posted in organizations and venues frequented by MSM, and announcements on MSM Internet sites. In some cities, market research firms contacted gay and bisexual men who had previously agreed to be informed about future research opportunities.

Potential participants were screened by telephone to determine eligibility. Eligibility criteria were reporting: (1) male gender, (2) HIV-seropositive status or never having been tested for HIV, (3) sex with one or more male partners in the prior 6 months, and (4) anal sex without a condom in the prior 6 months. Potential participants were excluded at screening if they: (1) had participated in another HIV-related study in the prior year, (2) worked or volunteered in an HIV prevention program in the prior year, or (3) did not speak English. Potentially eligible participants were scheduled for an in-person assessment visit. HIV serostatus was confirmed at the in-person visit. Individuals who could not provide evidence of their seropositive HIV status (e.g., HIV test results, HIV medications prescribed in their name, etc.) were not eligible.

A total of 393 men satisfied all eligibility criteria. For this chapter, analyses were limited to 202 participants (51%) who reported one or more acts of insertive or receptive anal sex with at least one non-main partner during the 30 days prior to interview. The average age of participants ranged from 21 to 68 years ($M = 42.1$, $SD = 7.5$). On average, participants have been living with HIV for 10.1 years ($SD = 5.6$ years, range = 3.7 months to 19.6 years) Other selected demographic characteristics of study participants are shown in Table 11–1.

Procedures

The in-person assessment consisted of: (1) written informed consent, (2) baseline assessment, (3) exposure or no exposure to an HIV prevention message, and (4) immediate post-test assessment. All data were collected using audio computer-assisted self-interview (A-CASI). After all study activities were completed, participants received HIV information, local referrals, and $75.

Measures

This study used data from the baseline assessment and post-test assessments. Demographics and risk behavior were assessed at pre-test. Intention, subjective norm, and perceived behavioral control were assessed at post-test.[1] The baseline and post-test assessments took a combined average of 43 minutes to complete (SD = 15, range = 21–137).

Sexual practices.   Data on sex behavior reported in this chapter were collected for the 30 days prior to interview using items adapted from prior research with HIV-seropositive MSM (Wolitski et al., 2004). Participants were asked separate sets of questions about sexual practices with their main partner and HIV-seropositive, HIV-seronegative, and unknown serostatus non-main partners. Vaginal intercourse, insertive anal intercourse, and receptive anal intercourse were assessed separately for the main partner and separately for HIV-seropositive, HIV-seronegative, and unknown HIV-serostatus non-main partners. For each behavior, participants were asked the number of times they engaged in the

---

[1]With one exception (intention to use condoms during receptive anal sex with a new HIV-seropositive male partner), message exposure was not associated with significant differences in variables that were examined in relation to behavior in the present study (i.e., intention and perceived behavioral control).

TABLE 11-1.
Demographic characteristics of HIV-seropositive MSM recruited from 12 U. S. cities (n = 202).

	N	%
Region of United States		
Midwest	29	14.4
Northeast	92	45.5
South	60	29.7
West	21	10.4
Race/Ethnicity		
Black or African American	84	41.6
Hispanic or Latino or Chicano	19	9.4
White	87	43.1
Asian, American Indian, Alaskan Native, Other	12	6.0
Sexual Orientation		
Gay or homosexual	170	84.2
Bisexual, straight, unsure, or other	32	15.8
Education		
Did not complete high school	15	7.4
High school diploma or GED	30	14.9
Some college or associates degree	82	40.6
Bachelor's degree	54	26.7
Master's, doctoral, or other advanced degree	21	10.4
Employment Status		
Employed full or part-time	86	42.6
Unemployed-permanent or temporary disability	69	34.2
Unemployed-other	47	23.3

behavior with a condom and the number of times they engaged in the behavior without a condom. Frequency data were used to compute the proportion of sexual acts that were condom protected for each sexual behavior assessed (e.g., number of condom-protected insertive anal sex acts with HIV-seropositive non-main partners/number of condom-protected insertive anal sex acts with HIV-seropositive non-main partners + number of unprotected insertive anal sex acts with HIV-seropositive non-main partners). The resulting values ranged from 0 (no condom use) to 1 (consistent condom use).

Intentions to use condoms. Intentions to use condoms during anal sex with a new non-main male partner were assessed using 6 items adapted from the CDC AIDS Community Demonstration Projects (CDC AIDS Community Demonstration Projects Research Group, 1999; Corby et al.,1996). Intention to use condoms was assessed separately for insertive and receptive anal sex with a new non-main male partner of each HIV serostatus. For instance, respondents were asked, "How sure are you that you would use a condom for *receptive anal sex* with this HIV-negative new male partner?" Responses were scored on a 7-point scale ranging from 1 (very sure I will not) to 7 (very sure I will).

Attitudes toward condom use.   Four semantic differential items that were adapted from prior research (Corby et al.,1996) were used to provide a direct measure of attitude toward condom use. Like the intention measures, this set of items was administered six times to assess attitude toward consistent condom use during insertive and receptive anal sex with a new non-main male partner whose HIV status was described by the respondent as either HIV-seropositive, HIV-seronegative, or of unknown HIV status. The following attitudinal dimensions were assessed: pleasant/unpleasant, wise/foolish, good/bad, and healthy/unhealthy. Each item was measured using a 7-point scale that ranged from 1 (e.g., very unpleasant) to 7 (e.g., very pleasant). A scale score was computed for insertive vs. receptive anal sex with each serostatus of non-main partner. Internal consistency for these scales was good for both the full sample (N = 393, alphas = 0.70 to 0.79) and the present subsample (n = 202, alphas = 0.68 to 0.78).

Subjective norm.   A single item adapted from prior research (Jamner et al., 1998) was used to assess subjective norms regarding consistent condom use for the six behavior–partner serostatus combinations. For example, participants were asked to respond to items such as "Most people who are important to me think that I should use a condom for *receptive anal sex* with this new male partner whose HIV status I do not know." Responses were recorded using a 5-point Likert-type scale that ranged from 1 (strongly disagree) to 5 (strongly agree). Motivation to comply with the perceived social norm was not assessed.

Perceived behavioral control.   A single-item measure of perceived behavioral control (Corby et al., 1996) was used for each of the six behavior–partner serostatus combinations. For example, "If you wanted to use a condom every time you have *insertive anal sex* with this HIV-positive new male partner, how sure are you that you could use one?" Responses were recorded using a 7-point scale that ranged from 1 (very sure I could not) to 7 (very sure I could).

Statistical Analyses

Descriptive statistics were generated for demographics and all TRA/TPB variables by type of sex and partner serostatus. Path analysis was conducted in order to determine the goodness of fit of the TRA/TPB model. Fit indices included a chi-square *p*-value, chi square/degrees of freedom, Bentler Comparative Fit Index (CFI) and Goodness-of-Fit Index (GFI). A chi-square p-value of greater than 0.05 or chi square/df < 2 is considered indicative of excellent model fit. It is considered acceptable if chi square/df < 3. Values greater than 0.90 indicate good fit for the CFI and GFI statistics (Norris, 2005).

Regression analysis was used to compute the path coefficients. The significance of the predicted direct associations with behavior were first assessed by regressing intention, perceived behavioral control, attitude, and subjective norm on behavior. The indirect effects of attitude, subjective norm, and perceived behavioral control on behavior were assessed by regressing these variables on intention. Six models were tested. Each model evaluated a separate set of variables representing one of two sexual behaviors (insertive vs. receptive anal intercourse) and one of three categories used to classify non-main partners by their HIV serostatus (HIV-seronegative, HIV-seropositive, and unknown HIV status).

RESULTS

Within this subsample of men who had anal sex with one or more non-main partners in the 30 days prior to interview, 75% of men reported at least one act of unprotected anal sex. The proportion of condom-protected acts ranged from 0.47 to 0.75 of acts (see Table 11–2). In general, the highest rates of condom use were observed for HIV-seronegative partners, the lowest rates were observed for HIV-seropositive partners, and intermediate rates were observed for partners of unknown HIV serostatus. However, the use of condoms was nearly identical for receptive anal sex with HIV-seropositive and HIV-unknown partners. For the most part this same pattern was observed for TRA/TPB variables measured for insertive anal sex (Table 2). This pattern was also present with regard to receptive anal sex for the intention to use condoms, but not the other TRA/TPB variables.

Based on the criterion of goodness of fit statistics, the six models provided a very good description of the relationship between the TRA/TPB variables. The fit indices for each model were as follows: insertive anal sex with HIV-seronegative partner ($X^2 = 2.07$, $p = 0.13$, X^2 /df = 0.69, GFI = 0.98, CFI = 1.00), receptive anal sex with HIV-seronegative partner ($X^2 = 1.86$, $p = 0.60$, X^2 /df = 0.62, GFI

TABLE 11–2.
Condom use and TRA/TPB variables by type of sex and partner HIV serostatus among HIV-seropositive MSM from 12 U.S. cities (n =202).

| | Type of Sex | | | |
| | Insertive Anal | | Receptive Anal | |
	M	SD	M	SD
HIV-Seronegative Partner(s)	n = 46		n = 56	
Proportion of condom-protected acts	0.75	0.33	0.65	0.39
Intention	5.9	1.6	5.4	1.8
Attitude	5.7	1.1	5.6	1.3
Subjective norm	4.4	0.8	4.3	0.9
Perceived behavioral control	5.8	1.6	5.9	1.5
HIV-Unknown Partner(s)	n = 96		n = 90	
Proportion of condom-protected acts	0.59	0.39	0.53	0.34
Intention	5.3	1.8	5.0	1.9
Attitude	5.6	1.2	5.7	1.2
Subjective norm	4.4	0.8	4.3	0.9
Perceived behavioral control	5.5	1.6	5.7	1.5
HIV-Seropositive Partner(s)	n = 93		n = 89	
Proportion of condom-protected acts	0.47	0.39	0.52	0.41
Intention	4.5	2.1	4.6	2.1
Attitude	5.3	1.3	5.4	1.3
Subjective norm	4.0	1.0	4.1	1.0
Perceived behavioral control	5.4	1.7	5.6	1.5

= 0.99, CFI = 1.00), insertive anal sex with unknown serostatus partner (χ^{-2} = 8.13, p = 0.04, χ^{-2} /df = 2.71, GFI = 0.97, CFI = 0.95), receptive anal sex with unknown serostatus partner (χ^{-2} = 2.84, p = 0.42, χ^{-2} /df = 0.95, GFI = 0.99, CFI = 1.00), insertive anal sex with HIV-seropositive partner (χ^{-2} = 5.45, p = 0.14, χ^{-2} /df = 1.81, GFI = 0.98, CFI = 0.99), and receptive anal sex with HIV-seropositive partner (χ^{-2} = 5.73, p = 0.13, χ^{-2} /df = 1.91, GFI = 0.97, CFI = 0.98).

There were significant associations between TRA/TPB variables and condom use for insertive and receptive anal intercourse with HIV-seronegative, HIV-seropositive, and unknown serostatus partners (see Figures 11–1, 11–2, and 11–3). The proportion of variance accounted for by these variables ranged from 0.21, for receptive anal intercourse with HIV-unknown status partners (p < .01), to 0.41 for both insertive anal sex with HIV-seronegative non-main partners (p < .01) and insertive anal sex with non-main partners of unknown serostatus (p < .001). For HIV-seronegative and HIV-unknown partners, the insertive anal sex models accounted for approximately twice the amount of variance in condom use compared to the corresponding receptive anal sex models. Interestingly, for HIV-seropositive partners, the proportion of variance accounted for by the insertive and receptive anal sex models was comparable.

The association between intention and behavior was significant for both insertive and receptive anal sex, regardless of partner serostatus. Attitude and perceived behavioral control were significantly associated with all six intention measures, but there was a significant direct association between perceived behavioral control and behavior for only insertive anal intercourse with a partner whose serostatus was not known by the respondent. For most behavior-partner combinations, subjective norm was not significantly associated with intention. A significant association between these two variables was observed for insertive anal sex with an HIV-seronegative partner and an association of borderline significance (p < .10) was observed for insertive anal intercourse with an HIV-seropositive partner.

CONCLUSION

The findings of the present study extend prior research and provide new evidence regarding the ability of the TRA/TPB to explain condom use among MSM living with HIV. Regardless of the HIV serostatus of the sex partner or the specific type of sex (insertive or receptive anal sex), attitudes and perceived behavioral control were associated with intention to use condoms with a new partner of a given serostatus in all of the models tested. This finding is consistent with the larger body of research that has examined the association between TRA/TPB variables and condom use intentions in a wide range of at-risk populations (Albarracín et al.,2001; Sheeran & Taylor, 1999). Consistent with this literature, we also found that attitude was the TRA/TPB construct most strongly associated with intention to use condoms.

The association between attitudes and intentions in the present study suggests that the failure of Godin and colleagues (1996) to find an association between these variables is likely due to specific characteristics of their study and not a pervasive difference in the role of attitudes in determining condom use intention for

Insertive Anal Intercourse (n = 46)

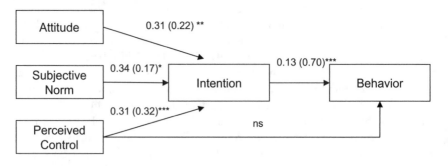

$R^2 = 0.41, p < .01.$

Receptive Anal Intercourse (n = 56)

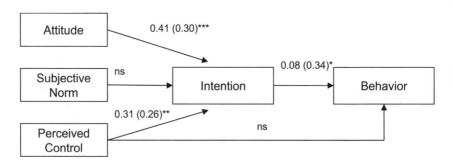

$R^2 = 0.23, p < .05$

Note: Standardized regression weights are shown in parentheses.

$^\dagger p < .10; * p < .05; ** p < .01, *** p < .001.$

FIGURE 11–1. Association of TRA/TPB Variables with Past Behavior: Condom Use
During Anal Intercourse with a New HIV-Negative Male Partner.

persons who are living with HIV versus those who are uninfected. One possible explanation for this difference is that Godin and colleagues used global measures of attitude and intention that did not take partner serostatus or the type of sex into account. As the present study illustrates, HIV-seropositive MSM hold different attitudes and intentions about condom use depending on partner serostatus and type of sex. It is likely that global measures would fail to adequately capture the complexity of HIV-seropositive MSM cognitive processes and obscure the more complex underlying associations. This explanation is supported by the present findings and other research indicating that HIV-seropositive MSM perceive the risks of sex differently for, and are much more likely to engage in unprotected sex

Insertive Anal Intercourse (n = 96)

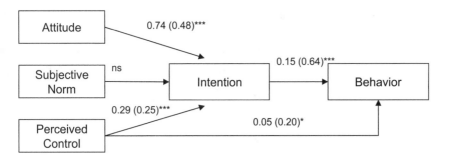

$R^2 = 0.41$, p < .001

Receptive Anal Intercourse (n = 90)

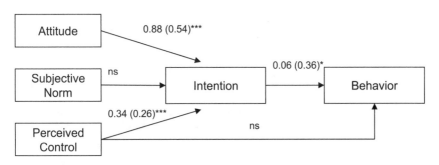

$R^2 = 0.21$, p < .01

Note: Standardized regression weights are shown in parentheses.

†p < .10; * p <.05; ** p < .01, *** p < .001

FIGURE 11–2. Association of TRA/TPB Variables with Past Behavior: Condom Use
During Anal Intercourse with a New HIV-Unknown Male Partner.

with, HIV-seropositive partners than with HIV-seronegative partners who are at
risk of contracting HIV (Halkitis et al., 2005; Parsons et al., 2005; Suarez &
Miller, 2001).

The present study provides only limited support regarding the predicted association between subjective norms and intentions. A significant association was
found in one model (insertive anal intercourse with HIV-seronegative partner) and
a marginally significant association ($p < .10$) was found in another model
(insertive anal intercourse with HIV-seropositive partner). Thus, an association
was observed for two of the three models assessing condom use during insertive
anal sex, but not for any of the three models for receptive anal sex. This pattern of

Insertive Anal Intercourse (n = 93)

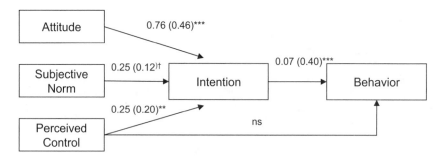

$R^2 = 0.34$, p < .001

Receptive Anal Intercourse (n = 89)

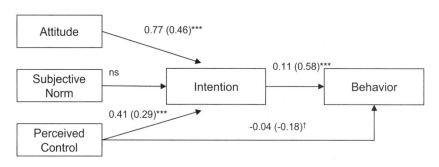

$R^2 = 0.41$, p < .001

Note: Standardized regression weights are shown in parentheses.

† p < .10; * p <.05; ** p < .01, *** p < .001

FIGURE 11–3. Association of TRA/TPB Variables with Past Behavior: Condom Use
During Anal Intercourse with a New HIV-Positive Male Partner.

results suggests that subjective norm may be a more important predictor of condom use when the individual has responsibility for wearing the condom than when
that responsibility rests with the partner. On the other hand, the lack of an association between subjective norms and intentions in most of the models may reflect
a true finding (i.e., that norms exert little influence over HIV-seropositive MSM
condom use behavior during receptive anal sex) or an inadequate specification of
the appropriate normative referents.

Sexual intercourse is a private behavior that requires interaction with another
person. As such, global measures of subjective norms may not be the best predictors of sexual behavior. Prior research with at-risk samples has shown that subjective norms are associated with condom use intentions, but that partner norms

(e.g., beliefs that one's sex partner desires condom use) are an even stronger predictor of condom use intention (Sheeran & Taylor, 1999). This is not surprising given the proximity of the partner to the behavior, the common motivation to please one's partner during sexual relations, and, if the partner is the insertive partner, the need for the partner to wear the condom. Further, some research suggests that factors outside of the TRA/TPB framework that are particularly relevant to intimate relationships may also affect condom use (Gebhardt, Kuyper, & Greunsven, 2003; Kashima, Gallois, & McCamish, 1993).

For HIV-seropositive persons in particular, global measures may fail to capture differences in the beliefs of referents who know that the respondent is HIV-seropositive and those who do not. Persons who are unaware of the respondent's HIV status may exert less influence over the respondent's condom use behavior than those who know that the respondent could transmit HIV to others. Similarly, other referents might be expected to exert differential normative influence including other HIV-seropositive persons (who understand the complexities of initiating and maintaining sexual relationships following an HIV diagnosis) and health care providers with whom respondents may have developed trusting relationships. In the present study, it is possible that assessing subjective norms differently (e.g., limiting the referents to those who were aware of the respondent's HIV-seropositive status or to the sex partner) would have improved the ability the normative component of TRA/TPB to explain condom use intention. These issues related to the measurement of normative influence should be examined in future research.

All six of the models tested in this study accounted for a significant proportion of the variance in condom use, ranging from 21% to 41% across the models. This compares favorably with the 41% of variance accounted for on average by the TPB for diverse health behaviors (Godin & Kok, 1996). Observationally, the proportion of variance accounted for was greatest for HIV-seropositive and HIV-unknown partners compared to HIV-seronegative partners. The reason for this pattern of results is not known, but it is possible that the TRA/TPB (or the measures of TRA/TPB variables used in this study) are better suited to explaining behaviors that pose a threat to oneself than behaviors that pose a risk to others. For HIV-seropositive and HIV-unknown status partners, some respondents may have been more motivated to adopt condom use to protect themselves from sexually transmitted infections and the possibility of superinfection with another strain of HIV (Schwartz & Bailey, 2005). The risks of unprotected sex with HIV-seronegative partners may have been viewed as largely accruing to the partner, not the respondent, and may be motivated by influences that were not specifically assessed in the present study. For example, attributions about one's own responsibility to protect others from HIV have been shown to be a predictor of sexual practices among HIV-seropositive persons (Wolitski et al., 2003; Wolitski, Flores, O'Leary, Bimbi, Gómez, in press). The potential role of such beliefs is not inconsistent with the TRA/TPB perspective as such beliefs likely to attitude formation. Future studies on sexual behavior among persons living with HIV should examine potential differences in beliefs regarding behaviors that may be viewed as serving to protect oneself versus one's partners from adverse consequences and the effects of these beliefs on condom use attitudes and intentions.

Although a significant proportion of the variance was accounted for in all of the models, the majority of variance was left unaccounted for. As discussed previously, specification and operationalization of TRA/TPB variables may have reduced the explanatory power of the models. One must also consider the possibility that other factors that are not accounted for by the TRA/TPB are important determinants of condom use. These factors may include individual-level influences that interact with TRA/TPB variables or directly affect the formation of intentions. For example, individual personality factors such as a tendency to seek novelty and increasingly heightened stimulation in sexual encounters (sexual sensation seeking) has been shown to affect sexual risk behavior (Kalichman & Rompa, 1995) and may operate by attenuating the influence of attitudes, norms, and perceived behavioral control on intention. Characteristics of the partner, such as partner attractiveness, may affect individuals' ability or willingness to follow through on previously formed intentions that were not partner-specific (Agocha & Cooper, 1999; Fishbein, Hennessy, Yzer, & Curtis, 2004). Substance use may directly affect risk (Leigh & Stall, 1993) by impairing the ability to act on intentions that are formed prior to a sexual encounter.

Factors that are external to individuals may also affect their ability to adopt and maintain consistent condom use. Obviously, social influences are one such factor and their importance is recognized by the TRA/TPB. However, this perspective addresses only the individual-level influence of norms and does not explicitly address the dynamics of sexual relationships or the development of community-wide norms and collective efficacy (Gebhardt et al., 2003; Kashima et al., 1993; Kippax, 1993). From a public health perspective it is critically important to gain a better understanding of the formation and evolution of community norms that affect sexual behavior among HIV-seropositive MSM. Changes in beliefs about the severity of HIV disease and attitudes toward condom use and intentional unprotected sex (barebacking) have emerged among gay and bisexual men and have been accompanied by increases in sexually transmitted infections and new HIV cases (CDC, 2005b; Fenton & Imrie, 2005; Wolitski, Valdiserri, Denning, & Levine, 2001). Better understanding of the development and diffusion of these community-wide changes in attitudes, norms, and behaviors, is a critical next step toward the development of effective strategies for avoiding a further resurgence of HIV in vulnerable communities.

An ecological perspective that views the individual as embedded within various social, community, and environmental/structural contexts may further improve the prediction of condom use. For example, the availability of condoms in the community and at the time that sex occurs affects whether or not condoms are used, but is often determined by factors that are beyond an individual's control (Blake et al., 2003; Cohen et al., 1999; Ibanez, Van Oss Marin, Villareal, & Gómez, 2005). Other factors, such as the organization of social groups, the physical environment in which sex occurs, and the broader community environment may also act on an individual's ability to use condoms (Fenton & Imrie, 2005; Frye et al., 2006). The linking of theory focused on individual decision making with approaches that address community-level and structural influences represents a promising direction for improving the prediction of condom use behavior that may have substantial public health benefits.

The present study was not originally designed as a test of the ability of TRA/TPB to predict condom use among HIV-seropositive MSM, and as a result it has a number of limitations. The sample is a convenience sample of HIV-seropositive MSM. The extent to which these results are generalizable to the populations from which these men were sampled is not known. Although the number of HIV-seropositive MSM recruited into the study was relatively large, the sample size for some analyses was much smaller due to the limited numbers of men reporting sex with a non-main partner of a given HIV serostatus.

Data that were collected in a single visit cannot reliably determine causality. (Author: or, is it "Data that were collected in a single visit cannot reliably…") For example, it is possible that past behavior was largely responsible for attitude formation and future intention. The correlations between intention and behavior in this study are associations between future intentions to use condoms with a new partner and past condom use behaviors with an unknown mix of new and established partners. The inconsistency in the measures and the cross-sectional nature of the study may have weakened associations between intentions and behavior. These associations may not have been observed at all (as was the case in Godin and colleagues' 1996 study) if future behavior had been assessed in a longitudinal design. Meta-analysis of TRA/TPB studies has previously shown that intentions are correlated more strongly with past behavior than with future behavior (Albarracín et al.,2001). Finally, the use of data collected before and after exposure to a brief HIV-prevention message may have affected the association between variables measured at the pre-test and those measured at the post-test. However, this concern is mitigated by the lack of significant post-test differences between message conditions for variables used in these analyses (data not shown).

The TRA and TPB have made numerous and important contributions to the prevention of HIV infection. These theories have provided important insights into the use of risk-reduction strategies that have formed the basis for successful HIV prevention interventions for many different at-risk populations (Albarracín et al., 2005). As the present data show, they also hold great promise for furthering our understanding of sexual practices among persons living with HIV. Not surprisingly, merely contracting a virus does not appear to fundamentally alter the underlying influences that affect sexual behavior, but it can affect how individuals perceive specific sexual practices depending upon the HIV status of their partners. There is a need for more effective interventions for people living with HIV, and the TRA/TPB will likely provide a useful theoretical foundation for these efforts. The prior contributions of the TRA/TPB to HIV prevention have been many, and the future contributions of these theories have the potential to be even greater as they are applied and extended in new arenas in an effort to meet the ever-changing challenges of the global HIV/AIDS epidemic.

ACKNOWLEDGMENTS

Richard J. Wolitski and Jun Zhang are with the Prevention Research Branch, Division of HIV and AIDS Prevention, National Center for HIV/AIDS, Viral Hepatitis, Sexually Transmitted Disease, and Tuberculosis Prevention, Coordinating Center for Infectious Diseases, Centers for Disease Control and Prevention, Atlanta, Georgia.

This research was supported by the Centers for Disease Control and Prevention and awarded to RTI International (contract number 200-2001-00123). The findings and conclusions in this report are those of the authors and do not necessarily represent the views of the Centers for Disease Control and Prevention.

The authors would like to acknowledge the following members of the Prevention Research Branch HIV Prevention Messages Study Team for their contributions to the development and implementation of this study: Carolyn Guenther-Grey, Jill Wasserman, Jennifer Uhrig, Jeff Henne, Barbara Burbridge, Lisa Belcher, Dogan Eroglu, Cari Courtenay-Quirk, Sherri Pals, Kristine Fahrney, Laxminarayana Ganapahti, Joseph Cappella, and Marty Fishbein.

REFERENCES

Agocha, V. B., & Cooper, M. L. (1999). Risk perceptions and safer-sex intentions: Does a partner's physical attractiveness undermine the use of risk-relevant information? *Personality and Social Psychology Bulletin, 25,* 746–759.

Ajzen, I. (1985). From intentions to actions: A theory of planned behavior. In J. Kuhl & J. Beckmann (Eds.), *Action control: From cognition to behavior* (pp. 11–39). Berlin, Germany: Springer-Verlag.

Ajzen, I. (1991). The theory of planned behavior. *Organizational Behavior and Human Decision Processes, 50,* 179–211.

Ajzen, I., & Fishbein, M. (Eds.). (1980). *Understanding attitudes and predicting social behavior.* Englewood Cliffs, NJ: Prentice Hall, Inc.

Albarracín, D., Gillette, J. C., Earl, A. N., Glasman, L. R., Durantini, M. R., & Ho, M. (2005). A test of major assumptions about behavior change: A comprehensive look at the effects of passive and active HIV-Prevention intervention since the beginning of the epidemic. *Psychological Bulletin, 131,* 856–897.

Albarracín, D., Johnson, B. T., Fishbein, M., & Muellerleile, P. A. (2001). Theories of reasoned action and planned behavior as models of condom use: A meta-analysis. *Psychological Bulletin. 127,* 142–161.

Bandura, A. (1986). *Social foundations of thought and action: A social cognitive theory.* Englewood Cliff, NJ: Prentice-Hall.

Bandura, A. (1994). Social cognitive theory and exercise of control over HIV infection. In DiClemente, R. J., & Peterson, J. L. (Eds.). *Preventing AIDS: Theories and methods of behavioral interventions* (pp. 25–59). New York, NY: Plenum.

Becker, M. H., & Joseph, J. (1988). AIDS and behavioral change to reduce risk: A review. *American Journal of Public Health, 78,* 394–410.

Blake, S. M., Ledsky, R., Goodenow, C., Sawyer, R., Lohrmann, D., & Windsor, R. (2003). Condom availability programs in Massachusetts high schools: Relationships with condom use and sexual behavior. *American Journal of Public Health, 93,* 955–962.

Buunk, B. P., & Bakker, A. B. (1997). Commitment to the relationship, extradyadic sex, and AIDS prevention behavior. *Journal of Applied Social Psychology, 27,* 1241–1257.

Centers for Disease Control and Prevention. (2003). Advancing HIV prevention: New strategies for a changing epidemic–United States, 2003. *Morbidity and Mortality Weekly Report, 52,* 329–332.

Centers for Disease Control and Prevention. (2005a). HIV prevalence, unrecognized infection, and HIV testing among men who have sex with men—Five U.S. cities, June 2004–April 2005. *Morbidity and Mortality Weekly Report, 54,* 597–601.

Centers for Disease Control and Prevention. (2005b). Trends in HIV/AIDS diagnoses—33 States, 2001–2004. *Morbidity and Mortality Weekly Report, 54,* 1149–1153.

Centers for Disease Control and Prevention AIDS Community Demonstration Projects Research Group. (1999). The CDC AIDS Community Demonstration Projects: A multi-site community-level intervention to promote HIV risk reduction. *American Journal of Public Health, 89,* 336–345.

Cohen, D. A., Farley, T. A., Bedimo-Etame, J. R., Scribner, R., Ward, W., Kendall, C., et al. (1999). Implementation of condom social marketing in Louisiana, 1993 to 1996. *American Journal of Public Health, 89,* 204–208.

Corby, N. H., Enguidanos, S. M., & Kay, L. S. (1996). Development and use of role-model stories in a community-level HIV risk-reduction intervention. *Public Health Reports, 111*(Suppl. 1), 54–58.

Corby, N. H., Jamner, M. S., & Wolitski, R. J. (1996). Using the theory of planned behavior to predict condom use among male and female injecting drug users. *Journal of Applied Social Psychology, 26,* 52–75.

Crepaz, N., & Marks, G. (2002). Towards an understanding of sexual risk behavior in people living with HIV: A review of social, psychological, and medical findings. *AIDS, 16,* 135–149.

Fenton, K. A., & Imrie, J. (2005). Increasing rates of sexually transmitted diseases in homosexual men in Western Europe and the United Status: Why? *Infectious Disease Clinics of North America, 19,* 311–331.

Fishbein, M. (1967). Attitude and the prediction of behavior. In M. Fishbein (Ed.), *Readings in attitude theory and measurement* (pp. 477–492). New York: John Wiley & Sons, Inc.

Fishbein, M., & Ajzen, I. (1975). *Belief, attitude, intention and behavior: An introduction to theory and research.* Reading, MA: Addison-Wesley.

Fishbein, M., Hennessy, M., Kamb, M., Bolan, G. A., Hoxworth, T., Iatesta, M., et al. (2001). Using intervention theory to model factors influencing behavior change. *Evaluation & the Health Profession, 24,* 363–384.

Fishbein, M., Hennessy, M., Yzer, M., & Curtis, B. (2004). Romance and risk: Romantic attraction and health risks in the process of relationship formation. *Psychology, Health & Medicine, 9,* 273–285.

Fishbein, M., Middlestadt, S. E., & Hitchcock, P. J. (1991). Using information to change sexually transmitted disease-related behaviors: An analysis based on the theory of reasoned action. In J. N. Wasserheit, S. O. Aral, & K. K. Holmes (Eds.), *Research issues in human behavior and sexually transmitted diseases in the AIDS era* (pp. 243–257). Washington, DC: American Society for Microbiology.

Fisher, J. D., & Fisher, W. A. (2000). Theoretical approaches to individual-level change in HIV risk behavior. In Peterson, J. L. &, DiClemente, R. J. (Eds.). *Handbook of HIV prevention* (pp. 3–55). Dordrecht, Netherlands: Kluwer.

Fleming, P. L., Byers, R. H., Sweeney, P. A., Daniels, D., Karon, J. M., & Janssen, R. S. (2002, February). *HIV prevalence in the United States, 2000.* Paper presented at the 9th Conference on Retroviruses and Opportunistic Infections, Seattle, WA.

Frye, V., Latka, M. H., Koblin, B., Halkitis, P. N., Putnam, S., Galea, S., et al. (2006). The urban environment and sexual risk behavior among men who have sex with men. *Journal of Urban Health, 83,* 308–324.

Gebhardt, W. A., Kuyper, L., & Greunsven, G. (2003). Need for intimacy in relationships and motives for sex as determinants of adolescent condom use. *Journal of Adolescent Health, 33,* 154–164.

Glynn, M., & Rhodes, P. (2005, June). *What is really happening with HIV trends in the United States? Modeling the national epidemic.* Paper presented at the National HIV Prevention Conference, Atlanta, GA.

Godin, G., & Kok, G. (1996). The Theory of Planned Behavior: A review of its application to health-related behaviors. *American Journal of Health Promotion, 11*(2), 87–98.

Godin, G., Savard, J., Kok, G., Fortin, C., & Boyer, R. (1996). HIV seropositive gay men: Understanding adoption of safe sexual practices. *AIDS Education & Prevention, 8*, 529–545.

Gold, R. S., & Skinner, M. J. (1992). Situational factors and thought processes associated with unprotected intercourse in young gay men. *AIDS, 6*, 1021–1030.

Gold, R. S., & Skinner, M. J. (1996). Judging a book by its cover: Gay men's use of perceptible characteristics to infer antibody status. *International Journal of STD and AIDS, 7*, 39–43.

Guinan, M. E., & Leviton, L. (1995). Prevention of HIV infection in women: Overcoming barriers. *Journal of the American Medical Women's Association, 50*(3–4), 74–77.

Halkitis, P. N., Gómez, C., & Wolitski, R. J. (2005). *HIV + Sex: The Psychological and Interpersonal Dynamics of HIV-Seropositive Gay and Bisexual Men's Relationships.* Washington, DC: American Psychological Association.

Hoff, C. C., Stall, R., Paul, J., Acree, M., Daigle, D., Phillips, K., et al. (1997). Differences in sexual behavior among HIV discordant and concordant gay men in primary relationships. *Journal of Acquired Immune Deficiency Syndromes, 14*, 72–78.

Hospers, H. J., & Kok, G. (1995). Determinants of safe and risk-taking sexual-behavior among gay men–A review. *AIDS Education & Prevention, 7*, 74–96.

Ibanez, G. E., Van Oss Marin, B., Villareal, C., & Gómez, C. A. (2005). Condom use at last sex among unmarried Latino men: An event level analysis. *AIDS and Behavior, 9*, 433–441.

Jamner, M. S., Wolitski, R. J., Corby, N. H., & Fishbein, M. (1998). Using the theory of planned behavior to predict intention to use condoms among female sex workers. *Psychology and Health, 13*, 187–205.

Janssen, R. S., Holtgrave, D. R., Valdiserri, R. O., Shepherd, M., Gayle, H. D., & DeCock, K. M. (2001). The serostatus approach to fighting the HIV epidemic: Prevention strategies for infected individuals. *American Journal of Public Health, 91*, 1019–1024.

Kalichman, S. C. (2000). HIV transmission risk behaviors of men and women living with HIV-AIDS: Prevalence, predictors, and emerging clinical interventions. *Clinical Psychology: Science and Practice, 7*, 32–47.

Kalichman, S. C., & Rompa, D. (1995). Sexual sensation seeking and sexual compulsivity scales: Reliability, validity, and predicting HIV risk behavior. *Journal of Personality Assessment, 65*, 586–601.

Kamb, M. L, Fishbein, M., Douglas, J. M., Jr., Rhodes, F., Rogers, J., Bolan, G., et al. (1998). Efficacy of risk-reduction counseling to prevent human immunodeficiency virus and sexually transmitted diseases: A randomized controlled trial. *Journal of the American Medical Association, 280*, 1161–1167.

Kashima, Y., Gallois, C., & McCamish, M. (1993). The theory of reasoned action and cooperative behaviour: It takes two to use a condom. *British Journal of Social Psychology, 32*, 227–239.

Kippax, S. (1993). Flaws in the theory of reasoned action. In D.J. Terry, C. Gallois, & M. McCamish (Eds.), *The theory of reasoned action: Its application to AIDS-preventive behaviour* (pp. 253–269). Elmsford, NY: Pergamon Press.

Kok, G. (1999). Targeted prevention for people with HIV/AIDS: Feasible and desirable? *Patient Education and Counseling, 36*, 239–246.

Leigh, B. C., & Stall, R. (1993). Substance use and risky sexual behavior for exposure to HIV. *American Psychologist, 48*, 1035–1045.

Marks, G., Burris, S., & Peterman, T. A. (1999). Reducing sexual transmission of HIV from those who know they are infected: The need for personal and collective responsibility. *AIDS, 13*, 297–306.

Misovich, S. J., Fisher, J. D., & Fisher, W. A. (1997). Close relationships and elevated HIV risk behavior: Evidence and possible underlying psychological processes. *Review of General Psychology, 1*, 72–107.

Norris, A. (2005). Path analysis. In Munro B. (Ed.), *Statistical methods for health care research* (4th ed., pp. 377–404). Philadelphia: Lippincott.

O'Leary, A. (2005). Guessing games: Sex partner serostatus assumptions among HIV-positive gay and bisexual men. In P. N. Halkitis, C. A. Gómez, & R. J. Wolitski (Eds.), *HIV + Sex: The Psychological and Interpersonal Dynamics of HIV-Seropositive Gay and Bisexual Men's Relationships* (pp. 121–132). Washington, DC: American Psychological Association.

O'Leary, A., Wolitski, R., J., Remien, R. H., Woods, W., Parsons, J. T., Moss, S., et al. (2005). Psychosocial correlates of transmission risk behavior among HIV-seropositive gay and bisexual men. *AIDS, 19*(Suppl. 1), S67–S75.

Ostrow, D. G, McKirnan D., Klein C., & DiFranceisco, W. (1999). Patterns and correlates of risky behavior among HIV+ gay men: Are they really different from HIV- men? *AIDS and Behavior, 3,* 99–110.

Parsons, J. T., Halkitis, P. N., Wolitski, R. J., Gómez, C. A., & the Seropositive Urban Men's Study (SUMS) Team. (2003). Correlates of sexual risk behavior among HIV+ men who have sex with men. *AIDS Education and Prevention, 15,* 383–400.

Parsons, J. T., Schrimshaw, E. W., Wolitski, R. J., Halkitis, P. N., Purcell, D. W., Hoff, C., et al. (2005). Sexual harm reduction practices of HIV-seropositive gay and bisexual men: Serosorting, strategic positioning, and withdrawal before ejaculation. *AIDS, 19*(Suppl. 1), S13-S25.

Rosenstock, I. M, Strecher, V. J., & Becker, M. H. (1994). The health belief model and HIV risk behavior change. In DiClemente, R. J. & Peterson, J. L. (Eds.). *Preventing AIDS: Theories and methods of behavioral interventions* (pp. 5–24). New York, NY: Plenum.

Schiltz, M. A., & Sandfort, T. G. (2000). HIV-positive people, risk and sexual behaviour. Social *Science and Medicine, 50,* 1571–1588.

Schwartz, D. J., & Bailey, C. J. (2005). Between the sheets and between the ears: Sexual practices and risk beliefs of HIV-positive gay and bisexual men. In P. Halkitis, C. Gómez, & R. J. Wolitski (Eds.), *HIV + Sex: The Psychological and Interpersonal Dynamics of HIV-Seropositive Gay and Bisexual Men's Relationships* (pp. 55–72). Washington, DC: American Psychological Association.

Sheeran, P., & Taylor, S. (1999). Predicting intentions to use condoms: A meta-analysis and comparison of the theories of reasoned action and planned behavior. *Journal of Applied Social Psychology, 29,* 1624–1675.

Simoni, J. M., & Pantalone, D. W. (2005). HIV disclosure and safer sex. In S. C. Kalichman (Ed.), *Positive Prevention: Reducing HIV Transmission among People Living with HIV/AIDS* (pp 65–98). New York, NY: Kluwer Academic/Plenum Publishers.

Suarez, T., & Miller, J. (2001). Negotiating risks in context: A perspective on unprotected anal intercourse and barebacking among men who have sex with men. *Archives of Sexual Behavior, 30,* 287–300.

United Nations Programme on HIV/AIDS (UNAIDS). (2006). *2006 Report on the Global AIDS Epidemic.* Geneva, Switzerland: UNAIDS. Retrieved May 30, 2006, from http://www.unaids.org/en/HIV_Data/2006GlobalReport/default.asp

Warner, L., Stone, K. M., Macaluso, M., Buehler, J. W., & Austin, H. D. (2006). Condom use and risk of gonorrhea and Chlamydia: A systematic review of design and measurement factors assessed in epidemiologic studies. *Sexually Transmitted Diseases, 33,* 36–51.

Weinhardt, L. S., Carey, M. P., Johnson, B. T., & Bickman, N. L. (1999). Effects of HIV counseling and testing on sexual risk behavior: A meta-analytic review of published research, 1985–1997. *American Journal of Public Health, 89,* 1397–1405.

Wolitski, R. J., Bailey, C., O'Leary, A., Gómez, C. A., Parsons, J. T., & the Seropositive Urban Men's Study Group. (2003). Self-perceived responsibility of HIV-seropositive men for preventing HIV transmission to sex partners. *AIDS and Behavior, 7,* 363–372.

Wolitski, R. J., Flores, S. A., O'Leary, A., Bimbi, D. S., & Gómez, C.A. (in press). Beliefs about personal and partner responsibility among HIV-seropositive men who have sex with men: Measurement and association with transmission risk behavior. *AIDS and Behavior.* DOI: 10.1007/s10461-006-9183-6.

Wolitski, R. J., Janssen, R. S., Onorato, I. M., Purcell, D. W., & Crepaz, N. (2005). A comprehensive approach to prevention with people living with HIV. In S. C. Kalichman (Ed.), *Positive Prevention: Reducing HIV Transmission among People Living with HIV/AIDS* (pp 1–28). New York: Kluwer Academic/Plenum Publishers.

Wolitski, R. J., Parsons, J. T., & Gómez, C. A. (2004). Prevention with HIV-seropositive gay and bisexual men: Lessons learned from the Seropositive Urban Men's Study (SUMS) and the Seropositive Urban Men's Intervention Trial (SUMIT). *Journal of Acquired Immunodeficiency Syndromes, 37*(Suppl 2), S101–S109.

Wolitski, R. J., Valdiserri, R. O., Denning, P. H., & Levine, W. C. (2001). Are we headed for a resurgence in the HIV epidemic among men who have sex with men? *American Journal of Public Health, 91,* 883–888.

CHAPTER 12

Through the Theoretical Microscope: Comments on Kasprzyk and Montaño, Wolitski and Zhang, and Middlestadt and Yzer

Lorraine Sherr

Royal Free and University College Medical School, London, United Kingdom

Theories provide the lens through which chaos makes sense. They set events in sharp focus and can highlight relationships that may otherwise be overlooked or blurred. Theory development and provision can operate at three levels. The first level is a descriptive one where the benefit of the theory is to allow for understanding of behavior. The theory gives an understanding of context and allows for behavioral clusters to be described, thereby shedding light on the relationship and the phenomenon. The second level is one of prediction. At this level the theory allows behavior to be predicted. Clearly this is a level of excitement. Knowledge of the elements of the theory would allow for accurate advance prediction and can anticipate human behavior. Indeed, when viewed backwards, such theory can be validated by measuring the predictors and assessing the extent to which they were, indeed, predictive. Both these levels are well established in the theory of reasoned action (TRA) and the theory of planned behavior (TPB; Fishbein 1975; Ajzen, 1985, 1991; Ajzen & Fishbein, 1980. The third level of theory, which dramatically changes its utility and importance, is the level where theory can be used to change behavior. This brings with it many issues: first, the moral and ethical issue of social engineering and behavior change, and second, the application of health imperatives where changing existing negative behaviors or influencing the adoption of new positive behaviors are the goal. There are good arguments in health, for example, that adopting healthy behaviors, and desisting from unhealthy behaviors (both behavior changes of a very different sort), contribute to a human good.

The test of a good theory, indeed, is when such crises can be avoided, and the application of the theory allows for behavioral good to prevail and behavioral harm to be minimized.

There is a role for all three levels of theory. However, the highest level, that of behavior change, is the one that has the most applied utility. The advent of the HIV/AIDS epidemic served as a wake-up call to behavioral scientists and provided a challenge to psychological behavioral theories. The urgency of the crisis, the lethality of the infection, and the direct control via behavioral management and change was the perfect platform to try out theories and see if they were worth their salt.

As with all new areas, some basic lessons are hard learnt. The sophistication of the TRA and TBA theories ensured that simplistic views on attitudinal–behavioral links did not persist. Even at the start of the HIV epidemic, there was overwhelming evidence that simplistic theories were inadequate and that theories needed to be complex if they were to be effective in any behavior change. At that early time, it was well established that behavioral intentions were better predictors of behavior than attitude. Yet initially, there was a knee-jerk return to the belief that simple knowledge and knowledge change, attitude and attitude change, was all that was required to avert infection. This was compounded by the belief that the best and only tool was fear arousal (Sherr 1990). In the early days of the HIV epidemic, many campaigns marked a regression in terms of theory, which did not help the cause of HIV prevention.

The chapters in this section of the book show the opposite movement—in contrast to that early regression, they demonstrate an elevation in thinking and the way things can move forward. They are not set out as tests of theory, but rather invoke theory to inform their interventions and to underpin their evaluations. The results, therefore, provide both proof of concept and also efficacy of intervention. More importantly, they ensure against complacency. Human behavior, like theories, evolves over time. As Fishbein himself stated in 2002 (AIDS Impact conference, Brighton), "if the theories are not working, it is time for new theories."

The chapter by Montano and Kaspryzk takes the utility of theory to an additional level. For the most part, theories have been implemented at the individual level. Their work sets out to explore the efficacy of community-level interventions and adapt the theory accordingly. They also raise the complex question of cross-cultural applicability. This may be particularly appropriate for epidemic-level challenges. The cross-cultural generalization is fascinating to unpick. Is it simply that the element of *normative* influences can be described differently in different cultures and contexts, or is it that the entire fabric of intention, cognition, and behavior is intrinsically bound up with culture to the extent that there is no generalizability of theories to such diverse cultures? This exciting chapter and research project has meticulously used qualitative techniques to understand and unpick these specific beliefs, and furthermore to incorporate them into instruments for subsequent behavior change measures. Their data seemed to support the idea that specific attitudes towards a specific behavior was the best indicator of behavioral intention. However, the chapter goes on to raise some issues in relation to application. The underlying intervention is based on a *popular opinion leader* model.

The aim here is, by recruiting popular opinion leaders, intervening with them, a drip down effect of change can be triggered in a community setting. However, this model may be more difficult to apply. It has been shown to have mixed efficacy (Kelly et al., 1991, 1992, 1997, 2004; Elford, Bolding, & Sherr, 2001, 2004; Elford, Hart, Sherr, Williamson, & Bolding, 2002; Elford, Sherr, Bolding, Serle, & Maguire, 2002; Flowers, Hart, Williamson, Frankis, & Der, 2002), and at times the very cultural variations may have either resulted in the concept not fully realized, in difficulties mounting the intervention to all specifications or the need to adapt to local culture which has negated efficacy (Elford et al. 2004, Hart, Williamson, & Flowers, 2004.) This also raises the question of manipulation of cultural norms and behavior by recruiting and training popular opinion leaders—an issue that has not been fully explored and will be further expanded when the final Montano and Kaspryzk trial is completed.

Yzer gives a thoughtful insight into the notion of perceived control. Is perceived control a prerequisite, how is it measured, and to what extent is it an overlooked concept in many of the applied studies? Although not specifically focused on HIV, this piece has important implications for much of the HIV/condom literature as well as other applied behavioral interventions. Yzer focuses on questions that advance the theories—notably the sufficiency of the proposed set of behavioral determinants as an account of behavior, the nature or conceptual meaning of the proposed constructs, and the causal relationships between these constructs (Ajzen & Fishbein, 2005). If behavioral control is out of the hands of the individual, then attitude and social norms are ineffective at predicting or influencing intentions. This means that improving perceived control, or even having a measure of it, may affect intentions or clarify the strength of intentions. On the other hand, if there is zero perceived control, the behavior may well become one not subject to intentional change. Indeed, a recent paper by Boily (Boily, Godin, Hogben, Sherr, & Bastos, 2005) has shown that non-volitional factors may have quite an impact on the way in which the HIV epidemic evolves. Yzer then raises the important questions of definition of perceived control, measurement of the construct and the nature of links between perceived control and intention/behavior. Yzer summarizes studies on the role of perceived control in determining intentions and also on the role of perceived control in behavior. The actual nature of the relationships has not been definitively described. Is it additive or is it interactive? Furthermore, is there a relative scale of volitional control or is it absolute? This fascinating concept, together with the empirical imperative to operationalize and quantify the role and mechanisms of perceived control, have been underinvestigated. Yzer summarizes the available studies and notes that despite the fact that the studies are few and the sample sizes are small, a consistent effect seems to be reported. Yet the methodology, measurement, and application of the concept may still form a challenge. Clearly the future lies in controlled studies where perceived control is moderated and the effects carefully monitored.

From these chapters there is a fascinating contemplation of concepts such as perceived control, but also the issue of quantum is raised. How much of an effect is needed? Is a stronger effect a stronger predictor? In field applications, what is enough? What is the cost benefit? This notion extends to all the concepts within the theories and is particularly relevant in intervention programs where change is sought. Many of the notions are measured by way of Lickert type scales and thus it is unclear what form of movement along these scales would be sufficient to alter the balance.

Middlestadt provides a detailed examination on the selection of specific behaviors to be targeted for intervention. The complexity of this task must not be undervalued. Indeed, efficacy of interventions, according to the theories, are based on the behavior rather than health status or health outcomes (these are much more complex and multifactorial). By way of example Middlestadt describes the complexity of such specific behavior selection. This highlights the meticulous planning and conceptual understanding needed to target, and subsequently affect, given behaviors. By way of example, HIV shows the complexity of the task, and the variety of interventions with vague and clear behaviors under study. Again this raises the issue of magnitude of the behavior and magnitude of the change—a concept rarely considered in much of the literature. How much change is needed to be effective? Is the same theory or intervention valid for minor change compared to major or total change? What is the quantum in terms of accomplishing these various degrees of change?

Wolitski and Zhang look specifically at the prevention of HIV transmission risk. They overview the key concepts in terms of the history of HIV, the need for behavior change, and the relevance of models to predict behavior such as TRA and TPB. There are a vast number of studies examining the efficacy of these models in predicting condom use, and these generally show the theories as effective (Albarracín et al., 2005; Albarracín, Johnson, Fishbein, & Muellerleile, 2001, 2005; Sheeran & Taylor, 1999). Furthermore, one of the most effective tests of the theory has been within project RESPECT, which provided randomized controlled methodology to test out an intervention based on TRA, a reduced counseling intervention, and a didactic message (Kamb et al., 1998). This study definitively showed a longer-term behavior change, and specifically was able to isolate the changes associated with targeted elements according to the TRA theory constructs (Fishbein et al., 2001). Yet Wolitski considers how this relationship may change if the trigger for behavior is not related to protection from infection (the case of the HIV negative or HIV untested), but into the protection of others from infection, that is, the desistance of transmission (the case of the HIV positive). For this group the use of condoms has a dual purpose, which can perhaps be rank ordered. One purpose is to ensure that others are not infected, and the second purpose is to self-protect against re-infection of resistant strains which may affect treatment options and, in addition, to protect against other sexually transmitted infections. The chapter reports on an intervention study with HIV-positive individuals with care to explore details of actual behaviors, partner type (casual or main), as well as partner status (HIV positive, HIV negative, and HIV status unknown). They found a significant association between intention and behavior for both insertive and receptive anal sex, regardless of partner serostatus. Attitude and perceived behavioral control were significantly associated with all intention measures, but perceived behavioral control related to behavior for only insertive anal intercourse with a partner whose serostatus was not known by the respondent (interesting findings in the light of the Yzer call to examine perceived control in systematic depth.) Of note in the study was the fact that much of the variance was not accounted for. This leaves open the need for growth in the theories to understand and accommodate additional factors that may not currently feature in existing models.

Although these empirical studies form the core of understanding, they also raise questions in relation to some of the limitations. In this particular study, sample size and the demerits of convenience samples may have a specific role to play. It, together with the cluster of chapters, raises a number of theoretical questions.

The first major question, which extends beyond the current studies, relates to the curious question of time and chronology. When is it appropriate to measure intention? Must it always precede the behavior? Can current intentions predict or at least explain previous behavior? Could behavior affect reported intentions (or even perceived intentions) under a self-perception type paradigm (I did it therefore I must believe…)? Could there be an ameliorating factor related to hindsight bias where knowing one's behavior affects one's recall and rating of intention. It seems that ideally there should be a chronology, especially in research where preexisting intentions are vital to measure, rather than a recall of both behavior and intention.

The second relates to the curious question of secrets and private (vs. public) behavior. Is there a grading of private/public behaviors? Is there universal agreement on the private/public distinction, or is this categorization subjective? Are some behaviors more social and some more secret than others? Does this affect the components of the theory and the predictive ability of theory? Sex and condom use may be particularly affected by these notions. This begs the very question as to whether theories apply generally or whether they are situational specific and specifically whether secretive, private, or sensitive behavior responds equally to the elements of a theory as public, shared behaviors.

The third curious question is in terms of individual versus interpersonal behaviors. Sex and condom use provide fascinating working examples of this dilemma. Given that there are at least two parties involved in a mutual behavior, the interactive dance between different norms, beliefs, intentions, and control may result in a behavior that is greater than the sum of the individual components. The nature of this interaction and the mechanisms of influence are yet to be understood. This is particularly relevant in imbalanced interactions (such as sexual behavior with differential power between the partners). Such a concept may be the true challenge to the applicability of these models in high HIV demand areas such as Sub-Saharan Africa. The models provide a two-dimensional look at behavior and its prediction, and this question raises a third dimensional need.

The chapter by Middlestadt gives very clear insight into the need to hone in on specific behaviors that refine the theory, but this focus may in itself mask the complexity of some human endeavors.

Volitional and non-volitional behavior, especially but not exclusively in relation to perceived control, may well be the next challenge for these theories. There is some clarity in applied situations where there is no volitional control (e.g., where condoms are simply not available; Boily et al., 2005). However, grading between the two and appraisal of how volitional a situation may be a future demand.

The question of quantum is a fascinating one for discussion. It is highly relevant in the applied field. If it is established that there is a link between intention and behavior change, how much intention is needed? How much change is needed?

Is there an absolute or variable level? Does it happen incrementally or catastrophically (sudden change)?

Finally, a discussion point raised specifically by the Wolitski chapter relates to the question of whether behaviors on one's own behalf differ from behavior on another's behalf. Is there a concept of consequence that backward drives the theory or its components? This is a new direction and is raised eloquently in the notion of positive prevention (Wolitski et al., this volume).

CONCLUSION

This series of chapters raise more questions than they answer, a true token of how an intriguing theory opens doors that were previously closed and also shows the way to pathways not hitherto encountered. The need to integrate concepts and move forward is a vital component of theory evolution. The reasoned action approach marks this out very clearly and reminds us to keep on our toes and to constantly question whether theories are doing their job, advancing the knowledge, or, as Fishbein (Fishbein, Hennessy, Yzer, & Douglas, 2003) put it, "when does the time come for us to need new theories?"

REFERENCES

Ajzen, I. (1985). From intentions to actions: A theory of planned behavior. In J. Kuhl & J. Beckmann (Eds.), *Action control: From cognition to behavior* (pp. 11–39). Berlin: Springer-Verlag.

Ajzen, I. (1991). The theory of planned behavior. *Organizational Behavior and Human Decision Processes, 50,* 179–211.

Ajzen, I., & Fishbein, M. (Eds.). (1980). *Understanding attitudes and predicting social behavior.* Englewood Cliffs, NJ: Prentice Hall.

Ajzen, I., & Fishbein, M. (2005). The influence of attitudes on behaviour. In D. Albarracin, B. T. Johnson, & M.P. Zanna (Eds.), *Handbook of attitudes and attitude change: Basic principles.* Mahwah, NJ: Lawrence Erlbaum Associates.

Albarracín, D., Gillette, J. C., Earl, A. N., Glasman, L. R., Durantini, M. R., & Ho, M. (2005). A test of major assumptions about behavior change: A comprehensive look at the effects of passive and active HIV-prevention intervention since the beginning of the epidemic. *Psychological Bulletin, 131,* 856–897.

Albarracín, D., Johnson, B. T., Fishbein, M., & Muellerleile, P. A. (2001). Theories of reasoned action and planned behavior as models of condom use: A meta-analysis. *Psychological Bulletin. 127,* 142–161.

Boily, M. C., Godin, G., Hogben, M., Sherr, L., Bastos, F. I. (2005) The impact of the transmission dynamics of the HIV/AIDS epidemic on sexual behavior: A new hypothesis to explain recent increases in risk-taking behavior among men who have sex with men. *Med Hypotheses. 65,* 215–226

Elford, J., Bolding, G., & Sherr, L. (2001). Peer education has no significant impact on HIV risk behaviors among gay men in London. *AIDS, 15,* 535–538.

Elford, J., Hart, G., Sherr, L., Williamson, L., & Bolding, G. (2002). Peer-led HIV prevention among homosexual men in Britain. *Sexually Transmitted Infections, 78*, 158–159.

Elford, J., Sherr, L., Bolding, G., Serle, F., & Maguire, M. (2002). Peer-led HIV prevention among gay men in London: Process evaluation. *AIDS Care, 14*, 351–360.

Elford J., Bolding G., & Sherr, L. (2004). Popular opinion leaders in London: A response to Kelly. *AIDS Care, 16*,151–158.

Fishbein, M., & Ajzen, I. (1975). *Belief, attitude, intention, and behavior: An introduction to theory and research.* Reading, MA: Addison-Wesley.

Fishbein, M., Hennessy, M., Yzer, M., & Douglas, J. (2003). Can we explain why some people do and some people do not act on their intentions? *Psychology Health and Medicine, 8*, 3–18.

Fishbein, M., Hennessy, M., Kamb, M., Bolan, G. A., Hoxworth, T., Iatesta, M., et al. (2001). Using intervention theory to model factors influencing behavior change. *Evaluation & the Health Profession, 24*, 363–384

Fishbein, M. (2002). Plenary Lecture AIDS Impact Conference Brighton. UK.

Flowers, P., Hart, G., Williamson, L., Frankis, J. S., & Der, G. J. (2002), Does bar-based, peer-led sexual health promotion have a community-level effect among gay men in Scotland? *International Journal of STD and AIDS, 13*, 102–108.

Hart, G. J., Williamson, L. M., & Flowers, P. (2004). Good in parts: The Gay Mens Task Force in Glasgow—a response to Kelly *AIDS Care, 16*, 159–166.

Kamb, M. L, Fishbein, M., Douglas, J. M., Jr., Rhodes, F., Rogers, J., Bolan, G., et al. (1998). Efficacy of risk-reduction counseling to prevent human immunodeficiency virus and sexually transmitted diseases: A randomized controlled trial. *Journal of the American Medical Association, 280*, 1161–1167.

Kelly, J. A. (2004). Popular opinion leaders and HIV prevention peer education resolving discrepant findings and implications for the development of effective community programmes. *AIDS Care,16*, 139–150.

Kelly, J. A., Murphy, D. A., Sikkema, K. J., McAuliffe, T. L., Roffman, R. A., Solomon, et al. (1997). Randomised, controlled, community-level HIV-prevention intervention for sexual-risk behavior among homosexual men in US cities. Community HIV Prevention Research Collaborative. *Lancet, 350*,1500–1505.

Kelly, J. A., St. Lawrence, J. S, Diaz, Y. E., Stevenson, L. Y., Hauth, A. C., Brasfield, et al. (1991). HIV risk behavior reduction following intervention with key opinion leaders of population: An experimental analysis. *American Journal of Public Health, 81*, 168–171.

Kelly, J. A., St. Lawrence, J. S., Stevenson, L. Y., Hauth, A. C., Kalichman, S. C., Diaz, Y. E., et al. (1992). Community AIDS/HIV risk reduction: The effects of endorsements by popular people in three cities. *American Journal of Public Health, 82*, 1483–1489.

Sheeran, P., & Taylor, S. (1999). Predicting intentions to use condoms: A meta-analysis and comparison of the theories of reasoned action and planned behavior. *Journal of Applied Social Psychology, 29*, 1624–1675.

Sherr, L. (1990). Fear arousal and AIDS—do shock tactics work? *AIDS, 4*, 361–364.

CHAPTER 13

Commentary on the Theories of Reasoned Action and Planned Behavior and Their Use in Health Promotion

Gerald Gorn

Department of Marketing
Hong Kong University of Science and Technology

The contributions of the theory of reasoned action (TRA) to our understanding of what motivates people to behave the way they do are manifold. First, a key element of the model is that it incorporates relevant social norms, in addition to attitudes. After the fact, the idea that a model of behavioral intentions needs to take salient social norms into account might be considered somewhat intuitive. To my knowledge, however, the TRA was the first model of behavioral intentions to incorporate social norms and do it in a structured way where a score for a person could be obtained for salient norms and that score could be combined with the person's attitude score. The way these norms were operationalized in the model represents a very important contribution. They were incorporated as *subjective* normative beliefs. As with attitude, the model considers important normative influences from the *actor's* point of view. Thus, although others might have recognized the importance of social norms, the TRA was the first to incorporate them into a formal model for predicting behavioral intentions.

Advertisers intuitively recognize the power of subjective norms. A number of years ago commercials were run for Stove Top Stuffing in which a mother was shown buying potatoes instead of stuffing. In the commercial, an interviewer asks her why she purchased potatoes rather than stuffing. She responded that it was because her husband wanted potatoes with his evening meal. In other words, she had a normative belief that her husband didn't want her to purchase stuffing. Rather, he preferred her to purchase potatoes. In the next scene in the commercial, the announcer proceeded to show her a videotape of her husband saying in an interview that he would prefer stuffing rather than potatoes with his evening meal. This was a clear example of an *intervention* trying to change a subjective normative belief.

Perhaps an even more important contribution of the TRA is the fundamental distinction between attitude towards a behavior and attitude towards an object. Think of this: attitude towards the behavior rather than the attitude towards the object should be used to predict behavioral intentions. Although this distinction between attitude towards a behavior and an object may also seem natural and intuitive, until Fishbein made the distinction, researchers had been trying to use attitude towards the object to try to predict single behaviors. One still sees researchers today unaware of the model, using attitudes towards the object when trying to predict and understand a particular behavior. Poor prediction will typically be the result?a point reinforced by Montano and Kasprzyk in their chapter. General condom attitude measures were poor predictors of condom use intentions in their study.

The behavioral focus of the model is probably a critical reason for its extraordinary impact in so many fields. Its contribution to our understanding of health-related behavioral intentions and behavior has been particularly heartening to so many people. The chapters in this section are fine examples of the information that can be learned and insight that can be gained about health behaviors from using the TRA and the theory of planned behavior (TPB), an extension of it.

Another reason for the exceptional impact of the TRA is that it is a structural model of behavioral intentions with clearly identifiable underlying components. The model specifies the component(s), that is, the reason(s) why a person intends to or does not intend to engage in a behavior. In other words, it specifies the underlying drivers and subdrivers of intentions. By isolating components that may potentially be in need of change, it offers guidance to a potential change agent as to how to proceed with an intervention.

Typically, intentions are changed by changing the belief components of the model. Although generally this might be true, I have a personal illustration of a situation in which another component of the model was the key to change, namely the evaluative aspect (e_i) of the model. I was a research assistant in a continuing education department when I was doing my PhD in psychology at Penn State. I was fresh out of my exposure to Prof. Fishbein and his approach. The department in which I was a research assistant was having the following problem. Registration was down in the management development courses they were offering in the various cities and towns in the state. I proceeded to use Fishbein's approach to try to understand why this was the case. It turned out that it wasn't because potential participants didn't believe that attending these courses would have the outcomes that were promoted. They believed they would. Interestingly and surprisingly, it was because they did not evaluate the evaluative aspects of these beliefs (the e_i s), very favorably. They already knew that attending these courses might, for example, raise their chances for a promotion, but they didn't evaluate being promoted very positively. They felt that a promotion would entail moving to headquarters, which was usually located in another town or city rather than the one they lived in, and they didn't want to move. In fact, in most cases, the truth was that they could be promoted without having to move. As a result, by isolating the drivers of intentions, the model diagnostically identified an intervention to make the courses more attractive. The strategy was to change the evaluative aspects of the beliefs?in this case the outcomes associated with *performing* the behavior of attending these courses—rather than the beliefs themselves.

Often salient outcomes reflect strong *visceral influences* (e.g., emotions/ drives) rather than attributes like increasing one's chances of promotion (see Lowenstein (1996) for a very interesting discussion of visceral influences on behavior). As an example, take the beliefs in the Montano and Kasprzyk chapter. Preliminary one-on-one, open-ended interviews and focus group discussions with the target population revealed that the salient beliefs associated with condom use intentions included such outcomes as "being embarrassing," "getting less pleasure," and "not having a sexual release."

Often these visceral influences will however go unmentioned when people are asked for important salient outcomes in the elicitation stage. For example, visceral influences associated with condom use—from sexual desire to embarrassment?may not be fully appreciated outside the situation in which they are experienced. In other words, people will tend to have difficulty anticipating the degree of influence of these visceral factors on their behavior; visceral influences are likely to be underappreciated until they are actually experienced (Lowenstein, 1996). This renders the task of assessment with any instrument removed from the actual situation very difficult. That said, there are perhaps a number of things that might be done to increase the likelihood of the elicitation of visceral factors in the elicitation stage of the application of the TRA/TRB models.[1] If elicitation is done in the actual situation in which we seek to predict behavior or behavioral intentions from attitude, then visceral influences associated with the behavior are more likely to be generated and thus more easily captured. For example, contrast the attributes that might be elicited regarding a hot sports car either via telephone interview or as the individual is actually in the car about to drive it. If eliciting attributes in the latter situation is not possible, then the elicitation might minimally be done close in time to the actual situation, for example, just before an individual is going to test drive the car. As we now know, behavioral intentions are better predictors of behavior if measured close in time to the behavior. The longer the time interval between the two, "the greater the likelihood that unforeseen events will produce changes in intentions" (Ajzen, 1988, p.115). Analogously, visceral influences on behavior are most likely to be captured if the elicitation is done proximate to the behavior.

One approach that might be effective in eliciting relevant visceral factors is encouraging people to project themselves into the situation. Encouraging projection during the elicitation phase might be effective in bringing relevant visceral

---

[1]See Ajzen and Fishbein (2005) for a discussion of some similar and different approaches for dealing with visceral influences.

influences to the surface. Take for example Wolitski and Zhang's chapter. They found that the TRA and TPB variables were significant predictors of condom use, but also that much variance was left unexplained. Perhaps some of this variance could be explained by visceral forces people only feel in the "heat of the moment." One way to capture these influences might be to encourage participants to literally visualize themselves in a specific sexual situation. MacDonald, Fong, Zanna, & Martineau (2000) used a hypothetical scenario with a sexually charged scene between a young man and woman to set the stage for the dependent measure: should the couple go ahead with unprotected sex or not? This same approach could readily be used to arouse the passions of the participants during elicitation.

Drinking alcohol is of course common in many cultures (see for example Montano and Kasprzyk chapter and their report of the percentage of men [56%] who drink in Zimbabwe: 74% get drunk monthly) and sexual behavior is commonly associated with drinking. Alcohol consumption leads to *alcohol myopia*, which when it comes to sexual behavior leads to a greater focus on the physical pleasures associated with having sex than on the costs (MacDonald et al., 2000). To pick up salient outcomes when people are drinking, perhaps elicitation could be done with participants after they have consumed a moderate amount of alcohol. It might even be possible to do the elicitation in a real situation like a bar. It is in more realistic sexual contexts that people ought to be sensitized to relevant factors and elicitation of these would be enhanced.

There may still remain emotional or other outcomes that are not mentioned by a person during elicitation because the person is unaware of them or cannot verbalize them. Under these circumstances, indirect techniques might be helpful. If hidden motivations, emotional or otherwise, are uncovered in this way, it might then be possible to assess their salience during elicitation.

I would like to use the research my colleagues and I have conducted on the acquisition of condoms as an example of an emotion whose significance at least some of the participants in our research did not fully appreciate. We found that quite a few people who at least said they were not embarrassed at all about purchasing condoms, nevertheless engaged in activities that suggested otherwise. They used what have been termed *coping strategies*. These coping strategies included engaging in behaviors like deliberately "spending as little time in the aisle as possible" or "buying other items with condoms," and "self-talking," such as saying to themselves, "I shouldn't be embarrassed because stores sell condoms every day" or "I go over in my mind what I will say or do." Eighty-four percent of participants who had indicated that they felt no embarrassment at all about purchasing condoms still used at least one of these coping strategies (Moore, Dahl, Gorn, & Weinberg, 2006). The coping activities of these supposedly unembarrassed respondents therefore suggested that they were not fully aware that they were at least somewhat embarrassed about purchasing condoms. Discussions with people who said they were not embarrassed at all revealed that it wasn't that they were reluctant to admit being embarrassed, rather, they were indeed just unaware of their actual embarrassment. One could speculate that if their (coping) strategies were pointed out to them, and they recognized that they did not engage in comparable coping strategies when buying everyday products like toothpaste, they might accept the fact that they were at least somewhat embarrassed when they purchased condoms.[2] Framing the elicitation this way should encourage this group of people to recognize their embarrassment. As a different example of how difficult it can be to elicit a significant but non-apparent motive, consider the power of attractive older models for kids who universally want to grow up as soon/fast as possible. Are kids aware of or can they verbalize this powerful influence/motivation? Perhaps and perhaps not. It would be up to the researcher to sensitively frame the elicitation context and procedure.

Now consider for a moment the dependent variable side of the TRA and TPB equations, the behavioral side. The Middlestadt chapter discusses the importance of identifying and selecting the right behavior to target in the health promotion area, the difficulty in doing so, and how to resolve (overcome) difficulties. Consistent with previous research, the determinants of behavior are seen to vary as a function of the particular behavior examined. Regarding sexual behavior, Middlestadt discusses her previous research showing that trust was a more important determinant of condom use with a steady partner than a non-steady or new partner. The Montano and Kasprzyk chapter provides additional evidence for this. In their study, the determinants of condom use intentions in their study varied as a function of the nature of the relationship between the person and their sexual partner.

The Yzer chapter takes a different tack and focuses on the moderating role of perceived control. In a very interesting chapter, Yzer goes through the intuitive logic for expecting perceived control interactions. Despite this logic, the amount of research examining them has been modest, with the results of the studies that have been carried out modest as well. The latter he primarily attributes to the constraints associated with the use of a correlational approach, and he notes that all of the previous research examining perceived control interactions has been correlational. Yzer calls for more research, particularly experimental research.

The modest variance explained in intentions by perceived control interactions in previous research raises an additional question. What criteria should be used in deciding what beliefs to target with an intervention? In addition to the variance explained by a predictor, the focus of the chapters in this book section, consideration might also be given to an intervention's likely success in influencing the predictor, or as Hornik and Woolf (1999) put it, "whether or not the predictor belief is 'movable.'" Here, previous research on the relevant target population, or similar ones, could provide some guidance. Some of a person's attitudinal or normative beliefs may be just too difficult to change. Perhaps the normative belief regarding whether the spouse wanted her husband to use a condom is such a belief. It might be very difficult to change the normative belief of a person who felt that his spouse would be suspicious if he used a condom; in other words, he believes that using a condom might spoil their relationship.

---

[2]Of course, this would have to be done carefully so as to increase condom purchase. One wouldn't want people to be less likely to purchase condoms because they were now aware that they were in fact embarrassed about purchasing them.

Finally, the Montano and Kasprzyk and Wolitski and Zhang chapters made me curious about the cultures in which the research was conducted. In their sample of high risk men in rural Zimbabwe, Montano and Kasprzyk found that subjective norms were less important than attitude in predicting condom use intentions with a spouse, but the reverse was true with regard to condom use intentions with a steady partner. Are there any aspects of the Zimbabwean culture that might help explain this finding? Similarly, in Wolitski and Zhang, could explanations, perhaps even hypotheses, be derived by considering some aspects of the culture of males who have sex with males?

CONCLUSION

The chapters in this section affirm the predictive power of the theories of reasoned action and planned behavior. They testify to the importance of isolating the different components underlying a particular health-related intention/behavior of interest. Doing so enables key drivers to be identified. This not only increases our understanding of the intention/behavior, but also provides areas of focus for an intervention effort as well. The knowledge gained regarding the behavioral intentions/behaviors associated with an increased risk of acquiring the HIV is a particular emphasis in two of the chapters.

In addition to discussing the chapters in this section, this commentary points out some of the more general and key contributions of the two models. Suggestions are also put forward regarding procedures for how they might better capture salient visceral outcomes.

ACKNOWLEDGMENTS

I would like to thank Marv Goldberg, Jaideep Sengupta, and Bob Wyer for their helpful comments.

REFERENCES

Ajzen, I., & Fishbein, M. (2005). The influence of attitudes on behavior. In D. Albarracín, B. T. Johnson, & M. Zanna (Eds.), *The handbook of attitudes* (pp. 173–221). Mahwah, NJ: Lawrence Erlbaum Associates.

Ajzen, I. (1988). *Attitudes, personality, and behavior*. Chicago: The Dorsey Press.

Hornik, R. & Woolf, K. D. (1996). Using cross-sectional surveys to plan message strategies. *Social Marketing Quarterly, 5,* 34–41.

Lowenstein, G. (1996). Out of control: Visceral influences on behavior. *Organizational Behavior and Human Decision Processes, 65*, 272–292.

MacDonald, T. K., Fong, G. T., Zanna, M. P., & Martineau, A. M. (2000). Alcohol myopia and condom use: Can alcohol intoxication be associated with more prudent behavior? *Journal of Personality and Social Psychology, 78,* 605–619.

Moore, S. G., Dahl, D. W., Gorn, G. J., & Weinberg, C. B. (2006). Coping with condom purchase embarrassment. *Psychology, Health, and Medicine, 11*, 70–79.

CHAPTER 14

Exploring HIV Serosorting as a Preventive Behavior Among Men Who Have Sex with Men, Using a Comprehensive Approach to Behavioral Science Theory

Emily Hopkins and Cornelis A. Rietmeijer

Denver Public Health Department, Colorado

Serosorting, defined as selecting sex partners and deciding on sexual practices based on perceived seroconcordance of partners, appears to be an increasingly adopted behavior among men who have sex with men (MSM) as a means to prevent the transmission and acquisition of HIV (Parsons et al., 2005). Recent reports have described the increase of this behavior both among persons known to be HIV seropositive (Elford, Bolding, Sherr, & Hart, 2005; McConnell & Grant, 2003), and HIV negative (Truong, McFarland, Kellogg, & Dilley, 2004). In a recent analysis of MSM visiting a sexually transmitted infection (STI) clinic in Denver, consistent serosorting was reported by 47% of HIV-positive men and by 38% of HIV-negative men, while 70% of men reported serostatus discussion with at least one partner during the previous 4 months. In this study, MSM who recruited sex partners on the Internet were more likely to serosort than MSM who recruited partners in other venues such as gay bathhouses.(Rietmeijer, Lloyd, & McLean, 2006). Thus, the increasing popularity of the Internet as a place where sex partners may be found (Elford, Bolding, & Sherr, 2001; McFarlane, Bull, & Rietmeijer, 2000; Rietmeijer, Bull, & McFarlane, 2001), may have been an important factor in the increase of serosorting as a preventive behavior. While one study has shown that serosorting was associated with lower risk of HIV acquisition (Golden, Brewer, Kurth, Holmes, & Handsfield, 2004), public health officials have been divided in sending messages to endorse this behavior. Some are supportive, believing that serosorting may be responsible for the paradoxical fact that while non-HIV STIs including gonorrhea and syphilis have been increasing among MSM since the mid-nineties, HIV incidence has not (Murphy, 2005). Others are more reserved, feeling that HIV serosorting can never be perfect, thus resulting in HIV transmission, while also expressing concern that serosorting may lead to transmission of other non-HIV STI and to superinfection with drug-resistant HIV among those already HIV positive (Simao, 2005). Clearly, more research is needed to inform this debate. In this chapter, we present an analysis of differences in psychological antecedents related to serosorting and condom use behaviors using concepts from a comprehensive approach to behavioral science theory as forwarded by Fishbein and Guinan (1996), which incorporates concepts from the Theory of Reasoned Action (Fishbein & Ajzen, 1975), Social Cognitive Theory (Bandura, 1986), the Health Belief Model (Rosenstock, Strecher, & Becker, 1994), and the Transtheoretical Model.(Prochaska & Velicer, 1997a).

Methods

This project was intended as a small, hypothesis-generating study among high-risk MSM. Thus, MSM who reported at least one occasional sex partner with whom they engaged in anal sex were eligible for this study. MSM were recruited from the Denver Public Health (DPH) Denver Metro Health Clinic, the largest STI clinic and HIV-testing site in the Rocky Mountain region; from the DPH Infectious Diseases/AIDS clinic; and from one of Denver's gay bathhouses, where DPH regularly conducts outreach activities. As the study was conducted anonymously, eligible men who agreed to be in the study were consented verbally. The study was comprised of an interviewer-administered, paper-based survey comprised of 45 items that typically took 20 minutes to complete. Study participants received a $25.00 reimbursement. The study was determined to be exempt from review by the Colorado Multiple Institutional Review Board.

Survey items were adapted from the Brief Street Intercept (BSI) survey that was used in the CDC AIDS Community Demonstration Projects (CDC AIDS Community Demonstration Projects Research Group, 1999). The BSI was based on a comprehensive approach to behavioral science theory specifically aimed at its utility for use in public health settings to inform the development of HIV prevention interventions (Fishbein & Guinan, 1996). Survey items analyzed for the purposes of this chapter are summarized in the Appendix.

We assessed condom use and serosorting behaviors and its determinants at three levels. First, we asked questions about consistency of current behaviors. We defined consistent condom use as reporting the use of condoms for anal sex with a new partner *every* time for at least 6 months. Likewise, consistent serosorting was defined as discussing HIV serostatus every time when having anal sex with a new partner for at least 6 months.

Next, we assessed long-term and short-term intentions to condom use and serosorting and combined this with reported behaviors in a stage of change model (Prochaska & DiClemente, 1993; Prochaska & Velicer, 1997b). We defined the following stages: (1) Precontemplation: no or infrequent condom use or serosorting and little or no intention to always use condoms/serosort in the future; (2) Contemplation: no or infrequent condom use or serosorting but intention to begin doing so consistently in the near future (6 months); (3) Preparation: infrequent condom or serosorting, but intention to do so in the immediate future; (4) Action: Consistent condom use/serosorting for less than 6 months; (5) Maintenance: Consistent condom use/serosorting for 6 or more months (CDC AIDS Community Demonstration Projects Research Group, 1999). The value given to the stage of change variable corresponded to the stage rank, that is "1" for precontemplation, "2" for contemplation, etc. Third, we assessed attitudes towards condom use and serosorting, beliefs about the positive and negative consequences of performing these behaviors, perception of social norms, and self-efficacy (Fishbein & Guinan, 1996). Attitudes, the overall positive or negative feelings about performing the behavior, were assessed by using questions about how wise/foolish, good/bad, important/unimportant, and pleasant/unpleasant the use of condoms and serosorting were felt to be as measured on 7-point Likert scales. Outcome expectations were also assessed on 7-point Likert scales, asking respondents how sure they were that consistently using condoms or serosorting would protect them from HIV or STIs. Perceived norms were assessed by asking how many people the respondent knew that consistently performed these behaviors (on a 5-point Likert scale) and whether people important to the respondent think that the respondent should or should not perform these behaviors (3-point Likert scale). Finally, using 7-point Likert scales, self-efficacy was assessed by asking how sure the respondent was that if they wanted to use a condom or serosort, they in fact could, and how much control they felt they would have over these behaviors when having anal sex with a new partner. More detail on the survey items are given in the Appendix.

For each of these detailed variables we were specifically interested in how these measures of cognitions would differ between the two behaviors, that is, condom use and serosorting, at the individual level. Assessing such differences would be important to increase understanding of the antecedents to these behaviors, and thus for the development of prevention interventions. Regardless of any differences, we were also interested to learn how these measures would be correlated between the two behaviors. We hypothesized that if a propensity to prevention-oriented behaviors would underlie both condom use and serosorting, then a strong positive association between these two behaviors would be observed at the individual level. If, by contrast, serosorting would be employed as a preventive behavior in lieu of or to avoid condom use, then a negative correlation would be observed. Statistical tests for differences and correlations included the McNemar and chi-square statistics for binominal data and Wilcoxon's signed rank and Spearman correlation for ordinal data, including those obtained from Likert scale measures. All analyses were conducted using the SAS statistical software package, version 8.1 (SAS Institute, Cary, NC).

Results

A total of 71 MSM were enrolled in the study. Of these, 38 (53.5%) were enrolled in the STI clinic and HIV-testing site, 30 (42.3%) in the bathhouse, and 3 (4.2%) in the ID/AIDS clinic. The demographic characteristics of the sample were very similar to the populations from which they were drawn: 71.9% Caucasian, 20.3% Hispanic, 4.7% African American, and 3.1% other. The mean age was 34.3 years (range: 19–63). Nine (12.7%) men were HIV-infected (by self-report). Respondents reported a mean of 7.7 (median 3.0) sex partners in the previous 2 months, and a mean of 4.0 (median 2.0) sex partners with whom they engaged in anal sex.

Of the 71 men, 37 (52.1%) reported consistent condom use or consistent serosorting; 27 (38.3%) men reported consistent condom use and 20 (28.2%) reported consistent serosorting. Seventeen (23.9%) reported consistent condom use alone, 10 (14.1%) reported consistent serosorting alone, 10 (14.1%) reported both consistent condom use and consistent serosorting, and 34 (47.9%) reported neither consistent condom use nor consistent serosorting. At the individual level, consistent condom use and consistent serosorting were neither significantly different nor associated. Thus, men were not more likely to be consistent condom users than to be consistent serosorters ($P = 0.25$, McNemar's test), and men who were consistent condom users were not more likely to be consistent serosorters ($P = 0.19$, Chi-Square test).

Stage of Change

The stage of change measure showed a difference in distribution between the two behaviors (Figure 14–1), with a shift towards higher stages when comparing condom use to serosorting. In fact, 34 (49.3%) men were in the precontemplation or contemplation stages for serosorting, compared to 14 (19.7%) men who were in these stages for condom use. On the 5-point continuum, respondents scored a mean of 3.42 for condom use (between preparation stage and action stage) and 2.76 for serosorting (between contemplation stage and preparation stage). This difference of 0.66 stage was significantly different ($P < 0.01$). However, stages for condom use and serosorting were not associated at the individual level (Rho = 0.16, $P = 0.22$).

Attitudes

Respondents scored high (i.e., lower scores) on the wise/foolish, good/bad, and important/unimportant scales indicating equally favorable attitudes toward condom use and serosorting. When comparing these measures for the two behaviors, we found that men scored slightly higher on each of these scales for condom use compared to serosorting and that these differences were significant. However, in comparing these measures for correlation, we found only the good/bad scale and the important/unimportant (STI) scale to be associated between behaviors. Generally less favorable scores were found on the pleasant/unpleasant scale for both behaviors, with serosorting found to be significantly more unpleasant than condom use ($P < 0.05$). This attitude was not correlated between the two behaviors (Table 14–1).

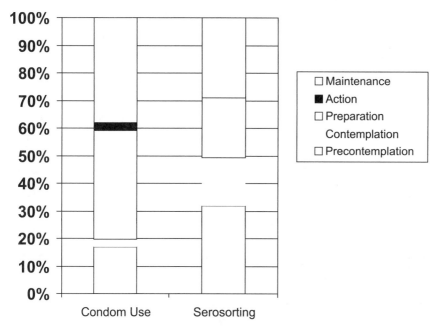

FIGURE 14–1.   Stage of change for condom use and HIV serosorting.

Outcome Expectancies

Outcome expectancies, that is, perceptions among respondents that condom use or serosorting will protect against the acquisition of HIV and other STI, were much more favorable for condom use than for serosorting. This difference was slightly stronger for STI other than HIV, but the differences were statistically significant for both. By contrast, there was no correlation when comparing the two behaviors (Table 14–1).

Perceived Social Norms

Men in the study perceived that people they know are more likely to use condoms when they have anal sex with a new partner than to serosort. They also perceived greater normative pressure for condom use than for serosorting. These differences were statistically significant. Normative pressure on condom use and serosorting was correlated, but perceived behavior performed by others was not (Table 14–1).

Self-Efficacy

Respondents scored equally high on the two self-efficacy measurements for condom use and serosorting, although a small, yet significant difference was found for how sure one could perform the behavior. However, there were statistically significant correlations when comparing these measures for condom use and for serosorting, indicating that men who had high levels of self-efficacy towards condom use also had higher levels of efficacy towards serosorting (Table 14–1).

TABLE 14-1.
Differences and Correlations Between Factors Influencing Condom Use and Serosorting Among High-Risk Men Who Have Sex with Men

	Item #*	Condom Use		Serosorting		Difference**		Correlation***	
		Mean	Median	Mean	Median	S	P	Rho	P
Attitudes									
Behavior is									
Wise/Foolish	7	1.14	1	1.36	1	52.50	<0.05	0.11	NS
Good/Bad	8	1.10	1	1.30	1	42.50	<0.05	0.25	<0.05
Important/Unimportant (for HIV)	9	1.47	1	1.92	1	173.50	<0.05	0.21	NS
Important/Unimportant (for STI)	10	1.55	1	2.05	2	183.00	<0.001	0.26	<0.05
Pleasant/Unpleasant	11	3.31	3	4.08	5	187.00	<0.05	0.12	NS
Outcome Expectancies									
Behavior will protect against:									
HIV	12	1.98	2	3.10	3	501.50	<0.0001	-0.01	NS
STI other than HIV	13	1.95	2	3.18	3	404.00	<0.0001	0.22	NS
Perceived Social Norms									
Behavior performed by others	14	2.67	3	3.22	3	215.00	<0.0004	-0.13	NS
Influence on behavior by others	15/16	1.21	1	1.50	1	-96.5	<0.0001	0.29	<0.05
Self-Efficacy									
How sure could perform behavior	17	1.51	1	1.77	1	91.5	<0.05	0.33	<0.01
How much control	18	6.38	7	6.21	7	21.5	NS	0.28	<0.05

*See Appendix
** Wilcoxon Rank Sum Test
*** Spearman Correlation

CONCLUSION

In a sample of high-risk MSM, we found that self-reports of consistent serosorting were slightly less common than reports of consistent condom use. However, when combining current behaviors with long-term and short-term intentions to perform these behaviors in a stage of change model, we found that respondents scored higher (i.e., further along in the stages of change) for condom use than for serosorting. When assessing factors theorized to influence these behaviors, this stage of change difference was reflected in generally lower favorable scores for attitudes, outcome expectancies, and perceived social norms when comparing serosorting to condom use.

There are a number of limitations to this study that prompt us to interpret these findings cautiously. Men in the study were recruited from high-risk venues and were selected on high-risk behavior (i.e., reporting anal sex with a new partner in the past 4 months) and are thus not representative of MSM in general, limiting the generalizability of our results. Furthermore, we have found in previous studies that men who recruit sex partners in bathhouses are less likely to serosort than MSM who recruit partners in other venues. Thus, the fact that more than 40% of study participants were recruited in a bathhouse may have biased our results toward less favorable assessment of serosorting. Due to our small sample size we were not able to conduct subanalyses to investigate this bias. Because of the small sample, the study may have also missed power to detect subtle differences. Differences may also have been obscured by the choice of measurements. For example, respondents invariably scored high on a number of variables, for example, the wise/foolish and good/bad constructs that suggested that these variables may not have been sufficiently discriminatory and that other attitudinal measurements may be needed.

With these caveats in mind, what do we conclude from our data? From a public health perspective, there are two findings that may assist us with the ongoing development and implementation of interventions aimed at HIV prevention. First, there was a clear difference when we compared outcome expectations among men in our study for consistent condom use versus serosorting. In other words, these men feel that serosorting is a less secure way of preventing HIV than condom use. If others in the respondent's social environment and sexual networks are perceived to feel the same way, than it is understandable that these men do not perceive much of a social norm for serosorting and may thus conclude that serosorting is of less importance to them, even though they feel quite capable of performing this behavior.

The relatively unfavorable outcome expectations for serosorting find a corollary in the ambivalence espoused by public health officials with some endorsing this behavior (Murphy, 2005) and others expressing concerns (Simao, 2005). Clearly, relying solely on serosorting comes with a certain risk, particularly among those who are not infected. Serosorting among HIV-infected individuals will likely result in an HIV-seroconcordant sexual encounter, given that lying about a positive serostatus is not that common. However, persons who indicate that they are not infected may be more likely to be untruthful about their status and, even if truthful, may have seroconverted since their last HIV-negative test. Still, it could be argued that while not fail-safe, any serosorting is probably better than no serosorting at all, assuming that serosorting itself does not increase high-risk behaviors. One study, conducted in a large urban STI clinic, found that after controlling for other risk factors, any unprotected anal sex with a partner of unknown or positive HIV status was the only factor associated with newly-diagnosed HIV infections. Moreover, HIV negative men in this study who reported unprotected anal sex with other men they perceived to be HIV-negative had similar risks for HIV infection as men who denied any unprotected anal intercourse (Golden et al.,2004).

A second finding in our study was the apparent lack of positive or negative correlation between condom use and serosorting stage of change and the cognitive factor that seemed to differentiate most strongly between the two behaviors, that is, outcome expectancies. This was somewhat surprising as we assumed that risk-averse persons might be more likely to combine risk-prevention strategies. On the other hand, a negative correlation might have suggested that persons who favor serosorting may less favor the use condoms, thus leading to the concern that more serosorting would come to the detriment of condom use. However, the absence of or weak correlations between the cognitions associated with the two behaviors indicates that serosorting and condom use behaviors and their behavioral antecedents may operate relatively independently. This is important because this would indicate that serosorting is not just another preventive behavior that is added to or comes in lieu of other preventive behaviors, but rather a behavior that may be considered regardless of other preventive behaviors, condom use in particular. This may also imply that serosorting messages may reach a different segment of the at-risk population.

While serosorting may prevent HIV transmission, there are other risks to this behavior when performed without concomitant condom use. These risks include the transmission of other non-HIV STIs and the possibility of superinfection with drug-resistant HIV strains among those who are HIV infected. More research is clearly needed to determine the pros and cons of serosorting and thus bolster the public health case for HIV serosorting as behavior for which interventions may be developed. Our study indicates that stronger and more unified public health messages may enhance outcome expectations of this behavior among MSM, and thus increase serosorting behaviors.

ACKNOWLEDGMENTS

The authors wish to thank Wayne Johnson, PhD, at the Centers for Disease Control and Prevention, for his advice on statistical methods.

REFERENCES

Bandura, A. (1986). *Social foundations of thought and action: A social cognitive theory.* Englewood Cliffs, NJ: Prentice Hall.

CDC AIDS Community Demonstration Projects Research Group. (1999). Community-level HIV Intervention in five cities: Final outcome data from the CDC AIDS Community Demonstration Projects. *American Journal of Public Health, 89,* 336–345.

Elford, J., Bolding, G., & Sherr, L. (2001). Seeking sex on the Internet and sexual risk behaviour among gay men using London gyms. *AIDS, 15*, 1409–1415.

Elford, J., Bolding, G., Sherr, L., & Hart, G. (2005). High-risk sexual behaviour among London gay men: No longer increasing. *AIDS, 19*, 2171–2174.

Fishbein, M., & Ajzen, I. (1975). *Belief, attitude, intention and behavior: An introduction to theory and research*. Reading, MA: Addison-Wesley.

Fishbein, M., & Guinan, M. (1996). Behavioral science and public health: A necessary partnership for HIV prevention [editorial]. *Public Health Rep, 111*(Suppl. 1), 5–10.

Golden, M. R., Brewer, D. D., Kurth, A., Holmes, K. K., & Handsfield, H. H. (2004). Importance of Sex Partner HIV Status in HIV Risk Assessment Among Men Who have Sex With Men. *Journal of Acquired Immune Deficiency Syndrome, 36*, 734–742.

McConnell, J., & Grant, R. (2003). *Sorting out serosorting with sexual network methods*. Paper presented at the 10th Conference on Retroviruses and Opportunistic Infections, Boston, MA.

McFarlane, M., Bull, S. S., & Rietmeijer, C. A. (2000). The Internet as a newly emerging risk environment for sexually transmitted diseases. *Journal of the American Medical Association, 284*, 443–446.

Murphy, D. (2005, August 18). A good report on AIDS, and some credit the Web. *The New York Times*.

Parsons, J. T., Schrimshaw, E. W., Wolitski, R. J., Halkitis, P. N., Purcell, D. W., Hoff, C. C., et al. (2005). Sexual harm reduction practices of HIV-seropositive gay and bisexual men: Serosorting, strategic positioning, and withdrawal before ejaculation. *AIDS, 19*(Suppl. 1), 13–25.

Prochaska, J. O., & DiClemente, C. C. (1993). Stages and processes of self-change in smoking: Towards an integrative model of change. *Journal of Consulting in Clinical Psychology, 51*, 390–395.

Prochaska, J. O., & Velicer, W. F. (1997). The transtheoretical model of behavior change. *American Journal of Health Promotion, 12*, 38–48.

Rietmeijer, C., Lloyd, L., & McLean, C. (2006). Discussing HIV serostatus with prospective sex partners: A potential HIV prevention strategy among high-risk men who have sex with men. *Sexually Transmitted Diseases*.

Rietmeijer, C. A., Bull, S. S., & McFarlane, M. (2001). Sex and the internet [comment]. *AIDS, 15*, 1433–1434.

Rosenstock, I., Strecher, V., & Becker, M. (1994). The health belief model and HIV risk behavior change. In R. DiClemente & J. Peterson (Eds.), *Preventing AIDS. Theories and methods of behavioral interventions*. New York: Plenum Press.

Simao, P. (2005). Internet fueling risky sex among gay men. Retrieved January 10, 2006, from http://www.msnbc.msn.com/id/8232157

Truong, H., McFarland, W., Kellogg, T., & Dilley, J. (2004). *Increases in "serosorting" may prevent further expansion of the HIV epidemic among MSM in San Francisco*. Paper presented at the 11th Conference on Retroviruses and Opportunistic Infections, San Francisco, CA.

Appendix - Survey Questions

Item #	Question	Response format
1.	When you have anal sex with a new male partner, how often do you use a condom/serosort?	1 - every time, 2 - almost every time, 3 - sometimes, 4 - almost never, 5 - never
2.	How long have you been using a condom (every time/almost every time) you have anal sex with a new male partner?	1 - in the last 30 days, 2 - more than 30 days - less than 6 months, 3-6 months ago or more
3.	In the next six months, how likely do you think it is that you will start using a condom/discuss serostatus every time you have anal sex with a new male partner?	1 - extremely sure I will; 2 - quite sure I will 3 - slightly sure I will; 4 - undecided; not sure if I will or won't; 5 - slightly sure I won't; 6 - quite sure I won't; 7 - extremely sure I won't
4.	How likely do you think it is that from now on you will use a condom/discuss serostatus every time you have anal sex with a new male partner?	1 - extremely sure I will; 2 - quite sure I will 3 - slightly sure I will; 4 - undecided; not sure if I will or won't; 5 - slightly sure I won't; 6 - quite sure I won't; 7 - extremely sure I won't
5.	How likely do you think it is that you could get HIV by having anal sex with a new male partner without using a condom/discussing serostatus?	1 - extremely likely; 2 - quite likely; 3 - slightly likely; 4 - undecided; not sure 5 - slightly unlikely; 6 - quite unlikely; 7 - extremely unlikely
6.	How likely do you think it is that you could get STIs, other than HIV, by having anal sex with a new male partner without using a condom/discussing serostatus?	1 - extremely likely; 2 - quite likely; 3 - slightly likely; 4 - undecided; not sure 5 - slightly unlikely; 6 - quite unlikely; 7 - extremely unlikely
7.	Do you think that using a condom/discussing serostatus every time you have anal sex with a new male partner would be extremely, quite, or slightly wise or foolish?	1 - extremely wise; 2 - quite wise; 3 - slightly wise; 4 - undecided; not sure 5 - slightly foolish; 6 - quite foolish; 7 - extremely foolish
8.	Do you think that using a condom/discussing serostatus every time you have anal sex with a new male partner would be extremely, quite, or slightly good or bad?	1 - extremely good; 2 - quite good; 3 - slightly good; 4 - undecided; not sure 5 - slightly bad; 6 - quite bad; 7 - extremely bad
9.	How important or unimportant is it to you to use a condom/discuss serostatus when you have anal sex with a new male partner in order to protect yourself from HIV?	1 - extremely important; 2 - quite important; 3 - slightly important; 4 - undecided; not sure; 5 - slightly unimportant; 6 - quite unimportant; 7 - extremely unimportant
10.	How important or unimportant is it to you to use a condom/discuss serostatus when you have anal sex with a new male partner in order to protect yourself from STIs other than HIV?	1 - extremely important; 2 - quite important; 3 - slightly important; 4 - undecided; not sure; 5 - slightly unimportant; 6 - quite unimportant; 7 - extremely unimportant

(continued)

Appendix—Continued

11.	Do you think that using a condom/discussing serostatus every time you have anal sex with a new male partner would be extremely, quite, or slightly pleasant or unpleasant?	1 - extremely pleasant; 2 - quite pleasant; 3 - slightly pleasant; 4 - undecided; not sure 5 - slightly unpleasant; 6 - quite unpleasant; 7 - extremely unpleasant
12.	How sure are you that always using a condom/discussing serostatus when you have anal sex with a new male partner will protect you from HIV?	1 - extremely sure it will; 2 - quite sure it will; 3 - slightly sure it will; 4 - undecided; not sure it will or won't 5 - slightly sure it won't; 6 - quite sure it won't; 7 - extremely sure it won't
13.	How sure are you that always using a condom/discussing serostatus when you have anal sex with a new male partner will protect you from STIs other than HIV?	1 - extremely sure it will; 2 - quite sure it will; 3 - slightly sure it will; 4 - undecided; not sure it will or won't 5 - slightly sure it won't; 6 - quite sure it won't; 7 - extremely sure it won't
14.	How many of the people you know use a condom/discuss serostatus every time they have anal sex with a new male partner?	1 - all or almost all; 2 - most; 3 - half do-half don't; 4 - very few; 5 - none or almost none
15.	Would you say that most of the people who are important to you think you should or should not use a condom/discuss serostatus every time you have anal sex with a new male partner? (By important people I mean people like friends, family, a social worker, someone at church or in a clinic, or anyone else who you feel is important to you).	1 - should; 2 - should not
16.	How strongly do you think they feel about that?	1 - strongly; 2 - somewhat strongly; 3 - not very strongly
17	Now this is just a "what if" question, but if you wanted to use a condom/discuss serostatus every time you have anal sex with a new male partner how sure are you that you could?	1 - extremely sure I could; 2 - quite sure I could 3 - slightly sure I could ; 4 - undecided; not sure if I could or couldn't; 5 - slightly sure I couldn't; 6 - quite sure I couldn't 7 - extremely sure I couldn't
18.	How much control do you believe you have in using a condom/discussing serostatus every time you have anal sex with a new male partner?	7-point Likert scale, ranging from 1 (not at all) to 7 (very much)

CHAPTER 15

Extension of Theory of Reasoned Action: Principles for Health Promotion Programs with Marginalized Populations in Latin America

Susan Pick[1]

Universidad Nacional Autónoma de México (UNAM) and Instituto Mexicano de Investigación de Familia y Población (IMIFAP), Mexico City

This chapter provides an account of an approach to health promotion programming developed and implemented at Instituto Mexicano de Investigación de Familia y Población (IMIFAP) a Non-Government Organization (NGO) in Mexico. Much of the approach has been inspired by the Theory of Reasoned Action (TRA). Specifically, programs and workshops are designed to produce changes in specific behaviors. At the same time, uncertainties in the functioning of key constructs, such as intentions and attitudes, among underprivileged groups in Latin America suggest a need for some extensions or adaptations in the use of the theory. A second issue addressed is how broader effects of programs, reported widely in the literature and compatible with IMIFAP's field experience, should be accounted for.

The chapter starts with an example of a program for promotion of health behavior among women in South Mexican communities and illustrates how participants attribute behavior changes to the program that go beyond the targeted behaviors. The next section discusses the implications for norms, attitudes, and intentions of conditions of economic and social adversity, where people have little control over their lives and perceived choices of action are few. The third section outlines the Framework for Enabling Agentic Empowerment (FENAE),

---

[1]Written during a fellowship at Harvard University School of Public Health.

which is a conceptual summary of IMIFAP's approach. The notion of agency is presented as a way to deal with the issue of generalization of program effects. In a brief concluding section some major points of convergence are mentioned not only between TRA and FENAE, but encompassing a wider range of perspectives, including development economics.

AN EXAMPLE OF A HEALTH PROMOTION PROGRAM FOR WOMEN

Let me start with a description of one program for health promotion. The program was originally called "*Si yo estoy bien, mi familia también*"[2] (If I am OK, so is my family; Venguer et al., 2002; Venguer, Pick, & Fishbein, 2005). It was developed for and implemented in the Mixteca region of the state of Oaxaca in Mexico, one of the poorest regions in entire Latin America. There is not only great economic poverty, but also much social inequality. Living conditions are especially adverse for women and children. The description follows the various stages that form IMIFAP's strategy of program development and implementation (Pick & Poortinga, 2005; Pick, Poortinga, & Givaudan, 2003).

Definition of Needs

The first stage of program development entails an analysis of the needs and problems facing the target population. In order to arrive at an inclusive description of the issues to be addressed, explorations at both the cultural context and the personal level are required. The main goal of this phase is to identify the structural, social, and psychological constraints that limit readiness for behavior change, as well as the opportunities enabling such change through development programs. In order to arrive at an inclusive description of the problems to be addressed, explorations of both the context and personal resources (see the following discussion on FENAE) are needed.

Government statistics contained mostly information for the entire state of Oaxaca. Thirty seven percent of the population earns less than the minimum daily wage (43.65 pesos, approximately US$ 4.30 in 2001), and only 4% earns more than five times that amount. Only 35% of the communities have a water distribution system, 75% of the homes have dirt floors, and the Mixteca region of the state has the highest malnutrition index in the country (Red Oaxaqueña de Derechos Humanos, 2001). In Oaxaca, the infant mortality rate is 25.6 deaths per 1000, while the national rate is 19.7 deaths per 1000 (Consejo Nacional de Población, nd). Undernourishment is present in 27% of the children between 0 and 5 years of age, and 34% of the population is illiterate (INEGI, 2000). Access to adequate schooling and health services is extremely difficult. In general, the structural context (i.e., the climate and economic conditions) is harsh.

To gather information at the individual level we conducted four focus groups and 60 semi-structured interviews with traditional healers, priests, midwives, teachers, students, local and federal authorities, and health professionals in 16 communities. Social norms and expectations were found often to amount to severe restrictions on the behavior of women. Girls tend to be kept from attending school,

---

[2]Has since changed its name to "I want to, I can...care for my health and exercise my rights."

because formal education is considered irrelevant for them and their services are more useful at home. Once a woman is married she is expected to stay at home most of the time; she will eat after her husband and abide by his decisions. Communication about any matter related to sexuality is usually absent; sexual hygiene is frowned upon because it amounts to touching one's body. Even going to a doctor is "not done" when this is likely to lead to exposure of intimate parts of the woman's body. Beliefs found include, for example, that a woman is there to serve her family and that her own health is secondary to this; taking contraceptive pills will lead to prospective babies piling up in the abdomen; putting crickets under a child's tongue will accelerate his speech development; use of contraceptives leads to unfaithfulness and increased risk of illness; and clean-looking people cannot be a source of sexually transmitted infections. A lack in social skills to make decisions, to communicate in a clear manner, and to be assertive was striking. Answers were common such as: "I cannot decide," "whatever God wants," "only if my husband says it is OK."

Development of Program Modules

The next stage was to develop the first version of a series of modules and supporting materials that were to be presented to the target women in weekly workshops. The title of the program, *Si yo estoy bien, mi familia también* (If I am OK so is my family) emphasizes that in order for families to be healthy, the women must take care of their own health first.

Each of the modules of the program, here to be referred to with the acronym *Syeb* included knowledge, myth clarification and skills, such as decision making, communication, and assertiveness. The program also had a gender perspective. All modules supported empowerment of women; more specifically they addressed (i) health and the right to health; (ii) nutrition and health, including dietary needs; (iii) hygiene and sanitation; and (iv) sexuality and reproductive health and rights[3] (Venguer et al., 2002).

Program Implementation

After all materials had been piloted, *Syeb* was administered to 39,000 women between the ages of 15 and 45. They attended workshops every week for about 2 hours. Each module took 15 sessions; the total number of contact hours for the four modules was 120 hours. The implementation of the program was realized through a closely supervised *cascade* with three levels of *replicators*. Twenty community action promoters of the national health agency *IMSS Oportunidades* were trained by IMIFAP staff. The community action promoters, using participatory workshops, trained 500 rural health assistants working in the Oaxaca health system. In turn, these assistants trained about 3,100 local social volunteer promoters. These social volunteer promoters worked with women whom they recruited in their own communities in groups of approximately 15 persons. IMIFAP staff controlled the quality of the program delivery by spot checks at workshops (Venguer, Pick, & Fishbein, 2005).

---

[3]After these four there were two further modules with workshops on the health of their children, dealing with early stimulation, vaccination, nutrition, and prevention of dehydration.

Scaling Up

The fourth and final stage of program development and implementation is the upscaling to large target groups after a program has been found to be successful. At the time of writing this chapter, the *Syeb* program has become part of a United Nations funded integral community development program for 160,000 women in the Mexican central state of Hidalgo and the southern Mexican state of Chiapas, and has been adopted by *IMSS-Oportunidades,* the national health agency for extreme poverty stricken communities.

Advocacy

Carefully planned advocacy with different level authorities took place at each stage of program development and implementation. Dissemination of results was also carried out, mainly for three reasons: (i) to make communities aware of the results being obtained, (ii) to influence social norms through that awareness, and (iii) to prepare for a future scaling-up phase (Venguer, Pick, & Fishbein, 2005).

The activities were not limited to individuals. Factors in the social context were addressed through mass media messages on indigenous radio stations as well as wall posters and pamphlets. For example, two radio stations broadcast messages with key elements from the program on women's empowerment for 9 months on an hourly basis. These were accompanied by a special jingle composed for the program.[4] During the development of the program, a series of posters and pamphlets was prepared, as well as buttons with the program logo. The posters all carried this program logo and one of several printed messages containing the key ideas from the program. Additionally, murals with the logo and program messages were painted on the walls of community centers in many villages.

Evaluation

At all stages process evaluation was carried out. One informal indicator of program success is that attendance rates stayed high throughout[5] (Venguer, Pick, & Fishbein, 2005). Program impact was analyzed in a questionnaire and observation study with a treatment sample and a control sample, each consisting of several hundred respondents. Data were collected on three occasions: prior to the start of the program, after the completion of the four modules, and 18 months later.[6] When

---

[4]Of course, the radio messages also reached the villages where respondents were recruited for the control sample of the impact evaluation study (see below). However, in all likelihood changes in the control villages due to the radio messages did not invalidate the results of this study, but raised the barriers for showing significant program effects.

[5]A notebook was given to all promoters to keep records of attendance. An analysis of a sample of 100 records showed that the average attendance in workshop sessions increased from 15.5 to 17.4 persons.

[6]Interviews were conducted with independently selected samples for each measurement occasion. Women were recruited from 165 of the treatment villages (only participants in the program) and 44 control villages. The smallest cell in the design numbered 178 interviews. Villages were chosen as the unit of analysis rather than the individual women because women-within-communities were considerably more homogeneous than women-between-communities and ignoring these within-community dependencies might render incorrect results (Goldstein, 1995).

comparing the data from the first and second occasion (period 1) and from the second and third occasion (period 2), a MANOVA (multivariate analysis of variance) showed significant overall effects (p < .001) for treatment, period, and treatment by period interaction. Specific examples of significant (p <.05) results include: defending one's opinion ($\beta_{Period1}$ = − 0.085, $\beta_{Period2}$ = − 0.163, $\beta_{Period1 \times Treatment}$ = 0.037, $\beta_{Period2 \times Treatment}$ = 0.467*), women having Pap smears ($\beta_{Period1}$ = − 0.246, $\beta_{Period2}$ = 0.419*, $\beta_{Period1 \times Treatment}$ = 0.234, $\beta_{Period2 \times Treatment}$ = 0.511*), consumption of vegetables and seeds ($\beta_{Period1}$ = 0.124, $\beta_{Period2}$ = 0.175*, $\beta_{Period1 \times Treatment}$ = 0.240*, $\beta_{Period2 \times Treatment}$ = 0.126*), and use of contraception ($\beta_{Period1}$ = − 0.004, $\beta_{Period2}$ = − 0.025, $\beta_{Period1 \times Treatment}$ = − 0.035, $\beta_{Period2 \times Treatment}$ = 0.085*) (see Venguer, Pick, & Fishbein, 2005 for more details, and Leenen et al., 2005 for an evaluation study on the *Syeb* program in Guatemala). It may be noted that significant effects found for the second period imply that program effects lasted at least up to 1.5 years after the program.

At the time of writing, 60 interviews are being held with former participants 3 years after completion of the program, for a follow-up assessment (IMIFAP, in preparation). These interviews are relevant for a point to be discussed later in this chapter, namely to what extent a program that was mainly targeting specific behaviors ends up having more general effects. Here follow some quotes and excerpts from the 35 interviews conducted so far.

Lourdes[7] mentioned: "In the course everyone talked, gave opinions. We had exercises in which we did things, we played, we were asked to answer, to jump, to talk, we did not just sit there to hear what others said. ... [W]hen I decided to start a business it was hard at first, but as I started selling the *pena* [shame] went away, now I even go out to the bus stops and sell without *pena*. I am also training my daughter to sell. She already goes house to house."

Raquel has organized a movement that led to the closure of the local brothel. She is in the process of organizing women to provide inexpensive low-cost, highly nutritional community breakfasts for the children and the elderly. She convinced the municipality to cover half of the food costs; others in the community will cook and cover the other half of expenses. She says these changes were made possible because, "the course and putting into practice what I learned helped me feel self-confident, to believe in myself, because people trusted me."

Ana, a rural community health worker who also participated in *Syeb*, has encouraged the women in the community to help organize village festivities, something both she and many of the women had previously been afraid to do; has gone to midwives and healers encouraging them to talk to their patients about sexuality, hygiene and nutrition; and is planning to start a small business selling the products that healers and midwives need.

Esther, now involved in a savings group, says she used to be scared "because I do not know how to make decisions, nor rules, I do not know how to add...and now I am the treasurer and put the dates down in the bookkeeping books and I add

---

[7]For reasons of privacy fictional names are used.

the amounts that come in and go out. ... The trainer was very good because she would say...the group has to solve it...that was new to us...we were accustomed to hearing "do this" or "do that" ... now *we* are the ones solving."

Maria: "[T]he PRI [a political party] wanted us to sign papers supporting them and I took from my money to go to T (the next village)...and talked to the municipal president and asked him what we would get in return of signing those papers. Since he did not offer anything I came back to tell all the people here and we did not sign. Now people listen to me when I give them advice. We are never going to sell ourselves so easily again."

Not all the women report changes such as mentioned here. However, they have been found in 90% of the 35 interviews held so far. In addition, during and just after the implementation of the program, physicians working at health clinics made comments to the effect that women who used to just sit quietly looking at the floor and agreed with whatever they were told had started to look doctors directly into the eyes, asked questions, and even negotiated when surgery should take place.

In summary, *Syeb* has been evaluated and significant changes were found in the target behaviors. But the follow-up interviews tell us something that goes beyond the usual evaluation of program efforts.

TRA PRINCIPLES AND IMIFAP PROGRAMS

In TRA an individual's behavioral intention is seen as the immediate precursor and main determinant of a behavior (Ajzen & Fishbein, 1980; Fishbein & Ajzen, 1975). Intention, in turn, is determined by two major factors, namely attitudes and subjective norms. Attitude refers to positive or negative feelings towards performing the behavior. It happens as a consequence of (i) the individual's behavioral beliefs, that is, what he/she thinks can be the outcomes of performing the behavior and (ii) the value of these outcomes for the individual. Subjective norms refer to the person's perception of other people's opinions regarding a behavior. They are determined by (i) normative beliefs which are the individual's perception about what other people think the person should do and (ii) the individual's motivation to comply with the opinion of others. Changes in attitudes and subjective norms will lead to changes in behavioral intentions.

Extending TRA, Ajzen and Madden (1986) added perceived behavioral control, to account for influences outside of the individual's control which may affect intentions/behavior. This extension, called Theory of Planned Behavior (TPB), was developed to achieve enhanced ability to predict, understand, and change behavior in domains that are not fully under a person's control. Perceived behavioral control is determined by: (i) beliefs regarding resources and impediments affecting the behavioral performance, and (ii) perceived power, that is, the impact of the resources and impediments to, respectively, facilitate or inhibit the behavior.

When IMFAP started to develop health promotion programs some 20 years ago, TRA was the point of departure. Field experience has led to some elaborations of relevance especially for illiterate populations.

Norms

Norms regulate behaviors everywhere. In traditional societies the need to follow norms appears to be stronger than in western urban societies. According to Sinha and Verman (1987), people in collectivist cultures "tend to behave according to social norms which are often designed to maintain social harmony among the members of the ingroup" (p.124). Cultural norms are more likely to become internalized and thus more consistent with attitudes in collectivist cultures (Bontempo, Lobel, & Triandis, 1990). Such findings imply that the two determinants of norms and attitudes are less distinguishable. Salience of norms can also be seen as part of the distinction by Pelto (1968) between *loose* and *tight* societies. According to Pelto, in tighter societies the pressure to carry out one's role is high, while in looser societies, there is less pressure to oblige. This point becomes clearer if one considers that the degree of choice, that is, the space for personal decisions, is more reduced than in urban societies in which there is a larger diversity of options. For example, if the only alternative one knows to assure a job for oneself is through supporting the local political party in power (and whether one does so or not is closely monitored), it is unlikely that one will risk not voting for this party. Likewise, if there is no social and economic recognition for an unmarried woman, one will be more tolerant of violence within the marriage than if one perceives to have several alternatives for gaining social recognition and acceptance.

Beliefs

Little formal education and very limited access to the media and other sources of information in which diversity of ideas and behavior patterns is found imply that established beliefs are rarely confronted with new evidence (Segall, Dasen, Berry, & Poortinga, 1999). In so far as factual knowledge is limited, beliefs will tend not to be "fact based," but based on "myths"[8] (Pick, Poortinga, et al., 2003). Factually correct knowledge is the first key ingredient in behavior change. It is not very likely that a woman is going to boil the drinking water for her children if she believes (that is, take for a fact) that boiled water has fewer vitamins, or have a Pap smear, if she thinks it is a sin to have her genitals touched, or that a young man will use condoms if he believes they have a high likelihood of breaking.

Attitudes

It stands to reason that TRA and TRB (Ajzen, 1991; Fishbein, & Yzer, 2003) apply universally. At the same time, there may be differences between how a theory works out in western students or among rural populations in Latin America. In research on attitudes the focus has been on literate and educated samples, and on behavior outcomes that are within the reach of the participants. Of course, in groups with little formal education ideas about outcomes exist, and about what are desirable and undesirable outcomes. Still, the question can be raised whether these

---

[8]The distinction between *facts* and *myths* is somewhat arbitrary, but generally facts have been more subject to reality testing, preferably by technological procedures.

are articulated and function as precursors of action to the same extent as in literate societies.

In TRA attitudes precede behaviors and are formed based on behavioral beliefs (Fishbein & Ajzen, 1975). The responses of women mentioned before suggest that the formation of attitudes towards desirable behaviors, except as vague and general likes or dislikes, implies both a certain level of knowledge and of control over the situation. Reactions that speak about the importance of control in the formation of attitudes are not uncommon, for example: "One cannot know if one really wants something....it does not depend on oneself; it is decided 'there'...by them or who knows by whom." In other words, women in the Mixteca may have a vague notion about a behavioral outcome that for educated urban westerners evidently is a matter of their own choice.

In addition, under such pressuring circumstances the expression of attitudes is likely not to be socially acceptable, leading to not allowing oneself the privilege of owning and expressing one's attitudes. The role that social approval plays can be illustrated with the following quotes from interviews: "To say what one thinks about doing something or not is badly taken, especially among youngsters and females"; "As women, we must keep our opinions to ourselves. We have been taught that if quiet, very quiet we look prettier."

Attitudes formation and behavior would seem to form an interactive ongoing process. Bandura (1997) has criticized theories such as those of Prochaska and DiClemente (1982) among other things because their stages of behavior are not clean cut, and there is a back and forth between them.

Intentions

Plans for the future in some of the follow-up interviews, mentioned before, are articulated in rather precise terms; these women actually described their intentions. This may be quite remarkable. According to TRA, intentions are plans to carry out specific behaviors. In the 1970s an exploratory study was conducted (Pick, 1978) to examine how intentions could best be measured among young men and women in marginalized areas of Mexico City. The sample was composed of about 150 individuals with a low level of schooling.

In interviews questions were asked to participants about the intentions they had to engage in specific behaviors, such as using contraceptives the next time they had sex, drinking less the next time they went out with their friends, vaccinating their children in the upcoming vaccination campaign, going out to look for a job during the next month. Phrases were used such as "do you have the intention to, the plan to, do you plan to..., will you do..., you think you will..., in what time period do you think you will be doing ..., if all goes well would you carry out this plan?, do you see yourself in ..., do you see yourself doing...." Reactions amounted to not giving a concrete answer. Phrases tended to be used such as "I am ashamed," "it is not for me to decide," "it depends if my man allows me," "If God wants," "How can I know, it is not in my hands," "yes one can have intentions but then what?; it is not a thing of one's own," "if the money is there." Smiles and laughter even pointed to feelings of discomfort.

In the same study a series of questions were designed to understand whether the concept of time was a factor in the formation of intentions. Participants were asked how long after a person had not arrived would they say that he/she was late. Many answered something like: "Well if the day is over and the person has not come I guess he is late." Such answers make sense in the light of the many imponderables in the lives of poor Mexicans, such as hardly passable roads; a boss who was supposed to pay and did not, preventing the person from having money for the bus; the relative who was sick and was to be taken to the doctor. All of these point to imponderables which limit the plausibility of someone actually arriving, let alone arriving on time.

Under dire economic and social conditions and strong pressure to conform to traditional social norms, the scope for forming realistic intentions is limited; in collectivistic communities one is more an object of change than an agent thereof, and the regulation of behavior is less a personal matter. As the Integrative Model of Behavioral Prediction (Fishbein & Yzer, 2003) has suggested, impediments to behavior change, especially among underprivileged groups can reside in the social context rather than in personal or situational impediments. Unavailability of contextual resources is a key class of barriers to healthful behaviors. In empirical studies based on TRA, the concept of intentions refers to specific behaviors. When life is uncertain and there is little predictability, it is hard to make concrete plans.

Control

Rotter (1966) argued that one can see events in one's life either as dependent upon one's own behavior or as contingent upon forces beyond one's control. In other words, the locus of control can be perceived as *internal* or *external* to oneself. Success in life can be due to *skill* or to *chance* and so can failure. Within the USA, where most research on locus of control has been conducted, African Americans are more external than European Americans (Dyal, 1984). In the case of other groups in the USA, such as Hispanics, the results depend on the level of education and socioeconomic status of the samples tested. Generally the results have been consistent with the explanation that the average scores on locus of control questionnaires correspond with the actual degree of control that people can exert on the course of their own lives in the real world (Berry, Poortinga, Segall, & Dasen, 2002). On the basis of cross-cultural evidence, these authors questioned whether locus of control is better viewed as a general tendency (as Rotter would have it) or as specific to certain situations (which would be more compatible with TRA's emphasis on situation specificity). In any case, locus of control seems to fit reasonable expectations of individuals belonging to certain groups, given their actual living conditions, which may imply limited control in many everyday life situations.

The introduction of perceived control in TPB addresses this point. Perceived behavioral control impacts the formation of intentions and can also directly impact behavior independently of intentions (Ajzen, 1991). It relates to how outside factors are perceived to influence a person's ability to carry out a behavior.

A further step might be contemplated. If it is difficult to have intentions without a certain level of control, the relationship between these two is conditional. In other words, intentions may presume some level of control, otherwise they are merely day dreams. Perhaps the two concepts are so closely tied that they are better placed in one box together in models like TRA and TBA (i.e., intentions/control) when these are applied in rural populations with low education. The unpredictable and constraining context amounts to low control, which makes it hard to form intentions. As opportunities arise and choices develop to engage in a behavior that is perceived as under one's control, a more self-regulating, self-determining orientation becomes possible.

Generalization of Behavior Changes

The generalization of changes in behavior has been a major concern of psychologists for a long time. In classical learning experiments the generalization of reinforcement generally was found to be rather limited. Reinforcement led to changes in reactions to specific stimuli, but changes in reactions to related stimuli were much weaker, unless these were very similar to the original. Thus, even by the strict standards of experimental behaviorists generalization effects invariably occur, but they are limited.

The effectiveness of health promotion and educational programs can be overrated (e.g., Eldering & Leseman, 1999). The history of the well-known Head Start program is a case in point. The initially spectacular claims of success could not be upheld. However, even if the effectiveness was grossly overestimated initially, the program has continued to exist, because ultimately there were good reasons to believe that there is a general effect on the intellectual development of disadvantaged children in the U.S. (Andersen et al., 2003).

Although effects of instruction and stimulated behavior changes due to programs easily can be overestimated, there is widespread opinion that they occur. There are extensive arguments and findings in the literature to the effect that programs promote health effects beyond the behaviors that were targeted (e.g., Abbott, O'Donnell, & Hawkins, Hill, Kosterman, & Catalano, 1998; Durlak & Wells, 1997; Elias, Gara, & Schuyler, Branden-Muller, & Sayette, 1991; Flay, 2002; Kellam & Anthony, 1998; Kellam, Rebok, Ialongo, & Mayer, 1994). To explain such findings most psychologists refer to some form of internalization (e.g., Baumeister, 1993; Rotter, 1966).

TRA is more explicit than most theories that behavior change should be targeted in specific situations. In the next section it will become clear that in the conceptual framework underlying programs like *Syeb*, the emphasis is on addressing concrete situations. However, this does not mean that behavior change outcomes are necessarily limited to the situations targeted in a program. As more and more situations come under the control of the person, they can be said to result in changes in general dispositions. Such changes appear to be facilitated by the experience of control. Successfully mastering change leads to a sense of accomplishment, an aspect in human learning underrated by classical learning theories, which by and large presupposed a passive rather than an active learning organism (Valsiner, 2000).

THE FRAMEWORK FOR ENABLING AGENTIC EMPOWERMENT (FENAE)

Many of the ideas touched upon in the previous sections are reflected in a conceptual framework, referred to as the Framework for Enabling (FENAE, see Figure 15–1). FENAE is a framework, it is not meant to be a theory or testable model. Rather it tries to systematize and guide IMIFAP's approach to health promotion and community development programs. FENAE includes four frames, labeled context, person, situation, and behavior, which are presented in the following paragraphs.

Context

The notion of context refers to the circumstances in which people are living. It includes the structural opportunities and constraints, which in more recent work Fishbein (2000) has addressed as environmental variables. Also included are variables such as social norms in the traditional TRA model (Fishbein & Ajzen, 1975; Ajzen & Fishbein, 1980). Often a distinction is made between material and sociocultural aspects. Central to material context are economic factors (Berry et al., 2002). The members of a wealthy group or society have access to all kinds of material and non-material resources that are not available in a poor society, like reliable sources of food, fresh water, and good medical care. Education is closely related to a country's economy. In poor societies the financial resources for formal education are limited, and the quality of education tends to be lower, in so far as it is present. Sociocultural variables that are (largely) shared within a society include values, norms, and beliefs. Through socialization and enculturation individuals acquire the rules that are prevalent in their social environment (Segall et al., 1999; Valsiner, 2000).

The program developer has to understand the rules that govern behavior, especially those with a normative character, in order to grasp the possible constraints on behavior changes, and thus the scope for intervention (Marín, 1993). Program contents should be compatible with the experiential world of the target group (Wholey, Harty, & Newcomer, 1994). This also helps to assure that program clients feel the program is theirs. A successful program leads to changes in behavior patterns over time in many individuals, which in turn should lead to a context more conducive to the new patterns. This is indicated by the feedback arrow from behavior to context in Figure 15–1.

Person

This component refers to behavior patterns that are consistent over time and situations, and as such are characteristic of a person. The emphasis in Figure 15–1 is on more general dispositions that are the outcome of long-time social learning processes and in principle can be modified even later in life, particularly if the individual is exposed to new experiences and encouraged to change. (Individual) attitudes and norms are included here, because these tend to be relatively stable

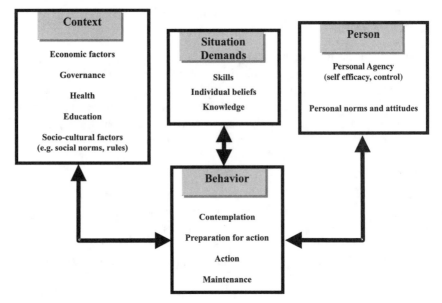

FIGURE 15–1.   A heuristic framework for health promotion programs (adapted from Pick, Poortinga, & Givaudan, 2003)

over time (Fishbein & Ajzen, 1975). Other terms listed include self-efficacy (Bandura, 1986, 1997, 2004) and agency (Kagitcibasi, 2005; Sen, 1999).

There are numerous concepts that refer to a person's general capability to deal with difficult situations in a socially competent and confident manner. Among these are agency (Kagitcibasi, 2005; Sen, 1999), self-efficacy (Bandura, 1997), self-esteem (Baumeister, 1993), self-determination (Deci & Ryan, 2000), self-regulation (Boekaerts, 1999), internal locus of control (Rotter, 1966), empowerment (Stein, 1997), autonomy (Assor, Kaplan, & Roth, 2002), and individualization (Crockett & Silbereisen, 2000). Of the concepts mentioned, *agency* has the advantage of being part of both the psychological literature and the literature on socioeconomic development. According to the economist Sen (1999), agency is the ability to define one's goals in an autonomous fashion and act upon them. Agency implies that one feels able to carry out behaviors of one's choice, monitor one's progress, and have the control over the decisions that generally precede a behavior. Personal agency is the recognition that people *can* be, and going a step beyond, *must* be agents of their own well-being. Only in this way can they be held responsible for the decisions they make regarding what behaviors they get involved in.

As people acquire the skills and knowledge that enable them to exercise control over their behaviors, they become agents of their behaviors. First this happens in concrete situations targeted in a program, such as going for a Pap smear. Such incidences of specific agency amount to small tangible achievements (e.g., a patient in therapy, a child in the classroom, a woman in her job). Gradually they extend not only through processes of passive generalization, but through the active extension of control over more situations, leading to a generalized sense of agency. Women in health promotion programs like *Syeb* become more open in communicating their needs, opinions, and interests not only with health providers or husbands who have been specifically targeted, but also in a broader sense. Thus, agency can extend to other areas of behavior even though these were not specifically addressed during the workshops and ultimately affect general behavior tendencies that constitute stable personality traits, such as self-worth, self-efficacy, etc.

Admittedly, agency is a tricky concept for reasons already indicated in the previous subsection. Any positive change reported by a program participant, a health professional or official, and any change observed by the program staff, can be attributed to changes in agency. However, such an explanation is largely post hoc. In experiments or quasi-experiments (Shadish, Cook, & Campbell, 2002) one can quite convincingly demonstrate changes in behavior and in skills, knowledge, and beliefs which are specific targets of a program, but this is much harder for generalized behavior tendencies. A sense of agency may show up in a variety of behaviors and these will differ from person to person. In the interviews with the women, mentioned previously, they expressed a range of different achievements and plans. Such broader effects of programs are hard to trace, exactly because they are so widely scattered—any specific effect will have a very small expected probability. When dealing with many possible effects at the same time, it is difficult to pinpoint which antecedent leads to what change.

The strength of evidence has to be balanced against the alternative that changes as reported in testimonials are *unrelated* to the program. Usually this is also hard to demonstrate. If clear experimental proof is outside our reach, we have to consider other standards of evidence, based on plausibility of relationship and, ultimately, common sense.

Please note the arrow in Figure 15–1 indicating that the person is supposed to change as a result of the program. Changes in the person are by and large an indirect consequence; they follow after changes in actual behavior. The person as defined in Figure 15–1 is not a primary emphasis in IMIFAP programs. The women attending the *Syeb* workshops are not told that the goal of the program is for them to change their norms and attitudes and acquire a higher level of agency. This would not be understood, and even if the women would understand, they would not be able to act on the basis of this understanding.

Situation

The third frame in Figure 15–1 refers to situations that an individual faces when others demand or expect a certain course of action, or when the person would like to realize something. The primary ingredients needed to address a situation are relevant knowledge and skills. Also placed in this frame are beliefs. Knowledge refers to facts (in the minds of the program developers). In *Syeb* knowledge concerns, for example, the advantages of boiling water, the need for proteins (beans) in the diet, human rights as reflected in the laws of the country, or how to prevent HIV/AIDS and unwanted pregnancies. Beliefs or myths include items of knowledge for which there is no empirical basis and that may even be demonstrably incorrect, for example, believing that women who enjoy having sex are less good wives and mothers (Pick, Givaudan, & Aldaz, 1996).

Appropriate skills allow the person to react optimally according to his or her own standards and desired outcomes. Examples of skills relevant to behavior change in health prevention are: being able to make one's own decisions; the use of direct, open, and assertive communication; and the expression of feelings. These are among the *life skills* that the World Health Organization has identified as a priority (World Health Organization, 1999) for health promotion programs.

It should be clear by now that the primary target of IMIFAP programs are concrete situations that have been selected on the basis of need analysis as being relevant to the target population and as offering scope for change. The emphasis on concrete situations is the clearest legacy of TRA manifest in IMIFAP's programs.

Evaluation studies of programs have shown that workshops need to be highly participatory in order to realize changes in behavior (Givaudan, Pick, Poortinga, Fuertes, & Gold, 2005; Pick et al., 1988; Pick & Givaudan, 1999). Skills are to be developed hand in hand with specific knowledge and rehearsed in various combinations so they can be applied under different situations and easily extended to new contexts. In this way multiple behaviors can be targeted that have the same skills in common.

Behavior

The main goal of IMIFAP programs is to encourage changes in target behaviors of individuals. Skills and knowledge lead to behaviors which are the actual manifestations of choice and intentions. This is in line with the assertion by Middlestadt et al. (1995) that the main outcomes of intervention programs at the individual level are changes in intentions and actual behavior. The concepts mentioned in the behavior frame of Figure 15–1 come from Prochaska and DiClemente (1982). They describe a gradual process of change; changes occur in steps, from contemplating change, to preparation for change, to making the change, and, finally, to maintaining the new behavior. This view is compatible with the recommendations of the World Bank (1997) on how to provide essential health, nutrition, and population preventive services, including raising awareness, identifying and overcoming barriers, motivating for change, providing information and skills, and providing the necessary reminders and social support to insure sustainability.

Ultimately behavior change can be seen as part of a spiral process. When a certain proportion of individuals in a community have changed a behavior, the context can be said to have changed. This in turn will influence the behavior of others. Similarly, after an individual has changed several practices, he or she can be said to have changed as a person, and this has consequences for future behavior. In Figure 15–1 these further connections are not represented by arrows. The reason is a simple one: Figure 15–1 has been construed from a perspective of programming, where concrete situations are the point of entry.

CONCLUSION

FENAE has much in common with TRA. This is not surprising since TRA was the starting point of the work that led to the FENAE framework. Somewhat more surprising is that FENAE also seems largely compatible with later theoretical developments (Ajzen, 1991; Fishbein & Ajzen, 2005; Fishbein & Yzer, 2003). This chapter has particularly referred to the addition of control as a parameter (Ajzen, 1991), and a greater emphasis on environment (Fishbein, 2000).

For the broader field of human development or social development probably the most important point of TRA is the emphasis that concrete behaviors have to be targeted for change (in this volume see e.g., Middlestadt, 2006). A similar point is made in Social Cognitive Theory when Bandura (1986) states that skills are necessary to translate risk knowledge to preventive behavior and that practicing of the newly acquired behavior in progressively more difficult contexts leads to increases in skills and self-efficacy. Furthermore, this point has been emphasized outside of psychology by at least two global institutions concerned with human development and health, namely the World Bank and the World Health Organization. As mentioned before, among the life skills that the World Health Organization (WHO, 1999) has identified as a priority are the ability to make one's own decisions, the use of direct, open and assertive communication, and the expression of feelings. Similarly, the World Bank (1997) has mentioned providing information and skills as part of health, nutrition, and population preventive services as means to overcome barriers.

The first and foremost contribution of psychology to human development lies in the expertise of our discipline concerning behavior change. In some respects this contribution is a sobering one: why change is difficult to realize, especially in groups with low education living in a *tight* environment, and why the lifting of constraints has to be targeted in concrete situations by means of concrete knowledge and skills rather than by addressing broader domains and trait-like characteristics of the person. The theoretical precision of models such as TRA, including subsequent versions, and the scope for experimental analysis make a unique contribution to the field of human development where the enthusiasm of grass root NGOs and naïve beliefs in grand schemes of policy makers often lead to disappointment and waste of resources, because changes are far more difficult to realize than imagined.

The strength of psychology at the same time is its weakness. The success of theories like TRA lies in predicting outcomes in target behaviors. Human development as a field is characterized by much broader perspectives, even if the validity of these broader ideas is hardly ever examined in a way satisfying to experimentally minded psychologists. Psychology has to learn from other fields when it comes to this broader perspective on human development.

From such a more encompassing idea on development, the United Nations Development Program published the first *Human Development Report* in 1990. It defines human development as "...a process of enlarging people's choices. In principle, these choices can be infinite and change over time. But at all levels of development, the three essential ones are for people to lead a long and healthy life, to acquire knowledge and to have access to resources needed for a decent standard of living. If these essential choices are not available, many other opportunities remain inaccessible" (p. 10).

Amartya Sen, who was awarded the Nobel Prize in Economics in 1998, argues in his book *Development as Freedom*: "Expansion of freedom is viewed...

both as the primary end and as the principal means of development. Development consists of the removal of various types of unfreedoms that leaves people with little choices and little opportunity of exercising their reasoned agency. The removal of substantial unfreedoms… is constitutive of development" (1999, p. xii).

A World Bank report on sustainable development beyond economic growth states: " 'Development' is really much more than simple economic growth. The understanding of development can differ among countries and even among individuals, but it usually goes far beyond the objectives of increased average income to include things like freedom, equity, health, education, safe environment, and much more" (Soubbotina, 2004, p. 1).

These quotes show that recent approaches to human development go well beyond economics. They address concerns that are at the heart of applied psychology.

The concepts of agency and context can have a bridging function between the individual level on which psychologists as behavior scientists tend to focus and the societal or group level that is the primary perspective of the social sciences. As mentioned, in FENAE agency reflects people's ability to make choices; it is the ability to define one's goals and act upon them. Agency develops within a sociocultural context that stimulates autonomy; it suffers in contexts where there is an emphasis on constraints rather than opportunities.

People are influenced and controlled by their psychological barriers and the constraints present in their context. To be able to exert influence on the social environment and respond to the controls it imposes requires the potential to perform considered or reasoned action. As Fishbein and his colleagues have pointed out repeatedly, such action is taken in concrete situations. That is where the understanding of human development has to begin.

REFERENCES

Abbott, R. D., O'Donnell, J., Hawkins, J. D., Hill K. G., Kosterman, R., & Catalano, R. F. (1998). Changing teaching practices to promote achievement and bonding in school. *American Journal of Orthopsychiatry, 68*(4):542–552.

Ajzen, I. (1991). The theory of planned behavior. *Organizational Behavior and Human Decision Processes, 50,* 179–211.

Ajzen, I., & Fishbein, M. (1980). *Understanding attitudes and predicting social behavior.* Englewood Cliffs, NJ: Prentice Hall.

Ajzen, I., & Madden, T. J., (1986). Prediction of goal-directed behavior: Attitudes and perceived behavioral control. *Journal of Experimental Social Psychology*, 22: 453–474.

Andersen, L. M., Shinn, C., Fullilove, M. T., Scrimshaw, S. C., Fielding, J. E., Norman, J., & Carande-Kulis, V. G. (2003). The effectiveness of early childhood development programs: A sympathetic review. *American Journal of Preventive Medicine, 24,* 32–46.

Assor, A., Kaplan, H., & Roth, G. (2002). Choice is good, but relevance is excellent: Autonomy-enhancing and suppressing teacher behaviors predicting students' engagement in schoolwork. *British Journal of Educational Psychology, 72,* 261–278.

Bandura, A. (1986). *Social foundations of thought and action: A social cognitive theory.* Englewood Cliffs, NJ: Prentice Hall.

Bandura, A. (1997). *Self-efficacy: The exercise of control.* New York: Freeman.

Bandura, A. (2004). Health promotion by social cognitive means. *Health Education and Behavior, 31,* 143–164.

Baumeister, R. F. (Ed.). (1993). *Self-esteem: The puzzle of low self-regard.* New York: Plenum Press.

Berry, J. W., Poortinga,Y. H., Segall, M. H., & Dasen, P. R. (2002). *Cross-cultural psychology: Research and applications.* Cambridge: Cambridge University Press.

Boekaerts, M. (Ed.). (1999). Self-regulated learning. *International Journal of Educational Research, 31,* 445–551.

Bontempo, R., Lobel, S., & Triandis, H. C. (1990). Compliance and value internalization in Brazil and the U.S.: Effects of allocentrism and idiocentrism. *Journal of Cross-Cultural Psychology, 21,* 200–213.

Consejo Nacional de Población (no date). *Indicadores demográficos básicos.* http://www.conapo.gob.mx/00cifras/00indicadores.htm

Crockett, L. J., & Silbereisen, R. K. (Eds.). (2000). *Negotiating adolescence in times of social change.* New York: Cambridge University Press.

Deci, E. L., & Ryan, R. M. (2000). The "what" and "why" of goal pursuits: Human needs and the self determination of behavior. *Psychological Inquiry, 11,* 227–268.

Dyal, J. A. (1984). Cross-cultural research with the locus of control construct. In H. M. Lefcourt (Ed.), *Research in locus of control* (Vol. 3, pp. 209–306). New York: Academic Press.

Durlak, J. A., & Wells, A. M. (1997). Primary prevention mental health programs for children and adolescents: A meta analytic review. *Journal of Community Psychology. 25,* 115–152.

Eldering, L., & Leseman P. (Eds.). (1999). *Effective early education: Cross-cultural perspectives.* New York: Garland.

Elias, M. J., Gara, M., Schuyler, T. F., Branden-Muller, L. R., & Sayette, M. A. (1991). The promotion of social competence: Longitudinal study of a preventative school-based program. *American Journal of Orthopsychiatry, 61,* 409–417.

Fishbein, M. (2000). The role of theory in HIV prevention. *AIDS Care. 12,* 273–278.

Fishbein, M., & Ajzen, I. (1975). *Belief attitude, intention and behavior: An introduction to theory and research.* Reading, MA: Addison-Wesley.

Fishbein, M., & Ajzen, I. (2005). Theory-based behavior change interventions: Comments on Hobbis and Sutton. *Journal of Health Psychology, 10,* 27–31.

Fishbein , M., & Yzer, M. C. (2003). Using theory to design effective health behavioral interventions. *Communication Theory, 13,* 164–183.

Flay, B. R. (2002). Positive youth development requires comprehensive health promotion programs. *American Journal of Health Behavior, 26,* 407–424.

Givaudan, M., Pick, S., Poortinga, Y. H., Fuertes, C., & Gold, L. (2005). A cervical cancer prevention program in rural Mexico: Addressing women and their context. *Journal of Community & Applied Social Psychology, 15,* 338–352.

Goldstein, H. (1995). *Multilevel Statistical Models* London: Arnold.

IMIFAP (in preparation). *Follow-up of a gender, empowerment and health program in indigenous areas of Mexico.* Mexico: IMIFAP.

INEGI (2000). *XII Censo General de Población y Vivienda 2000. Tabulados Básicos y Síntesis de Resultados por Entidad Federativa.* Mexico City: Instituto Nacional de Estadística Geografía y Informática/Gob. de México. http://www.inegi.gob.mx/inegi/default.asp

Kagitcibasi, C. (2005) Autonomy and relatedness in cultural context. *Journal of Cross-Cultural Psychology, 36,* 403–422.

Kellam, S. G., & Anthony, J. C. (1998). Targeting early antecedents to prevent tobacco smoking: Findings from an epidemiologically based randomized field trial. *American Journal of Public Health, 88*(10), 1490–1495.

Kellam, S. G., Rebok, G. W., Ialongo, N., & Mayer, L. (1994). The course and malleability of aggressive behavior from early first grade into middle school: Results from a developmental epidemiologically based preventive trial. *Journal of Child Psychology. 35,* 259–281.

Leenen, I., Venguer, T., Vera, J., Givaudan, M., Pick, S., & Poortinga, Y. H. (2006). *Effectiveness of an Integral Health Education Program in a Poverty Stricken Rural Area of Guatemala.* Manuscript submitted for publication.

Marín, G. (1993). Defining culturally appropriate community interventions: Hispanics as a case study. *Journal of Community Psychology. 20,* 375–391

Middlestadt, S. E. (in press). What is the behavior? Strategies for Selecting the Behavior to be Addressed by Health Promotion Interventions.

Middlestadt, S. E., Fishbein, M., Albarracín, D., Francis, C., Eustace, M. A., Helquist, M., et al. (1995). Evaluating the impact of a national AIDS prevention radio campaign in St. Vincent's and the Grenadines. *Journal of Applied Social Psychology, 25,* 21–34.

Pelto, P. J. (1968). The difference between "tight" and "loose" societies. *Transaction, 5,* 37–40.

Pick, S. (1978). *A social psychological study of family planning in Mexico City.* Doctoral thesis, University of London, London, UK.

Pick, S., Aguilar, J., Rodríguez, G., Reyes, J., Collado, M. E., Pier, D., et al. (1988). *Planeando tu vida.* Mexico City: Ariel.

Pick, S., & Givaudan, M. (1999). *Yo quiero, yo puedo Series of 10 interactive workbook from preschool through 9th globle.* Mexico City: Ideame.

Pick, S., Givaudan, M., & Aldaz, E. (1996). Adolescent sexuality: A qualitative study in Mexico City. Report presented to USAID, Washington, DC, USA. Mexico City: IMIFAP.

Pick, S., & Poortinga, Y. H. (2005). Marco conceptual y estrategia para el diseño e instrumentación de programas para el desarrollo: Una visión científica, política y psicosocial. *Revista Latinoamericana de Psicologia, 37,* 445–460.

Pick, S., Poortinga, Y.H., & Givaudan, M. (2003). Integrating intervention theory and strategy in culture-sensitive health promotion programs. *Professional Psychology: Research and Practice, 34,* 422–429.

Prochaska, J. O., & DiClemente, C. C. (1982). Transtheoretical therapy: Toward a more integrative model of change. *Psychotherapy: Theory, Research and Practice, 20,* 161–173.

Red Oaxaqueña de Derechos Humanos. (2001). *Secundo informe: Los derechos humanos en el estado de Oaxaca.* Report, January 2001. http://derechoshumanos.laneta.org/documentos/infooax.htm

Rotter, J. B. (1966). Generalized expectancies for internal versus external control of reinforcement. *Psychological Monographs, 80,* 1–28.

Segall, M. H., Dasen, P. R., Berry, J. W., & Poortinga, Y. H. (1999). *Human behavior in global perspective.* Boston, MA: Allyn and Bacon.

Sen, A. (1999). *Development as freedom.* Oxford: Oxford University Press.

Shadish, W. R., Cook, T. D., & Campbell, D. T. (2002). *Experimental and quasi-experimental designs for generalized causal inference.* Boston: Houghton Mifflin.

Sinha, J. B. P., & Verman, J. (1987). Structure of collectivism. In C. Kagitcibasi (Ed.), Growth and progress in cross-cultural psychology (pp. 123–129). Lisse, Netherlands: Swets & Zeitlinger.

Soubbotina, T. P. (2004). *Beyond economic growth—Introduction to sustainable development* (2nd ed.). Washington DC: World Bank.

Stein, J. (1997). Empowerment and women's health, London: Zed Books.

United Nations Development Programme (1990). *Human Development Report, 1990.* New York: Author.

Valsiner, J. (2000). *Culture and human development.* London: Sage.

Venguer, T., Leenen, I., Morales, N., Givaudan, M., Pick, S., Poortinga, Y. H., et al. (2002). *Multiplication of an integral health-education program for young women in the Oaxaca region of Mexico.* Report presented to GlaxoSmithKline, London, England. Mexico City: IMIFAP.

Venguer, T., Pick, S., & Fishbein, M. (2007). Health Education and Empowerment. A comprehensive Program for Young Women in the Mixteca Region & Mexico. *Psychology, Health and Medicine (in press)*

Wholey, J. S., Harty, H. P., & Newcomer, K. E. (Eds.). (1994). *Handbook of practical program evaluation.* San Francisco: Jossey-Bass.

World Health Organization (1999). *Partners in life skills education–Conclusions from a United Nations Inter-Agency Meeting* (WHO/MNH/MHP/99.2). Geneva, Switzerland: Author.

World Bank (1997). *World development report. The state in a changing world.* New York: Oxford University Press.

CHAPTER 16

Applying the Theory of Reasoned Action to HIV Risk-Reduction Behavioral Interventions

Loretta Sweet Jemmott and John B. Jemmott, III

University of Pennsylvania

HIV/AIDS is increasing among adolescents, particularly African American adolescents. Engaging in unprotected sexual intercourse is the main route of transmission for HIV/AIDS among adolescents. Without a cure or vaccine available for HIV, the best way to curtail this disease is to prevent it. Hence, HIV risk-reduction interventions are needed to assist adolescents to reduce their risk for HIV infection. The best method for developing an effective HIV prevention intervention is to use theoretical models to design it. In this light, the Theory of Reasoned Action, and its extension the Theory of Planned Behavior, might be a solution. This chapter will describe HV/STD risk behavior among teens, review the Theory of Reasoned Action/Planned Behavior, describe our use of these theories in designing HIV risk-reduction interventions, and the outcomes of those research studies.

THE RISK OF SEXUALLY TRANSMITTED HIV INFECTION AMONG ADOLESCENTS

Evidence from several sources indicates that adolescents are at high risk for sexually transmitted disease (STD), including HIV, which causes AIDS. Individuals 15 to 24 years of age accounted for 15% of the cumulative HIV infections confidentially reported as of December 2003 (Centers for Disease Control and Prevention [CDC], 2004a). From 2000 through 2003, the estimated number of HIV/AIDS cases in the U.S. increased among young people 13 to 24 years of age (CDC, 2004a). The HIV/AIDS epidemic has had an especially devastating impact on African American and Latino adolescents. For instance, in 2003, 15% of the adolescents in the United States were African American, but 66% of reported AIDS cases were in African Americans (CDC, 2004b).

About 62% of adolescents have had sexual intercourse by the time they are in the 12th grade according to the 2003 Youth Risk Behavior Surveillance Survey (Grunbaum et al., 2004), a nationally representative survey of students in grades 9 to 12. Older students, that is, those in higher grades, were more likely to report sexual experience. Overall, there was little difference in the prevalence of sexual intercourse between boys and girls in grade 10 and higher. However, among 9th grade students, a greater percentage of boys (37%) as compared with girls (28%) reported sexual intercourse. Similar to many other national surveys (e.g., Kann et al., 1996; Sonenstein, Pleck, & Ku, 1989), a greater percentage of African American (67.3%) and Latino (51.4%) students compared with White (41.8%) students reported sexual experience.

Statistics on STD and unintended pregnancy provide clear evidence of the consequences of unprotected sexual intercourse among adolescents. Each year 1 in 4 sexually active adolescents—3 million adolescents—contracts a STD (Eng & Butler, 1997). Women and African Americans are especially at risk. For instance, data from a nationally representative sample of young people ages 18 to 26 years found that 4.2% tested positive for chlamydia (Miller et al., 2004). Women (4.7%) were more likely to be infected than were men (3.7%). The prevalence of chlamydia was highest among African American women (14.0%) and African American men (11.1%); lowest prevalence rates were among Asian men (1.1%), White men (1.4%), and White women (2.5%). This survey also revealed that among young people 18 to 23 years of age, those who initiated sexual intercourse at younger ages had a greater risk of testing positive for an STD (Kaestle, Halpern, Miller, & Ford, 2005).

Despite recent drops in the adolescent birth rate, substantial morbidity and social problems still result from the approximately 870,000 pregnancies that occur each year among girls 15 to 19 years of age (Ventura, Abma, Mosher, & Henshaw, 2003). Nationwide, 4.2% of students in grades 9 to 12 were pregnant or had gotten someone pregnant in 2003 (Grunbaum et al., 2004). The prevalence of pregnancy was higher among African American (10.4%) and Latino adolescents (7.3%) than among their White counterparts (2.8%). In addition, studies of sexual behavior seem to suggest that failure to use condoms is a pervasive risk behavior among adolescents—more common than anal sex or having multiple partners.

Taken together, these data suggest that adolescents are at risk for sexually transmitted diseases, including HIV. Interventions to reduce HIV risk-associated sexual behavior are urgently needed for adolescents, particularly African American adolescents. Efforts to find a cure or a vaccine for HIV have not been successful. However, HIV can be prevented by changes in personal sexual behavior. The important question is how to effect changes in HIV risk-associated sexual behavior. To answer that question, one can consider the use of the Theory of Reasoned Action, and its extension the Theory of Planned Behavior.

The identification of the correlates and predictors of HIV risk-associated sexual behaviors, particularly condom use, is central to efforts to develop and implement effective interventions to change such behaviors. Interventions that are based on a systematic understanding of the causes of behavior they seek to change and are based on a solid theoretical foundation are most likely to be effective. Systematic understanding of the causes of behavior flows from a theoretical model of behavior and empirical tests of theory-based hypotheses. The Theory of Reasoned Action (Ajzen & Fishbein, 1980; Fishbein & Ajzen, 1975), and its extension the Theory of Planned Behavior (Ajzen, 1985; 1991), provide a conceptual framework within which to consider condom use. Following is a description of the Theory of Reasoned Action and the Theory of Planned Behavior.

The Theory of Reasoned Action/Theory of Planned Behavior

Our HIV risk-reduction research has drawn upon the Theory of Reasoned Action (Ajzen & Fishbein, 1980; Fishbein & Ajzen, 1975), and its extension the Theory of Planned Behavior (Ajzen, 1985, 1991; Madden, Ellen, & Ajzen, 1992). According to these theories, specific behavioral intentions are the determinants of behaviors. Consider, for instance, condom use. Based on these theories, it might be predicted that condom use among adolescents is a function of their intentions to use condoms. The theories further hold that a behavioral intention is determined by attitudes toward the specific behavior, subjective norms regarding the behavior, and perceived behavior control over the behavior. Perceived behavioral control reflects past experience as well as anticipated impediments, obstacles, resources, and opportunities. It has affinity with the Social Cognitive Theory construct of perceived self-efficacy (Bandura, 1982, 1986, 1989; O'Leary, 1985). If people believe that they have little control over performing a behavior because of a lack of requisite skills or resources, their intentions to perform the behavior may be low, even if they have favorable attitudes or perceive supportive subjective norms regarding it (Ajzen & Madden, 1986). Thus, people intend to perform a behavior when they evaluate that behavior positively, when they believe significant others think they should perform it, and when they feel confident in their ability to perform the behavior. The theory holds that the relative predictive power of attitude, subjective norm, and self-efficacy can vary from behavior to behavior and from population to population.

A valuable feature of the theory is that it directs attention to the basis of people's attitudes, subjective norms, and perceived behavioral control. Different types of salient beliefs underlie each of these constructs, and the theory holds that the nature of the beliefs can vary from population to population. Attitudes toward behavior are seen as reflecting salient behavioral beliefs about the consequences of performing the behavior weighted by evaluations of those outcomes. Thus a person who holds strong beliefs that positively valued outcomes will result for using condoms will have a positive attitude toward using condoms. Conversely, a person who holds strong beliefs that negatively valued outcomes will result from using condoms will have a negative attitude toward using condoms. Subjective norms are seen as reflecting salient normative beliefs about whether specific reference persons or groups would approve or disapprove of the behavior weighted by motivation to comply with those referents. Thus, a person will hold a positive subjective norm when he/she believes that certain referents (e.g., girlfriend or boyfriend) think he or she should use a condom, and is motivated to meet the expectations of those referents. Conversely, a person will perceive less normative support to use condoms when s/he believes these referents think he or she should not use condoms or who is less motivated to comply with those referents who approve condom use. Perceived behavioral control is determined by salient control beliefs about obstacles, impediments, resources, and opportunities weighted by evaluations of the extent which the factor would inhibit or facilitate the behavior. The salient beliefs specific to a behavior in a population can be identified through qualitative research, including elicitation surveys, focus groups, and interviews with members of the population.

For those who are interested in behavior change interventions, it may be possible to change behavioral intentions and therefore behavior by targeting the salient beliefs in a population that underlie attitudes, subjective norms, and perceived behavior control. In the case of condom use, perhaps the most obvious is the behavioral belief concerning prevention, that the use of condoms can prevent pregnancy, STD, and HIV infection (Jemmott, Jemmott, Spears , Hewitt, & Cruz-Collins, 1992). Another key consideration has been *hedonistic beliefs* (Jemmott, Jemmott, Spears et al., 1992) or beliefs about the consequences of condom use for sexual enjoyment. Several studies have tied such beliefs to condom use or intentions to use condoms (Catania et al., 1989; Hingson, Strunin, Berlin, & Heeren, 1990; Jemmott & Jemmott, 1992a; Valdiserri, Arena, Proctor, & Bonati, 1989). A third type of behavioral beliefs is partner reaction beliefs, whether people believe their partners would react favorably to their effort to use condoms (Jemmott & Jemmott, 1992b). The key referents for condom use often include sexual partners. Other referents who are sources of normative influence, at least in the case of adolescents, include peers, parents, and other family members (Fox & Inazu, 1980; Furstenberg, 1971; Handelsman, Cabral, & Weisfeld, 1987; Hofferth & Hayes, 1987; Milan & Kilmann, 1987; Morrison, 1985; Nathanson & Becker, 1986). Several types of control beliefs are relevant to perceived behavioral control regarding condom use. Availability beliefs concern confidence that condoms will be available when needed. Impulse control concerns the person's confidence that they can control themselves enough to use condoms when sexually excited. Perhaps most emphasized in HIV prevention research are negotiation beliefs which concern the person's confidence that they can persuade their sexual partners to use condoms. Technical skills concern the person's ability to use condoms with facility, and without ruining the mood.

The Theory of Planned Behavior does not include many variables that traditionally have been studied in attempts to understand preventive health behavior (i.e., SES, education level, and family structure). Attitudes, subjective norms, and perceived behavioral control are viewed as the sole determinants of intentions and behaviors. The effects on intentions and behaviors of other variables are seen as mediated by their effects on the attitudinal component, the normative component, the perceived control component, or all three. In this way, the theory can accommodate variables that are external to it (Ajzen, 1991; Fishbein & Middlestadt, 1989). Consider ethnicity, for instance. Different ethnic groups might vary in how strongly they hold particular beliefs and in the strength of the relation between such beliefs and intentions. In this view, attitudes and beliefs may be more important predictors than normative beliefs for one ethnic group, whereas normative beliefs may be more important predictors than attitudes and beliefs in another ethnic group (Jemmott & Jones, 1993). Other external variables that are not in the theory but have been linked to heightened sexual activity include low socioeconomic background, low parental education, residing in a female-headed household, and residing in households with a large number of children (Brown, 1985; Hofferth & Hayes, 1987; Hogan, Astone, & Kitagawa, 1985; Hogan & Kitagawa, 1985); age and sexual experience (CDC, 1998a & b; DiClemente et al., 1996; Jemmott & Jemmott, 1990;); race and ethnicity (CDC, 1998a & b); gender (e.g., CDC, 1998b; Leigh, Morrison, Trocki, & Temple, 1994); involvement in a steady relationship (Plichta, Weisman, Nathanson, Ensminger, & Robinson, 1992; Soskolne, Aral, Magder, Reed, & Bowen, 1991), and alcohol and drug use (e.g., Hingson et al., 1990; Jemmott & Jemmott, 1993; MacDonald, Zanna, & Fong, 1996).

One important external variable in our research is a behavioral intervention, which is designed to have an impact on salient behavioral beliefs. The Theory of Planned Behavior holds that interventions and other external variables affect specific behavioral intentions and behaviors by influencing attitudes toward those behaviors, subjective norms regarding them, or perceptions of control over them. In other words, the effects on intentions and behaviors of other variables are seen as mediated by their effects on the attitudinal component, the normative component, the perceived control component, or all three. In this way, the theory can accommodate variables that are external to it (Ajzen, 1991; Fishbein & Middlestadt, 1989).

Designing HIV Risk-reduction Interventions: Application of the Theory Reasoned Action/Planned Behavior

The Use of Focus Groups in Designing Interventions

Designing effective HIV risk-reduction interventions using the Theory of Reasoned Action/Planned Behavior as a framework first requires conducting open-ended elicitation interviews to identify the salient beliefs regarding the behavior of interest in the specific target population. This procedure also provides an opportunity to spend time with the population, taking time to get to know them and understand them. This will include assessing their knowledge, attitudes, beliefs, concerns, skills, needs and resources. This can be accomplished via elicitation surveys, focus groups, or individual interviews. This qualitative research is conducted with samples of 15–20 individuals from the population under investigation, half of whom have performed or intend to perform the behavior under investigation and half of whom have not performed the behavior. These individuals are asked to provide information regarding three types of beliefs. First, to assess salient behavioral beliefs, they are asked to describe any positive or negative outcomes of performing the behavior. Second, to assess normative beliefs, they are asked to describe any individuals or groups to whom they might listen, who are either in favor of or opposed to their performing the behavior. Third, to assess control beliefs, they are asked to describe any factors that might affect how hard or easy it is to perform the behavior. The collected information is then content analyzed to identify the relevant attributes or outcomes of the behavior and the relevant social referents. This phase is very crucial because it will provide valuable information that will assist in the development of measures and an intervention that is tailored to the salient beliefs about the behavior in the specific population.

Designing the intervention. We designed our interventions (Jemmott, Jemmott & Fong, 1992, 1998; 1999; Jemmott, Jemmott, Braverman, & Fong, 2005) to change behavioral beliefs about the consequences of protective and risky sexual behaviors and control beliefs about factors that would facilitate or thwart adolescents' performance of such behaviors. We used information gathered from elicitation surveys and focus groups conducted with members of the study population to identify these potential mediators of behavior change. In addition, we took into account the reactions of participants in pilot tests of the intervention. We reasoned that it is necessary to give adolescents not only information, but also skills and confidence in their ability to act safely. Another consideration was the kinds of activities that would be developmentally appropriate, especially for younger adolescents. We reasoned that adolescents would benefit most from short activities that involve active participation, concrete concepts, sufficient variation to keep their interest, and sufficient repetition to ensure integration of the most important beliefs about reducing sexual risk behaviors. In addition, we imbedded in the interventions themes such as "Be Proud! Be Responsible!" that emphasize personal pride and responsibility for not only oneself, but also one's family and community.

Overview of the Curriculum

The first curriculum we developed was called "Be Proud! Be Responsible! Strategies to Empower Youth to Reduce Their Risk for AIDS." It involved the use of audiovisuals, role-playing, skill-building activities, group discussion and other interactive activities designed to influence: (a) HIV risk-reduction knowledge, (b) behavioral beliefs about the consequences of condom use for sexual enjoyment, and (c) behavioral skills and self-efficacy regarding practicing abstinence and using condoms. In addition, it encouraged the adolescents to make proud and responsible decisions to protect themselves and their community. It consisted of six 50-minute modules. A typical module has several developmentally appropriate activities. This included videos, small group discussions, experiential exercises, and role-play scenarios. Each activity was of short duration (i. e., most lasted 25 minutes or less) and most were active exercises in which the adolescents got out of their seats and participated. In this way, it was possible to maintain interest and attention, which might fade if lecturing or lengthy group discussions were used. The activities were designed to provide information and to build skills in entertaining ways.

Curriculum activities are also designed to help participants recognize that faulty reasoning and decision making can increase their risk of HIV infection. The activities help the participants understand the adverse consequences of participating in unsafe sexual activity and the positive consequences of safer sexual practices, including abstinence. The participants engage in activities to increase comfort with condom use and to allay common concerns about the negative effects of condom use on sexual enjoyment and spontaneity. Participants handle condoms and learn to use condoms correctly. The current generation of young people has had substantial exposure to television, movies, and videos, and is accustomed to learning through such media. Throughout the curriculum culturally relevant videos depicting adolescents in various realistic situations are included to increase variety in the methodology, increase interest, repeat information in an entertaining way and permit a visual mode of learning. These videos evoke feelings, thoughts, attitudes, and beliefs about HIV infection, AIDS, and sexual risk behavior while highlighting prevention skills. The adolescents also participate in role-playing scenarios that allow them to observe, analyze, and practice the skills of negotiating abstinence or condom use in a variety of circumstances. The facilitator and the other participants provide constructive feedback and support during and after each role-play scenario. The later modules build on material presented in earlier modules and introduce new material. The initial modules focus more on information and motivation, whereas subsequent modules focus more on skill building. Closure activities review information in fun and interactive ways.

HIV Risk-Reduction Randomized Controlled Trials: Application of the Theory of Reasoned Action/Planned Behavior

Our research on inner-city African American adolescents documented early initiation of sexual intercourse, negative hedonistic beliefs regarding condom use, and the protective effect of parental strictness (Jemmott & Jemmott, 1990, 1992a). We also reported evidence on the utility of the Theory of Reasoned Action, Theory of Planned Behavior, and Social Cognitive Theory for understanding sexual risk behavior among inner-city African American adolescents and women (Jemmott & Jemmott, 1991; Jemmott & Jemmott, 1992b; Jemmott, Jemmott, & Hacker, 1992; Jemmott, Jemmott, Spears et al., 1992). This research showed that condom use intentions were associated with hedonistic beliefs about the effects of condoms on sexual enjoyment, normative beliefs regarding partners' and mothers' approval, and control beliefs regarding technical skill at using condoms, and self-efficacy to use condoms. This work supported the development of HIV/STD risk-reduction interventions evaluated in a series of randomized controlled trials.

Interventions Focusing on Adolescents

Intervening with Black male adolescents.   Our initial intervention study was a field experiment designed to test the effectiveness of "Be Proud! Be Responsible!" on African American male adolescents (Jemmott, Jemmott, & Fong, 1992). The study also addressed an important practical question regarding the implementation of HIV interventions with inner-city African American male adolescents. It might be hypothesized that a Black male educator would be a good role model for African American male adolescents. Hence, the second issue the study addressed was whether intervention effects would be enhanced if the facilitator was a Black man as opposed to a Black woman. The participants were 157 African American male adolescents from Philadelphia who volunteered for a "Risk-Reduction Project" designed to reduce important risks faced by African American youth, including unemployment, pregnancy, and AIDS. They were recruited from a local medical center, community-based organizations, and a local high school and assigned randomly to an HIV risk-reduction condition or a control condition on career opportunities and to a small group of about 6 boys led by a specially trained male or female Black facilitator. Few participants reported *ever* sharing needles (4%), *ever* having receptive anal intercourse (2%), having sexual relationships with males exclusively (2%), or having sexual relationships with both males and females (1%). Their chief HIV risk was from sexual relationships with women. Although the mean age of the sample was only 14.6 years, about 83% of the adolescents reporting having had coitus at least once. About 21% of respondents who had coitus in the past 3 months reported that they *never* used condoms during those experiences, and only 30% reported *always* using condoms.

Adolescents in the HIV risk-reduction condition received a 5-hour intervention involving videotapes, games, and exercises aimed at increasing AIDS-related knowledge, weakening problematic beliefs and attitudes toward HIV risk-associated sexual behavior, and increasing skill at negotiating safer sex. To control for Hawthorne effects, to reduce the likelihood that effects of the HIV risk-reduction intervention could be attributed to nonspecific features, including group interaction and special attention, adolescents randomly assigned to the control condition also received a 5-hour intervention. Structurally similar to the HIV risk-reduction intervention, it involved culturally and developmentally appropriate videotapes, exercises, and games, but regarding career opportunities. This control intervention was designed to be both enjoyable and valuable. Although career opportunity subjects did not learn about AIDS, given the high unemployment among inner-city Black adolescents, the goal was to provide information that would be valuable to them as they plan their future.

Adolescents in both conditions completed questionnaires before, immediately after the intervention, and 3 months after the intervention. Analyses of covariance, controlling for pre-intervention measures, revealed that adolescents who received the HIV risk-reduction intervention subsequently had greater AIDS knowledge, less favorable attitudes toward risky sexual behavior, and reduced intentions for such behavior compared with adolescents in the control condition. Responses to debriefing questions on the post-intervention questionnaire indicated that participants in the two conditions were equally involved in their respective activities and felt that they had a valuable and enjoyable experience. Of the original participants, 150 (96%) completed follow-up questionnaires 3 months after the intervention. Adolescents in the HIV risk-reduction condition reported less risky sexual behavior in the 3 months post intervention than did those in the control condition. For instance, they reported having coitus less frequently and with fewer women, they reported using condoms more consistently during coitus, and fewer of them reported engaging in heterosexual anal intercourse. Moreover, the AIDS-intervention participants still had greater AIDS knowledge and weaker intentions for risky behavior in the next 3 months than did the other participants. The study revealed scant evidence that the use of Black male facilitators would enhance intervention effects on Black male adolescents. Although analyses on the post-intervention questionnaire revealed a Condition x Gender of Facilitator interaction such that the HIV risk-reduction intervention caused a greater increase in AIDS knowledge among participants who had a male facilitator than among those who had a female facilitator, this interaction was not evident on other post-intervention measures or at the 3-month follow-up. In fact, the effects of the HIV risk-reduction intervention on attitudes and sexual behavior measured at the 3-month follow-up were significantly stronger with *female* facilitators than with male facilitators.

Intervening with Young Inner-city Black Adolescent: Testing the Generality of Effects. Jemmott, Jemmott, and Fong (1999) conducted a second study using the "Be Proud! Be Responsible!" curriculum, this time focusing on male and female African American adolescents. The study was designed not only to test the efficacy of the curriculum, but also to pursue further, practical questions about how interventions are implemented with inner-city African American adolescents. The study was designed to test whether intervention effects varied depending on whether the facilitator was African American or White, whether the gender of the facilitator and the gender of the adolescent were matched or different, whether the adolescents in the small group were homogeneous or heterogeneous on gender, and theoretically and practically important combinations of these factors. The participants were 506 7th and 8th graders (mean age, 13.1 years) recruited from the public junior high schools and elementary schools of Trenton, New Jersey for a study designed to discover ways to reduce important health risks that African American youths face. About 55% of respondents reported having experienced coitus at least once, and about 31% of all respondents reported having coitus in the past 3 months. About 25% of those reporting coitus in the past 3 months indicated that they never used condoms during those experiences, whereas 30% indicated they always used condoms during those experiences.

The adolescents were assigned randomly to either an HIV risk-reduction condition or a control condition and to a small group that was either homogeneous or heterogeneous in gender and that was led by a specially trained male or female facilitator who was African American or White. Adolescents in the HIV risk-reduction condition received the "Be Proud! Be Responsible!" curriculum. As in our previous intervention study, participants in the control condition also received an intervention. However, instead of an intervention on career opportunities, this control group received an intervention targeting behaviors (e.g., dietary and exercise habits and cigarette smoking) that affect the risk of certain health problems other than AIDS. These health problems, including cardiovascular disease, hypertension, and certain cancers, are leading causes of morbidity and mortality among

African Americans (Gillum, 1982; Ibrahim, Chobanian, Horan, & Roccella, 1985; Page & Asire, 1985). Structurally similar to the HIV risk-reduction intervention, the general health promotion intervention also lasted 5 hours and used culturally and developmentally appropriate videotapes, exercises, and games to reinforce learning and to encourage active participation.

After the interventions, the participants completed the post-intervention questionnaires. Adolescents in the HIV risk-reduction condition subsequently expressed stronger intentions to use condoms; had more favorable beliefs about the effects of condoms on sexual enjoyment and about the ability of condoms to prevent pregnancy, STD, and AIDS; had greater perceived self-efficacy to use condoms; and had greater knowledge about AIDS than did those in the control condition, controlling for pre-intervention measures of the particular dependent measure. Responses to debriefing questions indicated that participants in the HIV risk-reduction and general health promotion conditions did not differ in ratings of how much they talked during the interventions, liked the intervention activities, or learned from the activities.

Of the original participants, 489 (97%) took part in the 3-month follow-up and 469 (93%) took part in the 6-month follow-up. The effects of the HIV risk-reduction intervention on the motivational variables were sustained over the 6-month time interval. At both follow-ups, participants in the HIV risk-reduction intervention scored higher on intentions to use condoms, AIDS knowledge, hedonistic beliefs, and perceived self-efficacy to use condoms than did the participants in the health promotion condition. Although there were no significant effects of the HIV risk-reduction intervention on self-reports of unprotected coitus at the 3-month follow-up, at the 6-month follow-up adolescents who had received the HIV risk-reduction intervention reported fewer days on which they had coitus without using a condom in the past 3 months than did those who had received the health promotion intervention, controlling for pre-intervention self-reports.

There was evidence for the generality of the effects of the intervention across race of the facilitator, gender of the facilitator, gender of the participants, and gender composition of the intervention groups. Despite the relatively large number of interactions tested—which would have increased the likelihood of a Type I error—these factors did not moderate facilitators' reports of how the participants reacted to the intervention or participants' own reports of their reactions to the interventions: how much they liked it, how much they talked, and how much they felt they learned. In addition, these factors did not moderate effects of the intervention on AIDS knowledge, prevention beliefs, hedonistic beliefs, perceived self-efficacy, intentions, or self-reports of unprotected coitus. The effects of the HIV risk-reduction intervention were about the same irrespective of the race of the facilitator, the gender of the facilitator, the gender of the participants, and the gender composition of the intervention group. Our initial study on Black male adolescents (Jemmott, Jemmott, & Fong, 1992) also found that matching the gender of participant and facilitator did not enhance intervention effects. The lack of effects of race of facilitator may reflect the fact that the facilitators received common training in the intervention that was culturally appropriate. It may well be that if an intervention is culturally appropriate and the facilitators are well trained, the characteristics of the facilitators are not important determinants of the efficacy of intervention implementation. This, of course, is an empirical question.

Testing Abstinence and Safer-Sex HIV Intervention Strategies.   In another randomized controlled trial, we examined the efficacy of two types of HIV risk-reduction messages, abstinence and safer sex, delivered by two types of messengers, adult and peer facilitators, in reducing sexual risk behavior (Jemmott et al., 1998). The participants, 659 sixth- and seventh-grade Black adolescents (mean age = 11.8 years) from Philadelphia, were randomly assigned to 1 of 3 interventions and to a small group led by an adult facilitator or two peer co-facilitators. "Making a Difference!" was an abstinence intervention designed to encourage middle school students to delay initiation of sex, abstinence from sex, or reduce frequency of sex. "Making Proud Choices!" was a safer-sex intervention designed to encourage middle school students to use condoms if they have sexual intercourse. A health-promotion intervention served as the control. Each intervention consisted of eight 1-hour modules implemented over two consecutive Saturdays. About 98% of participants attended the second day of the interventions and 93% were retained at 12-month follow-up.

The "Making a Difference!" abstinence intervention participants were less likely to report having sexual intercourse in the 3 months after intervention than were control condition participants, but not at the 6- or 12-month follow-up. The "Making Proud Choices!" safer sex intervention participants reported more fre-quent condom use than did control condition participants at all follow-ups. The effects of the interventions did not vary significantly with adult facilitators and peer co-facilitators. However, there were interactions between pre-intervention sexual experience and the safer-sex intervention. Among adolescents who reported sexual experience at baseline, safer-sex intervention participants reported less frequent unprotected sexual intercourse at all follow-ups than did health con-trol intervention participants. The efficacy of the abstinence intervention did not vary depending on participants' baseline sexual experience.

Reducing Risk Behavior and STD Rates among Adolescent Medicine Clinic Female Clients.   In another randomized controlled trial, we focused on adolescent girls and the question of whether HIV risk-reduction interventions could reduce the incidence of STDs (Jemmott et al., 2005). We examined the efficacy of two types of risk-reduction interventions. An information-based HIV/STD intervention provided information necessary to use condoms, but did not provide skills practice. A skill-based HIV/STD intervention provides information and the opportunity for practice in the skills necessary to use condoms or to negotiate condom use. There was also a control condition that included a general health promotion intervention. The participants were 682 low-income African American and Latino adolescent girls recruited from the adolescent medicine clinic in Philadelphia (mean age = 15.5 years). The girls were randomized to one of the three interventions. The results revealed that only the skill-based intervention had significant effects on self-reported sexual risk behavior or STD rates. About 89% of participants were retained at 12-month follow-up and skills-intervention participants reported less unprotected sexual intercourse and fewer sexual partners and were less likely to test positive for an STD as compared with health control intervention participants. Few studies have examined the effects of interventions on sexual behavior in conjunction with alcohol and drug use. This study found that the skills participants reported a significantly lower frequency of sexual intercourse while intoxicated compared with the health control and information interventions at 3-month follow-up and compared with the health control intervention at 6-month follow-up.

HIV Risk-reduction Interventions for Women

Reducing Risk Behavior and STD Rates among Black Women's Health Clinic Clients.   Jemmott, Jemmott, and O'Leary (in press) have conducted a randomized controlled trial evaluating the effects of brief nurse-led HIV risk-reduction interventions for inner-city Black women. The objective was to identify effective interventions that can be implemented in clinics and other primary health care facilities. The efficacy of four theory-based interventions that contrasted two methods of intervention delivery—group versus individual—and two kinds of intervention content—information versus skill building— was tested. The participants were 564 Black women (mean age = 27.2 years) seeking care at the outpatient Women's Health Clinic of a large hospital in Newark, NJ. The participants were randomly assigned to 1 of 5 single-session interventions: 20-minute one-on-one HIV information intervention, 20-minute one-on-one HIV behavioral skill training intervention, 3.33 hour group HIV information intervention; 3.33 hour group behavioral skill-training HIV intervention; 3.33-hour health promotion control intervention. The study had excellent return rates, with 87% retained at 12-month follow-up. Generalized estimating equations analyses, controlling for baseline measures, revealed that considering the three follow-up periods together, the women who received the skill-training interventions compared with the control group were more likely to report using a condom the last time they had sexual intercourse, were more likely to report consistent condom use, and reported having unprotected sexual intercourse on fewer occasions. Although the interventions did not reduce STD incidence at 6-month follow-up, the women in the skill-training interventions were less likely to have a STD at 12-month follow-up than were those in the control group

Dissemination: Working with Community-based Organizations

Translating findings into community-based programs.   Often the results of intervention research remain buried in the pages of scientific journals, where they are unlikely to come to the attention of the community people who could make the best use of them. Unfortunately, the ideal of translating research results into practical community-based programs is seldom realized. We attempted to address this issue by adapting our HIV risk-reduction interventions for use in a program implemented by a community-based organization, the Urban League of Metropolitan Trenton, New Jersey (Jemmott & Jemmott, 1992).(a or b?)

The AIDS prevention program drew upon our experiences with the Jemmott, Jemmott, and Fong (1992) study and the Jemmott, Jemmott, Spears et al. (1992) study and used many of the same activities. It was designed to be meaningful and culturally appropriate for the specific population of inner-city African American adolescent women who would receive it. Prior to implementing the program, individual and focus group interviews were conducted with adolescents from Trenton. These interviews suggested that many of the adolescents had a strong sense of identification with Africa. Posters used to advertise the program were colored red, black, and green (the Black liberation colors) and bore a map of Africa and the motto "Respect Yourself, Protect Yourself—Because You Are Worth It." When the adolescents completed the program they were given T-shirts with the phrase "Respect Yourself, Protect Yourself" and a map of Africa colored in red, black, and green on the front and the phrase "Because I am worth it" on the back.

The program was 6 hours long. Taking into account the constraints within which the community-based organization had to work, however, it was designed to be implemented in three 2-hour sessions, which included 30-minute pre-intervention and post-intervention assessments, rather than our usual one session. The first session focused on factual information about the cause, transmission, and prevention of AIDS and the risks faced by Black women of childbearing age in New Jersey. The second session focused on beliefs regarding partner reactions and hedonistic beliefs. The third session focused on skill building and self-efficacy to use condoms. Videotapes, games, and exercises were used to reinforce learning and to encourage active participation. The participants received the intervention in small groups of 6 to 10 adolescents led by a specially trained African American female health educator who was a native Trenton resident.

The participants in the program were 109 sexually experienced African American female adolescents (mean age = 16.8 years). About 72% reported that they had had coitus in the past 3 months. As in previous research on inner-city African American adolescents, the chief risky sexual behavior was the failure to use condoms. About 19% of those who had coitus in the past three months reported that condoms were never used on those occasions, and only 29% reported that condoms were always used on those occasions. Analyses revealed that the adolescents scored higher in intentions to use condoms, AIDS knowledge, hedonistic beliefs, prevention beliefs, and self-efficacy to use condoms after the intervention compared with before the intervention (Jemmott & Jemmott, 1992a). In addition, increased self-efficacy and more favorable hedonistic beliefs and beliefs regarding a sexual partner's support for condom use were significantly related to increased condom-use intentions, but increases in general AIDS knowledge and specific prevention-related beliefs were not.

An Effectiveness Trial with Community-Based Organizations (CBOs).   On a broader scope, Jemmott, Jemmott, Hines, and Fong (2001) conducted a NIH-funded phase-IV trial involving 86 CBOs and 3,448 African American and Latino adolescents 13 to 18 years of age to test the effectiveness of the "Be Proud! Be Responsible!" curriculum when implemented by CBOs and to identify the amount of training they need to implement the intervention effectively. The study was a cluster randomized controlled trial. One-half the CBOs were randomized to implement Be Proud! Be Responsible! HIV/STD risk-reduction and one-half were to implement a health promotion intervention, which served as the control. Across several measures, adolescents in CBOs that implemented "Be Proud! Be Responsible!" reported significantly greater condom use than did those in CBOs that implemented the health-promotion control intervention. GEE analyses revealed that during the follow-up period, the mean proportion protected sexual intercourse, the rated frequency of condom use, and the percentage consistent condom use (P = .03) were significantly higher among the adolescents from the CBOs in the HIV/STD risk-reduction condition than among those in the health-promotion control condition. This is the first behavioral intervention randomized controlled trial to report intervention-induced increases in condom use when interventions were implemented by CBOs.

The CDC National Dissemination Project.   Once effective interventions are identified there is always the possibility that they will remain buried in the scientific and medical literature, unavailable to those who would be in the best position to use them. The CDC initiated a dissemination project, "Research to Classrooms: Programs that Work," which identified HIV-prevention curricula with credible scientific evidence of effectiveness with adolescents and that are user friendly and brought them to the attention of educators. Our curriculum, "Be Proud! Be Responsible!" was among the first three curricula selected for dissemination across the nation by the CDC. The CDC sponsored several national train-the-trainer sessions for school, clinic, and CBO personnel. As of October 2000, two other curricula we have developed were selected for the dissemination project: "Making a Difference" and "Making Proud Choices"—the two HIV/STD curricula tested in the Jemmott et al. (1998) study.

Culturally Adapting Effective Theory-Based HIV Risk-reduction Interventions

Puerto Rican adolescents in Philadelphia.   Villarruel, Jemmott, Jemmott, and Ronis (2006) tested the efficacy of "¡Cuídate!" (or "Take Care of Yourself") an adapted version of the "Be Proud! Be Responsible!" Curriculum for Latino adolescents. "¡Cuídate!" incorporated salient aspects of Latino culture, specifically familialism and gender-role expectations. We conducted a randomized controlled trial with 553 Latino high school students in Philadelphia who were randomized to "¡Cuídate!" or a culturally tailored general-health-promotion intervention. A unique feature of the trial is that half the students were monolingual in Spanish and received the interventions in Spanish, whereas the others received the interventions in English. GEE(explain acronym?) analyses over the 12-month follow-up period revealed that adolescents in "¡Cuídate!" were less likely to report sexual intercourse, multiple partners, and unprotected intercourse, and more likely to report using condoms consistently than were those who received the control intervention. There was some evidence that the efficacy of the intervention was greater with the adolescents who received the intervention in Spanish compared with those who received the intervention in English. Thus, the intervention was more efficacious in increasing condom use at last sex and increasing the proportion of protected sexual intercourse compared with a health promotion intervention among Spanish speakers than among English speakers.

Xhosa adolescents in South Africa.   Jemmott, Jemmott, and colleagues are currently conducting a randomized controlled trial of an HIV/STD risk-reduction intervention in South Africa with Xhosa-speaking sixth-grade adolescents. As part of this trial, we are translating the interventions into Xhosa and to be appropriate for Xhosa culture. This involves gathering information about common beliefs regarding HIV/AIDS among Xhosa people and any additional information that might be relevant to implementation of an HIV/STD risk-reduction intervention study. We implemented focus group sessions with sixth-grade adolescents, parents of sixth-grade adolescents, and teachers of sixth-grade adolescents. We held meetings with senior primary school principals from Mdantsane, an urban area, and Berlin, a more rural area. In the focus group sessions, adolescents provided feedback about health concerns. They also expressed an interest in talking to their parents about health-related issues. During these sessions, the adolescents recommended that the name of the project should be "Let Us Protect Our Future." In the parent focus group sessions, parents expressed a desire to talk to their children about preventing AIDS and other health problems. We developed the study questionnaire and conducted pilot questionnaire sessions with 63 sixth-grade adolescents from Mdantsane (urban) and Berlin (rural). We solicited their feedback and finalized the questionnaire.

We developed the two HIV/STD risk-reduction curricula and the general health-promotion curriculum, which will serve as the control. They are based on the information gathered in the focus groups, meetings, and questionnaire sessions, the input from South African consultants and co-investigators, and our previous experience in developing curricula for adolescents. Each curriculum consists of 12 one-hour modules to be implemented over 6 two-module sessions. Each curriculum is designed to be implemented by specially trained male and female adults from the community who will work in co-facilitator pairs. The curriculum includes take home assignments for the participants to complete with their parents. The goal of these homework assignments is to increase parent-child communication. The intervention implementation phase has been completed. The program is now in the follow-up data collection phase. The results of this project will contribute to the development of effective sustainable HIV/STD risk-reduction programs for South African adolescents.

CONCLUSION

There is ample evidence that adolescents are at high risk of sexually transmitted HIV infection. In this light, the results of our research are encouraging: they suggest that theory-based interventions can curb HIV risk-associated sexual behavior among adolescents in a variety of settings. Reductions in HIV risk-associated sexual behaviors were demonstrated across several populations of adolescents: male and female adolescents, younger and older adolescents, and African American and Latino adolescents. They were demonstrated across different facilitator characteristics: male and female facilitators, African American and white facilitators, adult facilitators and peer co-facilitators. They were demonstrated in single-gender and mixed-gender intervention groups. Moreover, the findings cannot be explained as a simple result of Hawthorne effects (Cook & Campbell, 1979) among the adolescents who received the HIV risk-reduction interventions. Several studies included comparison groups that provided controls for Hawthorne effects so that the effects of the HIV interventions could not be attributed to special attention or group interaction. These studies also demonstrated that participants in HIV risk-reduction interventions reported less HIV risk-associated sexual behaviors than did those in structurally similar interventions that concerned other issues (e.g., Jemmott, Jemmott & Fong, 1992, 1998; Jemmott et al, 1999, 2005; Villarruel et al., 2006).

One important challenge of HIV sexual risk-reduction research has been the fact that, by its very nature, risky sexual behavior is private behavior and consequently must be assessed with self-report measures. Thus, these studies examined not risky sexual behaviors, but self-reports of risky sexual behaviors. There is the lurking possibility that the participants' reports of their sexual practices might have been unintentionally or intentionally inaccurate. On several grounds, however, confidence about the accuracy of self-reports in the studies is warranted. To reduce problems in memory, researchers have typically asked adolescents to recall their sexual behaviors over a relatively brief period, which would enhance their ability to recall their behavior (Kauth, St. Lawrence, & Kelly, 1991). It is more difficult to recall accurately behavior over a 12-month period as compared with the 2- or 3-month period typically used in studies of adolescents. To increase further the accuracy of recall, studies have provided participants calendars with the dates clearly marked. This makes salient to respondents the dates that are included when they are asked to recall their behavior over a specific temporal interval.

We have employed several techniques to make it less likely that participants would minimize or exaggerate reports of their sexual experiences. In some studies, demand characteristics were reduced because the facilitators who implemented the interventions were not involved in any way in the data collection. Participants have been told that their responses would be used to help improve HIV-prevention programs for other youths like themselves, and that optimum programs would be created only if they answered the questions truthfully. Here, the attempt is to arouse the "social responsibility motive" to counteract any possible social desirability motive (e.g., Jemmott et al., 1998). In addition, participants have been assured that their responses would be kept confidential. Such assurances have been shown to increase frank responses to sensitive questions among adolescents (Ford, Millstein, Halpern-Felsher, & Irwin, 1997).

Another approach was to use indirect measures of sexual behavior that do not share the same problems as self-report measures. For instance, Jemmott et al. (2005, in press) utilized biologically confirmed STDs as an outcome. Some studies employed objective tests of whether the adolescents acquired the knowledge to perform safer behavior, for example, knowledge of how to use a condom (Jemmott et al., 1998).

Researchers have also addressed the issue of socially desirable responding statistically—by testing hypotheses about its impact. If participants' concern about how they would be viewed by others influenced their reports of their sexual behavior, the effects of HIV risk-reduction interventions should be stronger among participants who were higher in the need for social approval than among other participants. However, three studies examining this issue (Jemmott, Jemmott, & Fong 1992; 1998, Jemmott et al., in press) have found that the changes in reported behavior were unrelated to social desirability response bias (Crowne & Marlowe, 1964). Confidence in self-reported behavior is also based on studies demonstrating significant relations between self-reports of condom use and the incidence of clinically documented sexually transmitted infections among people who had sexual intercourse with partners known to have an STD (Warner, Stone, Macaluso, Buehler, & Austin, 2006).

Additional research is needed into interventions that stress abstinence from sexual intercourse. Although the correct and consistent use of latex condoms can sharply reduce the risk of HIV infection, abstinence is the only way to eliminate the chance of sexually transmitted HIV infection. Abstinence is a reasonable risk-reduction strategy for adolescents, especially young adolescents, who may not have the capacity to negotiate condom use or to grapple with the adverse consequences of unprotected sexual intercourse. There is a considerable body of research demonstrating that interventions emphasizing abstinence and condom use if adolescents choose to have sex can reduce HIV risk-associated behavior. There is far less evidence on the effectiveness of interventions stressing abstinence only, and most of the evidence comes from studies designed to prevent pregnancy. To our knowledge, only one HIV-intervention study has tested an abstinence intervention (Jemmott et al., 1998). It found that the abstinence intervention was effective at 3-month follow-up, but not at 12-month follow-up. We need a better understanding of what kinds of interventions are most effective in encouraging abstinence.

There is also a need for more research on the effects of behavioral interventions on health outcomes. We now know that behavioral interventions can influence sexual risk behaviors and mediators of such behaviors. The next generation of research must establish whether changes in self-reported sexual behavior translate into changes in health outcomes such as the incidence of sexually transmitted infections. At the same time, it should be recognized that reducing the incidence of STDs may not be a reasonable goal for every study. It is unlikely that the incidence of STDs will be changed in a short-term study conducted in a population with little sexual activity or in a community with a low prevalence of STDs. Populations with a high degree of sexual activity and a high prevalence of STDs are ideal for studying the effects of behavioral interventions on STD incidence. Such studies should be conducted with samples that are large enough and follow-ups that are long enough to provide excellent statistical power.

The argument here is not that STD incidence should replace the assessment of self-reported sexual risk behavior. Rather, STD incidence should complement self-reports of behavior. This is because the relation between unprotected sexual intercourse and STDs is not perfect. The presence of STD suggests that the person has engaged in unprotected sexual activity, but the absence of a STD does not necessarily mean the person has practiced abstinence or safer sex. The test could be negative, not because the person practiced abstinence or used condoms, but because the person had unprotected sex with a partner who was not infected. A potential secondary advantage of testing for STDs should be noted. Such testing may encourage the adolescents to report their sexual behavior more accurately.

For theory to help drive intervention, it must focus attention on how to select the important factors we can influence from among many factors associated with the behavior. The Theory of Reasoned Action and its extension in the Theory of Planned Behavior seem particular useful in this regard. Application of these models to understand a particular behavior will identify underlying beliefs that determine one's attitude, subjective norm, and perceived behavioral control, and thereby affect the likelihood of performing the behavior. It is therefore critical to assess the effect of interventions on the beliefs targeted and on other components of the model. The Theory of Reasoned Action and the Theory of Planned Behavior provide a basis for evaluating behavior change interventions because they provide hypotheses about how the intervention targeting a set of beliefs will affect the model component that those items compose (for example, attitude) and thereby affect intention and behavior. Often, the important beliefs affecting behavior are different for different related behaviors and for different populations. We found this to be true in our studies.

In conclusion, the studies discussed in this chapter demonstrate that behavioral interventions using the Theory of Reasoned Action/Planned Behavior can significantly influence HIV risk-associated sexual behavior, including condom use, frequency of intercourse, and number of sexual partners, and can influence STD incidence. Future research must extend these findings by exploring intervention effects in other populations, including men of color who have sex with men, men of color who have sex with women, and people in developing countries where HIV is having its most devastating impact. It is also essential that future studies include appropriately large samples to achieve adequate statistical power, that a core set of mediators and behavioral outcomes be assessed, and that objective outcomes such as STD incidence be included in the mix. Although the expense of such studies may be considerable, the alternative is to continue to conduct studies that despite great cost and effort are not fully capable of answering some of the questions that are now of central interest to the field. By conducting research along these lines, it may be possible to identify the most effective strategies to curb the further spread of sexually transmitted HIV infection worldwide.

REFERENCES

Ajzen, I. (1985). From intentions to actions: A theory of planned behavior. In J. Kuhl and J. Beckmann (Eds.), *Action-control: From cognition to behavior* (pp. 11–39). Heidelberg: Springer.

Ajzen, I. (1991). The theory of planned behavior. *Organizational Behavior and Human Decision Processes, 50,* 179–211.

Ajzen, I. & Fishbein, M. (1980). *Understanding attitudes and predicting social behavior.* Englewood Cliffs, NJ: Prentice Hall.

Ajzen, I., & Madden, T. (1986). Prediction of goal-directed behaviour: Attitude, intentions, and perceived behaviour control. *Journal of Experimental Social Psychology, 22,* 453–474.

Bandura, A. (1982). Self-efficacy mechanism in human agency. *American Psychologist, 37,* 122–147.

Bandura, A. (1986). *Social foundations of thought and action: A social cognitive theory.* Englewood Cliffs, NJ: Prentice Hall.

Bandura, A. (1989). Perceived self-efficacy. In V. M. Mays, G. W. Albee, & S. F. Schneider (Eds.), *Primary prevention of AIDS: Psychological approaches* (pp. 128–141). Newbury Park, CA: Sage.

Brown, S. V. (1985). Premarital sexual permissiveness among Black adolescent females. *Social Psychology Quarterly, 48,* 381–387.

Catania, J. A., Dolcini, M. M., Coates, T. J., Kegeles, S. M., Greenblatt, R. M., Puckett, S., et al. (1989). Predictors of condom use and multiple partnered sex among sexually-active adolescent women: Implications for AIDS-related health interventions. *Journal of Sex Research, 26,* 514–524.

Centers for Disease Control and Prevention (CDC). (1998a). State-specific pregnancy rates among adolescents–United States, 1992–1995. *Morbidity and Mortality Weekly Report, 47*(24), 497–504.

Centers for Disease Control and Prevention (CDC). (1998b). Youth risk behavior surveillance–United States, 1997. *MMWR, 47*(No. SS–3).

Centers for Disease Control and Prevention. (2004a). HIV/AIDS surveillance report. Retrieved February 10, 2004, from http://www.cdc.gov/hiv/stats/2003SurveillanceReport.pdf

Centers for Disease Control and Prevention. (2004b). HIV/AIDS Surveillance in Adolescents: L265 slide series. Retrieved October 9, 2005, from http://www.cdc.gov/higraphics/adolesnt.htm

Cook, T. & Campbell, D. (1979). *Quasi-experimentation: Design and analysis for field settings.* Chicago. (Publisher?)

Crowne, D., & Marlowe, D. (1964). *The approval motive.* New York: Wiley.

DiClemente, R. J., Lodico, M., Grinstead, O. A., Harper, G., Rickman, R. L., Evans, P. E., et al. (1996). African-American adolescents residing in high-risk urban environments do use condoms: Correlates and predictors of condom use among adolescents in public housing developments. *Pediatrics, 98,* 269–278.

Eng, T. R., & Butler, W. T. (1997). *The hidden epidemic: Confronting sexually transmitted diseases.* Washington, DC: National Academy Press.

Fishbein, M. & Ajzen, I. (1975). *Belief, attitude, intention and behavior.* Boston: Addison-Wesley.

Fishbein, M., & Middlestadt, S. (1989). Using the theory of reasoned action as a framework for understanding and changing AIDS-related behaviors. In V. M. Mays, G. W. Albee, & S. Schneider (Eds.), *Primary prevention of AIDS: Psychological approaches* (pp. 93–110). Newbury Park, CA: Sage.

Ford, C. E., Millstein, S. G., Halpern-Felsher, B. L., & Irwin, C. E. (1997). Influence of physician confidentiality assurances on adolescents' willingness to disclose information and seek future health care. A randomized controlled trial. *Journal of the American Medical Association, 278,* 1029–1034.

Fox, G. L., & Inazu, J. K. (1980). Patterns and outcomes of mother-daughter communication about sexuality. *Journal of Social Issues, 36,* 7–29.

Furstenberg, F. F. (1971). Birth control experience among pregnant adolescents: The process of unplanned parenthood. *Social Problems, 19,* 192–203.

Gillum, R. F. (1982). Idiopathic cardiomyopathy in the United States, 1970–1982. *American Heart Journal, 111,* 752–5.

Grunbaum, J. A., Kann, L., Kinchen, S., Ross, J., Hawkins, J., Lowry, R., et al. (May 21, 2004). Youth risk behavior surveillance—United States 2003. In *Surveillance Summaries*, MMWR 2004;53(No. SS–2, pp.1–100).

Handelsman, C. D., Cabral, R. J., & Weisfeld, G. E. (1987). Sources of information and adolescent sexual knowledge and behavior. *Journal of Adolescent Research, 2,* 455–463.

Hingson, R. W., Strunin, L., Berlin, B., & Heeren, T. (1990). Beliefs about AIDS, use of alcohol and drugs, and unprotected sex among Massachusetts adolescents. *American Journal of Public Health, 80,* 295–299.

Hofferth, S. L., & Hayes, C. D. (Eds.) (1987). *Risking the future: Adolescent sexuality, pregnancy, and childbearing* (Vol. 2). Washington, DC: National Academy Press.

Hogan, D. P., Astone, N. M., & Kitagawa, E. M. (1985). Social and environmental factors influencing contraceptive use among Black adolescents. *Family Planning Perspective, 17,* 165–169.

Hogan, D. P., & Kitagawa, E. M. (1985). The impact of social status, family structure, and neighborhood on the fertility of black adolescents. *American Journal of Sociology, 90,* 825–855.

Ibrahim, M., Chobanian, A. V., Horan, M., & Roccella, E. J. (1985). Hypertension prevalence and the status of awareness, treatment, and control in the United States. *Hypertension, 7,* 457.

Jemmott, L. S., & Jemmott, J. B. (1990). Sexual knowledge, attitudes, and risky sexual behavior among inner-city Black male adolescents. *Journal of Adolescent Research, 5,* 346–369.

Jemmott, L. S., & Jemmott, J. B. (1992a). Increasing condom-use intentions among sexually active inner-city Black adolescent women: Effects of an AIDS prevention program. *Nursing Research, 41,* 273–279.

Jemmott, L. S., & Jemmott, J. B. (1992b). Increasing condom-use intentions among sexually active Black adolescent women. *Nursing Research, 41,* 273–279.

Jemmott, J. B., & Jemmott, L. S. (1993). Alcohol and drug use during sexual activity: Predicting the HIV-risk-related behaviors of inner-city Black male adolescents. *Journal of Adolescent Research, 8,* 41–57.

Jemmott, J. B., Jemmott, L. S., Braverman, P. K., & Fong, G. T. (2005). HIV/STD risk reduction interventions for African American and Latino adolescent girls at an adolescent medicine clinic. *Archives of Pediatric and Adolescent Medicine, 159,* 440–449.

Jemmott, J. B., Jemmott, L. S., & Fong, G. T. (1992). Reductions in HIV risk-associated sexual behaviors among Black male adolescents: Effects of an AIDS prevention intervention. *American Journal of Public Health, 82,* 372–377.

Jemmott, J. B., Jemmott, L. S., & Fong, G. T. (1998). Abstinence and safer sex HIV risk-reduction interventions for African American adolescents: A randomized controlled trial. *Journal of the American Medical Association, 279,* 1529–1536.

Jemmott, J. B., Jemmott, L. S., & Fong, G. (1999). Editorial response to: Abstinence vs. safer sex: Testing HIV prevention strategies for young African American adolescents. *Journal of American Medical Association (JAMA).*

Jemmott, J. B., Jemmott, L. S., & Hacker, C. I. (1992). Predicting intentions to use condoms among African American adolescents: The theory of planned behavior as a model of HIV risk associated behavior. *Journal of Ethnicity and Disease, 2,* 371–380.

Jemmott, J. B., Jemmott, L. S., Hines, P. M. & Fong, G. T. (2001). Testing the theory of planned behavior as a model of involvement in violence among African American and Latino adolescents. *Journal of Maternal Child Health, 5,* 253–263.

Jemmott, J. B., & Jones, J. M. (1993). Social psychology and AIDS among ethnic minority individuals: Risk behaviors and strategies for changing them. In J. B. Pryor & G. D. Reeder (Eds.), *The social psychology of HIV infection.* Hillsdale, NJ: Lawrence Erlbaum Associates.

Jemmott L. S., Jemmott, J. B., & O'Leary, A. (in press). A randomized controlled trial of brief HIV/STD prevention interventions for African American women in primary care settings: Effects on sexual risk behavior and STD rate. *American Journal of Public Health.*

Jemmott, J. B., Jemmott, L. S., Spears, H., Hewitt, N., & Cruz-Collins, M. (1992). Self-efficacy, hedonistic expectancies, and condom-use intentions among inner-city Black adolescent women: A social cognitive approach to AIDS risk behavior. *Journal of Adolescent Health, 13*, 512–519.

Kaestle, C. E., Halpern, C. T., Miller, W. C., & Ford, C. A. (2005). Young age at first sexual intercourse and sexually transmitted infections in adolescents and young adults. *American Journal of Epidemiology, 161*, 774–780.

Kann, L., Warren, C. W., Harris, W. A., Collins, J. L., Williams, B. I., Ross, J. G., et al. (1996). Youth risk behavior surveillance–United States, 1995. *Morbidity and Mortality Weekly Report, 45*, 1–65.

Kauth, M. R., St. Lawrence, J. S., & Kelly, J. A. (1991). Reliability of retrospective assessments of sexual HIV risk behavior: A comparison of biweekly, three-month, and twelve-month self-reports. *AIDS Education and Prevention, 3*, 207–214.

Leigh, B. C., Morrison, D. M., Trocki, K., & Temple, M. T. (1994). Sexual behavior of American adolescents: Results from a U. S. national survey. *Journal of Adolescent Health, 15*, 117–125.

MacDonald, T. K., Zanna, M. P., & Fong, G. T. (1996). Why common sense goes out the window: Effects of alcohol on intentions to use condoms. *Personality and Social Psychology Bulletin, 22*, 763–775.

Madden, T. J., Ellen, P. S., & Ajzen, I. (1992). A comparison of the theory of planned behavior and the theory of reasoned action. *Personality and Social Psychology Bulletin, 18*, 3–9.

Milan, R. J. & Kilmann, P. R. (1987). Interpersonal factors in premarital contraception. *Journal of Sex Research, 23*, 289–321.

Miller, W. C., Ford, C. A., Morris, M., Handcock, M. S., Schmitz, J. L., Hobbs, M. M., et al. (2004). Prevalence of Chlamydial and Gonococcal infections among young adults in the United States. *Journal of the American Medical Association, 291*, 2229–2236.

Morrison, D. M. (1985). Adolescent contraceptive behavior: A review. *Psychological Bulletin, 98*, 538–568.

Nathanson, C. A., & Becker, M. H. (1986). Family and peer influence on obtaining a method of contraception. *Journal of Marriage and the Family, 48*, 513–526.

O'Leary, A. (1985). Self-efficacy and health. *Behavioral Research Theory, 23*, 437–451.

Page, H. S., & Asire, A. J. (1985). *Cancer rates and risks*. Washington, DC: US Government Printing Office,.

Plichta, S. B., Weisman, C. S. Nathanson, C. A., Ensminger, M. E., & Robinson, J. C. (1992). Partner-specific condom use among adolescent women clients of a family planning clinic. *Journal of Adolescent Health, 13*, 506–513.

Sonenstein, F. L., Pleck, J. H., & Ku, L. C. (1989). Sexual activity, condom use and AIDS awareness among adolescent males. *Family Planning Perspectives, 21*, 152–158.

Soskolne, V., Aral, S. O., Magder, L. S., Reed, D. S., & Bowen, G. S. (1991). Condom use with regular and casual partners among women attending family planning clinics. *Family Planning Perspectives, 23*, 222–225.

Valdiserri, R. O., Arena, V. C., Proctor, D., & Bonati, F. A. (1989). The relationship between women's attitudes about condoms and their use: Implications for condom promotion programs. *American Journal of Public Health, 79*, 499–503.

Ventura, S. J., Abma, J. C., Mosher, W. D., & Henshaw, S. (2003). Revised pregnancy rates, 1990–97, and new rates for 1998–99: United States. *National Vital Statistics Reports, 52*(7), 1–15.

Villarruel, A. M., Jemmott, J. B., Jemmott, L. S., & Ronis, D. (2006). A randomized control trial testing a HIV prevention intervention for Latino youth. *Archives of Pediatric and Adolescent Medicine.*

Warner, L., Stone, K., Macaluso, M., Buehler, J., & Austin, H. (2006). Condom use and risk of gonorrhea and chlamydia: A systematic review of design and measurement factors assessed in epidemiologic studies. *Sexually Transmitted Diseases, 33*, 36–51.

CHAPTER 17

The Theory of Reasoned Action and Advances in HIV/AIDS Prevention

Seth C. Kalichman

University of Connecticut

The Theory of Reasoned Action has widespread influence on public health research. For instance, in 2006 the National Institutes of Health was funding research grounded in the Theory of Reasoned Action that focused on colorectal cancer screening, mammography maintenance, sun protection behaviors in children, organ donation, influenza vaccination among health care workers, and drug prevention media campaigns. In the area of HIV prevention, contemporary HIV/AIDS research includes interventions targeting mothers and their daughters, parents and children in Black churches, drug using women, and club drug-using gay men.

The Theory of Reasoned Action is rooted in the premise that conscious cognitive processes drive human behavior. Of greatest interest to this theory are attitudes and perceptions of social norms regarding performing specific behaviors. Attitudes and perceived norms formulate intentions to engage in behaviors under specified conditions and intentions are the most proximal cognitive processes in relation to performing behaviors. Behavioral intentions consistently predict future behavior. These cognitive and behavioral linkages have been reliable in the area of HIV/AIDS prevention. Remarkably, the association between intentions to use condoms and future condom use is consistent across numerous studies—correlations ranging between .40 and .60. The Theory of Reasoned Action is therefore parsimonious, predicting complex behavior from only a few well defined constructs. Research has repeatedly shown that the underlying structure of the Theory of Reasoned Action is robust and valid.

The field of HIV/AIDS prevention has been highly influenced by the Theory of Reasoned Action. Of particular importance is the utility that the theory has shown in developing behavioral prediction models. Studies that have been guided by the Theory of Reasoned Action have advanced our understanding of sexual risk and protective behaviors, especially condom use. Beyond empirical studies of behavioral prediction, the Theory of Reasoned Action has guided the development of effective interventions for HIV risk-reduction behavior change. Interventions delivered to individuals in counseling sessions, to small groups, and to communities have translated Theory of Reasoned Action constructs and predictive paths into pragmatic and meaningful interactive intervention activities. The findings from these interventions have been impressive and have had major influences on HIV prevention programming and prevention policy.

Here I briefly discuss three levels of HIV prevention interventions that have been shown effective. The interventions discussed have either explicitly used the Theory of Reasoned Action as the basis for their models or have integrated substantial elements of the theory into their content. I discuss interventions that have been delivered to individuals, small groups, and communities.

INDIVIDUAL RISK REDUCTION COUNSELING

As a result of the mixed evidence for behavioral effects of standard HIV counseling and testing, the CDC designed a large multisite study of a clinic-based, enhanced model of HIV counseling for use with testing. Project Respect was conducted between 1993 and 1996 at STD clinics in five U.S. cities: Baltimore, Denver, Long Beach, Newark, and San Francisco. The study randomly assigned 5,872 men and women who tested HIV seronegative to receive one of three models of HIV post-test counseling: (1) two sessions of HIV information and education that emphasized correct and consistent condom use delivered by a clinician, set forward as the standard of care; (2) two sessions of HIV risk-reduction counseling following the 1993 CDC guidelines for HIV counseling that emphasized client centered strategies to increase risk perceptions, and use specific, practical steps to achieve risk reduction; or (3) four sessions of enhanced counseling that included steps toward risk reduction based on theories of behavior change (Kamb et al., 1998). Participants who received pre-test counseling and had their blood drawn for HIV testing were randomly assigned to one of the three interventions conditions. The experimental risk-reduction interventions were derived from the Theory of Reasoned Action. The enhanced counseling intervention included multiple components and its development was particularly guided by principles of the Theory of Reasoned Action. For example, counselors challenged false beliefs about HIV transmission risks and worked to change negative attitudes toward condoms using behavioral rehearsal and desensitizing exercises. The enhanced counseling condition included a series of small group workshops designed to build risk-reduction supportive social norms. Project Respect contained exercises aimed to challenge risk-promoting beliefs, attitudes, and behavioral intentions, as well as skills-training activities to increase self-efficacy for making effective behavioral changes.

Study participants were reassessed at four time points, every three months for one year. Eighty four percent of participants completed the HIV education sessions and 86% completed the prevention counseling sessions, but significantly fewer, 71%, completed the enhanced intervention sessions, suggesting differential dropout due to participant burden from a four versus two session intervention (Kamb et al., 1998). Results of the outcome analyses showed that participants in the prevention counseling and enhanced counseling interventions both resulted in changes in HIV risk behaviors and reduced rates of STDs compared to health education in the standard care condition. However, the enhanced counseling condition resulted in greater increases in condom use for both men and women (Kamb et al., 1998). These findings support the potential benefits gained from intensive counseling in association with HIV testing and are consistent with the lack of positive outcomes observed from minimal counseling, suggesting that client centered counseling that actually follows CDC guidelines or more intensive counseling that directly challenges beliefs, changes attitudes, and enhances behavior change intentions in conjunction with HIV antibody testing can lead to reductions in HIV risk behaviors.

Although risk reduction counseling derived from the Theory of Reasoned Action can significantly impact sexual risk behaviors, the context of risk is dynamic and can influence the effects of counseling. As reported by Hopkins and Rietmeijer (in press, this volume), individuals at high risk for HIV invent behavioral practices to reduce their own personal risks. An emerging behavioral practice that must be considered in counseling today that was not an issue when Project Respect was conducted includes partner selection strategies (Parsons et al., 2005). Hopkins and Rietmeijer discuss one such strategy, where individuals select partners based on their perceived HIV status. Commonly referred to as *serosorting* (e.g., selecting sex partners based on serological status), this behavior can be practiced by both HIV positive and HIV negative persons. When two HIV positive persons agree to engage in unprotected sex there is no risk for transmitting the virus to an uninfected partner (although there are other health risks such as co-occurring sexually transmitted infections). In contrast, there are considerable risks for new infections when a person who does not have HIV has unprotected sex with another person they believe to be uninfected. People are known to assume that their partner is HIV negative based on perceptions and impressions. Even when a partner discloses being HIV negative there are risks that the person became infected between the time of their last HIV test and their current sexual encounter. Thus, serosorting is creating an entirely new context for theory-based risk reduction counseling, such as that tested in Project Respect.

SMALL GROUP INTERVENTIONS

HIV risk-reduction interventions delivered to small groups in workshop-like formats have demonstrated significant behavior change (Jemmott & Jemmott, in press). Jemmott, Jemmott, & Fong (1992) demonstrated that a single session workshop focusing on changing behavioral attitudes, beliefs, and cognitive-behavioral skills produced positive changes among African American adolescent males, including significant increases in HIV-related knowledge, reductions in risk-promoting beliefs, and lower frequencies of high-risk sexual behaviors. The curriculum from this intervention has been packaged as a program entitled "Be Proud! Be Responsible" and has been implemented in a variety of settings including schools and community centers (Jemmott, Jemmott, & McCaffree, 1994).

An example of a game developed for providing basic risk information illustrates Jemmott et al.'s (1994) "Be Proud! Be Responsible" is grounded in the Theory of Reasoned Action. AIDS education was placed in the context of a basketball game played by dividing the group into two teams, with members rotating answering questions about AIDS, scoring points for correct responses. Consistent with the Theory of Reasoned Action, couching educational concepts within the content of a game had the potential to build pro-risk reduction social norms and alter preventive attitudes. The game was developed following formative research with the target population. Using basketball as a vehicle for delivering educational messages shows how theoretically derived intervention components can be, and indeed should be, tailored to match the interests of target populations. Jemmott et al. (1994) also provided a good example of how open discussions can be incorporated into educational activities. Jemmott et al. used AIDS basketball to describe the difference between HIV and AIDS, explain how the human immune system functions and how HIV disrupts immune processes, and the ways in which HIV is transmitted through blood, semen, vaginal secretions, and breast milk. Most importantly, peers influenced the transfer of information used for risk reduction. Jemmott et al. (1994) included several activities aimed to change adolescents' risk-related attitudes and beliefs.

Risk sensitization was also directed at enhancing behavior change intentions that occurred in Jemmott et al.'s intervention through the use of videotapes prompting discussions about personal risks. Videos that portray people living with HIV who share common characteristics with the intended audience may reduce the perception that "AIDS doesn't happen to people like me." Videotapes portraying people living with HIV telling their stories and sending prevention-related messages have been widely disseminated for specific populations.

HIV-prevention interventions based on sound theories of behavior change such as Theory of Reasoned Action, often measure relevant theoretical constructs, typically referred or as mediators of behavior change, even though mediating effects are not often tested. For example, Jemmott et al. (1992) showed that in HIV risk-reduction interventions that target adolescents, the average effect size on behavioral intentions is .22, and that interventions that had greater effects on mediating variables, such as attitudes, norms, and intentions, demonstrated the greatest effect sizes on risk-reducing behaviors. However, these findings were reported from a quantitative literature review that was unable to test for mediation per se. In fact, there are very few examples in the HIV-prevention literature of interventions that were grounded in the Theory of Reasoned Action and showed intervention effects on Theory of Reasoned Action constructs as well as behavior change, that actually test for mediation. In a rare example, Bryan, Aiken and West (1996) demonstrated that social cognitive theoretical constructs, including perceived benefits of condom use, self-efficacy for condom use, and attitudes toward condoms, mediated the effects of a brief behavioral intervention designed to increase condom use among young women on intentions to use condoms and condom use. These results are encouraging in that they support the notion that intervention designed to influence theoretical mediators of behavior change may exert their effects through these constructs.

COMMUNITY-LEVEL INTERVENTIONS

The AIDS Community Demonstration Projects were initiated in 1989 to evaluate the effects of street outreach to reduce risk for HIV infection (Guenther-Grey, Johnson, Higgins, Fishbein, Moseley, & The National Center for HIV, STD, & TB Prevention, 1996). Five cities participated, each targeting persons at risk: high-AIDS prevalence census tracts in Dallas; injection drug users and men who have sex with men in Denver; injection drug users and their female sex partners, and female commercial sex workers in Long Beach; female partners of injection drug users in New York City; and non-gay identified men who have sex with men, female commercial sex workers, and street youth in Seattle. Each city identified two distinct geographical areas for the project. Thus, a total of 10 geographic areas were identified across the five cities, one to serve as the intervention community and the other as a comparison community. Each city implemented a common intervention protocol that was tailored to fit the city and target population subcultures. In each case, the intervention was guided by the transtheoretical, stages of change model, as well as influence from the health belief model, and social cognitive theory. However, the Theory of Reasoned Action was particularly salient in this intervention (Fishbein & Rhodes, 1997). As instructed by the Theory of Reasoned Action, each site performed extensive formative research to identify the determinants of risk in their subpopulations and used these data to develop informational materials for distribution through outreach activities. The printed small media campaign consisted of brochures, flyers, and newsletters that were crafted around local culture, and served as a major component of the intervention.

The formative research phase was designed to reach persons who would be unlikely to attend facility-based interventions. Each city defined their target population based on characteristics of the local epidemic and prevention needs. It was necessary to determine the geographic boundaries within which at-risk individuals congregated and where the intervention activity could be conducted and evaluated. Over the course of six months, project staff performed interviews with local health department personnel and community gatekeepers in each city for each target population. Field observations were also performed in areas where the target population was identified to determine their accessibility and the layout of the environment. The project staff used this information to create localized intervention materials to address the attitudes, social norms, beliefs, behaviors, and stages of change of their target population.

At the heart of the Community Demonstration Projects were locally tailored role model stories disseminated through small printed media, including brochures, flyers, pamphlets, trading cards, and newsletters (Corby & Wolitski, 1997). Stories were derived directly from members of the targeted community and were presented in materials which depicted first-hand accounts of persons who were at various stages of behavior change. Guided by the Theory of Reasoned Action, each story highlighted motivations, attitudes, beliefs, and behaviors of persons who were at various stages of change. The role-model stories were aimed at underlying beliefs as well as perceived social norms, with the ultimate aim to enhance behavior change intentions. The role-model stories illustrated challenges of behavior change but also positively reinforced for performing(is this correct?) risk-reduction behaviors.

Role-model stories were approximately 200 to 250 words in length and included a photo or illustration depicting the role model. The printed materials were distributed along with condoms and bleach kits within community networks identified by the project staff. These networks consisted of peers, merchants, community leaders, and others who regularly interacted with the target population. Outreach workers recruited identified members of the networks to participate in training sessions, which included basic HIV-AIDS education, an explanation of role-model stories, and instruction in how the materials could be used to initiate conversations about HIV risk reduction and positively reinforce efforts to change risk behaviors. The sessions also included role-play practice interactions between members of identified networks and recipients of the materials. The cities varied widely in the number of persons who distributed materials, ranging from 4 to 85 across sites. The number of materials distributed through outreach also varied, from 800 to 6,350 per month. In addition, three cities, Dallas, Denver, and New York, established storefront locations to serve as hubs for the outreach activities.

The Community Demonstration Projects were evaluated through surveys administered on the streets of the targeted communities. Using a street intercept survey method, persons on the street identified as members of the target population were stopped and asked to complete a brief interview assessing among other things their exposure to intervention materials and stage of HIV risk-behavior change. Street intercept surveys showed that exposure rates to the intervention materials increased over time, from an average of 9% of interviewed persons reporting exposure during the first distribution periods, to 38% during early implementation phases. In addition, each intervention community was matched to a comparison community for evaluation purposes. Only in Dallas, however, were intervention and comparison interventions randomly assigned to conditions. In the other cities, assignment of community pairs to conditions was based on pragmatic and logistic considerations. Using a stages of change algorithm to characterize attitude and behavior change (Schnell, Galavotti, Fishbein, & Chan, 1996), results showed movement across the stages of change at the community level, with respondents reporting advances along the stages of change continuum toward ready for action and action following the implementation of the intervention. The effects were particularly meaningful when considered within the context of community-level interventions (Fishbein, 1996). The effects were greatest among persons who reported exposure to the intervention materials relative to persons who were not exposed. The Community Demonstration Projects therefore provide evidence for community-level changes resulting from an intensive outreach intervention.

More recently, Pick et al. (Pick, Poortinga, & Givaudan, 2003; Pick, this volume) have described how the Theory of Reasoned Action constructs can be applied cross-culturally to develop community-level HIV-prevention services. In this case, the premise that attitudes precede behavior was used to guide a series of health promotion activities for women living in an impoverished area of Mexico. The health promotion intervention was comprehensive and included increased service utilization. As suggested by the Theory of Reasoned Action, formative work was conducted to define concepts and identify needs. The program implementation suggested a successful translation of theoretical constructs and their articulation into health promotion program components. Thus, on a smaller and more concentrated scale than seen in the Community Demonstration Projects, Pick et al. showed similar capacity for the Theory of Reasoned Action to guide behavioral interventions at the community level.

CONCLUSION

HIV-prevention interventions derived from the Theory of Reasoned Action focus on changing attitudes and beliefs to facilitate intentions to practice specific behaviors. The theory has been particularly useful in interventions that focus on increasing condom use to reduce sexual risks. Contemporary HIV-prevention research must now move beyond focusing on condoms to other risk-reducing practices, including partner selection strategies (e.g., serosorting) and sexual practices that are alternatives to anal and vaginal intercourse. The Theory of Reasoned Action applies equally well to these behaviors and should be just as useful as it has been with condoms. In addition, HIV-prevention research is a global priority, and the Theory of Reasoned Action has been demonstrated valid in multiple cultures. The Theory of Reasoned Action therefore offers an elegant and productive framework for continuing to guide HIV-prevention research.

ACKNOWLEDGMENTS

Preparation of this chapter was supported by the National Institute of Mental Health (NIMH) Grant R01-MH71164.

REFERENCES

Bryan, A. D., Aiken, L. S., & West, S. G. (1996). Increasing condom use: Evaluation of a theory-based intervention to prevent sexually transmitted diseases in young woman. *Health Psychology, 15*, 371–382.

Corby, N. H., & Wolitski, R. (1997). *Community HIV prevention: The Long Beach AIDS Community Demonstration Project.* Long Beach, CA: University of California Press.

Fishbein, M. (1996) Editorial: Great expectations, or do we ask too much from community-level interventions? *American Journal of Public Health, 86,* 1075–1076.

Fishbein, M., & Ajzen, I. (1975). *Belief, attitude, intention, & behavior: An introduction to theory and research.* Reading, MA: Addison Wesley.

Fishbein, M., Middlestadt, S., & Hitchcock, P. (1994). Using information to change sexually transmitted disease-related behaviors: An analysis based on theory of reasoned action. In R. DiClemente & J. Peterson, *Preventing AIDS: Theories, methods, and behavioral interventions* (pp. 61–77). New York: Plenum.

Fishbein, M., & Rhodes, F. (1997). Using behavioral theory in HIV prevention. In N. Corby and R. Wolitski (Eds.). *Community HIV prevention: The Long Beach AIDS Community Demonstration Project.* Long Beach, CA: University of California Press.

Guenther-Grey, C. A., Johnson, W. D., Higgins, D. L., Fishbein, M., Moseley, R. R., & The National Center for HIV, STD, & TB Prevention. (1996). Community-level prevention of human immunodeficiency virus infection among high risk populations: The AIDS Community Demonstrations Projects. *MMWR, 45,* (RR–6).

Jemmott, J. B., & Jemmott, L. S. (in press). Applying the Theory of Reasoned Action to HIV Risk Reduction Behavioral Interventions. In Ajzen et al. *Prediction and Change of Health Behavior: Applying the Reasoned Action Approach.* Mahwah, NJ: Lawrence Erlbaum Associates.

Jemmott, J. B., Jemmott, L. S., & Fong, G. T. (1992). Reductions in HIV risk-associated sexual behaviors among Black male adolescents: Effects of an AIDS prevention intervention. *American Journal of Public Health, 82,* 372–377.

Jemmott, L. S., Jemmott, J. B., & McCaffree, K. A. (1994). *Be Proud! Be Responsible: Strategies to empower youth to reduce their risk for AIDS.* New York: Select Media.

Kamb, M., Fishbein, M., Douglas, J., Rhodes, F., Rogers, J. Bolan, G., Zenilman, J., et al. (1998). Efficacy of risk-reduction counseling to prevent Human Immunodeficiency Virus and sexually transmitted diseases. *JAMA, 280,* 1161–1167.

Parsons, J. T., Schrimshaw, E. W., Wolitski, R. J., Halkitis, P. N., Purcell, D. W., Hoff, C. C., & Gomez, C. A. (2005). Sexual harm reduction practices of HIV-seropositive gay and bisexual men: Serosorting, strategic positioning, and withdrawal before ejaculation. *AIDS, 19*(Suppl. 1), S13-S25.

Pick, S. (in press,). Extension of Theory of Reasoned Action principles for health promotion programs with marginalized populations in Latin America. In Ajzen et al. *Prediction and Change of Health Behavior: Applying the Reasoned Action Approach.* Mahwah, NJ: Lawrence Erlbaum Associates.

Pick, S., Poortinga, Y. H., & Givaudan, M. (2003). Integrating intervention theory and strategy in culture-sensitive health promotion programs. *Professional Psychology: Research and Practice, 34,* 422–429.

Schnell, D. J., Galavotti, C., Fishbein, M., Chan, D. K-S., & The AIDS Community Demonstration Projects. (1996). Measuring the adoption of consistent use of condoms using the stages of change model. *Public Health Reports, 111*(Suppl. 1), 59–68.

CHAPTER 18

Applied Aspects of Health Promotion Interventions Based on Theory of Reasoned Action and Theory of Planned Behavior

David Holtgrave

Johns Hopkins University

The three previous chapters demonstrate that the Theory of Reasoned Action and the Theory of Planned Behavior (TRA/TPB) have inspired the development of interventions that have successfully impacted health behaviors of major public health import (including but not limited to HIV-related risk behaviors). In this chapter, we attempt to expand on the applied aspects of TRA/TPB research in four specific ways. To structure our comments, we employ a conceptual model of science/policy linkages developed by Holtgrave (2004); it is recognized that this conceptual model is normative (or idealized) rather than purely descriptive of complex and sometimes subjective policy-making processes.

The science/policy linkage model depicted in Figure 1 posits that scientists and policy makers (including program managers) ideally should interface in a bidirectional dialogue, with scientific findings informing policy setting and decision making in real time. The model asserts that policy makers should express their information needs in a way that maximizes the opportunities for informing the research agenda of scientists. However, policy makers often must make financial decisions, and scientific studies often do not include intervention cost or cost-effectiveness information that is needed by policy makers. Hence, quantitative policy analysis techniques of cost, cost of unmet needs, decision, cost-effectiveness and cost-utility analysis may be employed as a type of bridge to better link scientists and policy makers. For instance, a behavioral scientist might conduct a prevention intervention study, but adding cost per client and cost-effectiveness

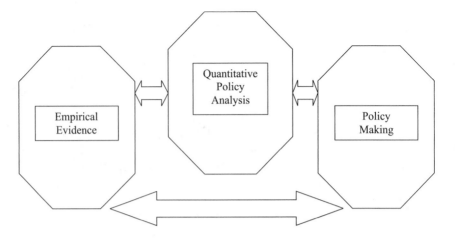

FIGURE 18–1.   An idealized model of the linkages between scientific evidence, policy making, and quantitative policy analysis (adapted from Holtgrave, 2004).

information to the study might make it more relevant to a Congressperson on an appropriations committee.

The science/policy linkage conceptual model may be used to highlight four aspects of the previous chapters of this book. First, we ask whether any of the interventions described by Jemmott and others have been subjected to cost-effectiveness analysis. Second, we ask whether the previous chapters address policy-relevant issues in a real time frame suitable for informing policy making. Third, we examine whether broad social constructs of governmental, health care, educational and other systems of interest to policy makers can be illuminated by TRA/TPB. And finally, we inquire as to whether TRA/TPB might be used to study the behavior of policy makers themselves.

Cost-effectiveness of Behavioral Interventions.   Jemmott and Jemmott make a compelling case for the efficacy of TRA/TPB-inspired HIV-prevention interventions as studied by university researchers, and for the effectiveness of these interventions when delivered by community-based organizations in the field (Jemmott and Jemmott, in press). Clearly the Centers for Disease Control and Prevention (CDC) has been impressed by these studies and it has placed the Jemmotts' intervention work in the forefront of its technology transfer efforts (CDC, 2006).

However, funders deciding whether or not to put more resources into HIV-prevention efforts desire further information about the cost-effectiveness of this intervention (Holtgrave, 1998; Holtgrave and Curran, 2006). In particular, decision makers at the White House Office of Management and Budget, and in Congressional appropriations committees, may be interested in the results of cost-utility analysis which determine the cost-per-QALY (quality adjusted life year) saved; cost-utility analyses can be used to compare the efficiency of medical and public health interventions across a wide variety of disease, injury, and wellness areas. The OMB Web site makes clear an emphasis on economic evaluation in the budget-setting process (Office of Management and Budget, 2006).

There is a relatively large and rapidly growing literature on the cost-utility of HIV-prevention interventions (Holtgrave; 1998; Holtgrave and Curran, 2006; Pinkerton, Johnson-Masotti, Holtgrave, & Farnham, 2002). This literature includes one study on an intervention developed by the Jemmott research team (Pinkerton, Holtgrave and Jemmott, 2000). Pinkerton, Holtgrave and Jemmott determined that the cost of a TRA/TPB-inspired cognitive-behavioral HIV-prevention intervention for African American male adolescents was approximately $89 per client to deliver. Of this amount, approximately $26 per client was devoted to food and monetary incentives. When the full sample of sexually active and not sexually active adolescents was considered, the cost-per-QALY saved for the intervention was about $57,000 ($41,000 if start-up, intensive training was excluded; $18,000 if training and participant costs were excluded). This means that the intervention compared very favorably to other medical and public health interventions (e.g., kidney dialysis costs very roughly $50,000 per QALY saved). If the intervention is targeted to just the sexually active adolescents, the cost per QALY saved drops to $28,000 ($19,000 without training costs, or $5,000 without training or participant costs). This study suggests that not only is a cognitive-behavioral intervention based on TRA/TPB effective, but also relatively cost-effective—especially if the intervention is targeted to adolescents who are already sexually active.

Timely Study of Policy Relevant Behavioral Selection.   Hopkins and Rietmeijer demonstrate that TRA/TPB can be used to understand how people make choices between the condom use and serosorting behaviors (Hopkins and Rietmeijer, in press). This is a very timely topic. Currently, the CDC is updating the national HIV-prevention plan, and of much of that strategic planning discussion is focused on what types of behaviors, populations, and interventions should receive priority consideration in the coming years (CDC, 2001)

It is also a revealed preference that in the recently unveiled President's budget for fiscal year 2007, there is an increase in funding of $93 million for domestic HIV-prevention efforts. However, this increased funding has an exclusive emphasis on HIV counseling and testing—not on any other type of effective behavioral intervention (I do not mean to downplay the importance of counseling and testing, rather I note that of the many other types of behavioral HIV-prevention intervention already shown effective, none receive additional funding in the proposed budget increase).

Further, discussions among HIV-prevention program managers, service providers, researchers, and policy makers have recently focused on a variety of ongoing and emerging behaviors including condom use, abstinence, serosorting, strategic positioning, use of highly active antiretroviral therapy as prevention, pre- and post-exposure prophylaxis, and HIV-prevention burnout leading to no precautionary measures whatsoever being taken (Holtgrave and Curran, 2006). Additionally, these discussions include consideration of the role of substance use behaviors in concert with (perhaps causing, accompanying, or following) unsafe sexual risk behaviors. HIV-related risk behavioral patterns have been continually changing and evolving over the course of the epidemic, as have the prevention services responses to them. Being able to monitor risk behaviors, and understand and modify their determinants in a rapid, *real-time* fashion provides the greatest opportunities for implementing successful HIV-prevention interventions.

Another example of this type of real-time research is a study of the potential impact of a proposed FDA change in condom labeling in the US. Fishbein and Holtgrave are investigating the impact of this recently proposed FDA condom labeling change, and this is being done so in a time frame that could inform policy making (at least inform the many discussions currently waging about this possible label change). In this study, Fishbein and colleagues are presenting respondents with either (a) the currently required condom label, (b) the FDA's proposed additional label language, or (c) the CDC's frequently used language describing condom effectiveness. Fishbein et al. are randomly displaying one of these three labels to respondents, then asking whether respondents would be interested in using condoms and whether they would recommend a condom to their friends. The analysis of the data is currently underway, and will hopefully be able to inform the current debate over whether the FDA's proposal is too stringent (as some AIDS advocates assert) or too weak (as some conservative legislators maintain). In this particular study, a null finding is also of policy relevance (provided there is sufficient statistical power) because it would appear to indicate that the reaction to the FDA's proposal is too strident and the proposed change is actually of little practical consequence.

Contextual Issues Operating Via TRA/TPB Constructs. Susan Pick's chapter (Pick, in press) reminds us that important contextual factors of interest to policy makers (e.g., economic, health care, education, and other societal-level systems) may exert their influence on key public health behaviors via the constructs embedded in TRA/TPB. This position is consistent with the writings of Montaño, Kaspryzk and Taplin (as well as Fishbein himself) who assert that factors not specifically demarcated in TRA/TPB may potentially act via constructs elucidated in the theory (Montaño, Kaspryzk and Taplin, 1997).

Indeed, policy makers responsible for a wide variety of areas of public interest would like to find societal-level interventions that can improve the public wellbeing in a number of areas at once. In this vein, we have been explored the empirical relationship between poverty, income inequality and social capital and several areas of infectious diseases (Holtgrave and Crosby, 2003, 2004; Crosby and Holtgrave, 2006; Crosby, Holtgrave, DiClemente, Wingood, & Gayle, 2003). At the outset of this line of research we entertained both the hypothesis that social integration could lead to social interactions that spread infectious diseases, and the hypothesis that social capital leads to stronger, more integrated communities that could mount successful defenses against the spread of infectious diseases. We found very strong, protective effects of social capital on STDs, AIDS, teen pregnancy, HIV-related risk behaviors, and TB at the state level. For instance, the bivariate Pearson Product Moment Correlation Coefficient between a state-level measure of social capital and AIDS case rates is −.50, and with teen pregnancy is −.78.

We are inspired by Pick's chapter to return to our social capital research and consider what type of evidence would be required to determine whether social capital is exerting influence over infectious disease rates via social norms, control, or other constructs from TRA/TPB. This can not be determined from the state-level data on social capital currently available, but perhaps could be ascertained from multi-level studies that simultaneously examine individual HIV-related risk behaviors, organizational existence and membership patterns, and selected attitudes toward behavioral engagement.

TRA/TPB Studies of the Behavior of Decision Makers Themselves. Throughout this volume, there appears to be a paucity of work on the use of TRA/TPB to study the behavior of policy makers themselves. It would be of theoretical interest to compare TRA/TPB to both linear and non-linear/dynamic models of policy making [such as multi-attribute utility theory (Ferrari et al., 2005) and the *garbage* can model (Cohen, March and Olsen, 1972)]. Do decision makers develop in a planful way behavioral intentions based on the constructs featured in TRA/TPB, or do they simply experiment with various policy positions ("float trial balloons"), get feedback, and modify their position accordingly?

Further, it may be of practical import to employ the constructs of TRA/TPB to conduct case studies of presidential decision making. Such case studies would allow a better understanding of how scientific data regarding intervention effectiveness is weighed by the most senior policy makers, and when and how it is trumped by political and/or other considerations. For instance, it would be of interest to study how for two decades U.S. presidents have made decisions to invoke or maintain a ban on the use of federal funds to support the scientifically sound HIV-prevention intervention of needle and syringe exchange services (Holtgrave, Pinkerton, Jones, Lurie, & Vlahov, 1998). The constructs of TRA/TPB might be able to help us understand these decisions, and to predict future presidential decision making in similar circumstances.

Also of interest would be TRA/TPB studies of well-specified groups of decision makers—such as a HIV-prevention community planning group or Ryan White planning group members (Holtgrave et al., 2000). Persons on these planning groups make important decisions about the prioritizing of populations to received HIV-prevention and treatment services, as well as prioritizing what specific types of services to deliver to each population. However, these group decision-making processes have received surprisingly little attention in the HIV literature (Rose, Gomez, and Valencia-Garcia, 2003). Understanding these group decision-making processes could lead to greater transparency, potentially help to resolve conflict, and perhaps allow scientists working on HIV-related studies to better dialogue with community planning decision makers.

CONCLUSION

In this chapter, we acknowledge and are inspired by the work of Pick, Rietmeijer, Hopkins, Jemmott and Jemmott. We embed their papers in a conceptual framework for linking science and policy making in the hopes of furthering a discussion of how to accelerate the already substantial practical utility of TRA/TPB. It does not appear to be an overstatement to say that TRA has already lead to the development of HIV-prevention interventions that have saved lives, and with further study and uptake, TRA/TPB will lead to even further public health impact in the future. Indeed, we appear to be closer to the beginning than the end of realizing the full public health benefits of Fishbein's seminal theoretical and empirical work.

REFERENCES

Centers for Disease Control and Prevention (CDC). (2001). *HIV Prevention Strategic Plan Through 2005.* Retrieved April 14, 2006, from www.cdc.gov

Centers for Disease Control and Prevention (CDC). (2006). *Compendium of HIV Prevention Interventions with Evidence of Effectiveness.* Retrieved April 14, 2006, from http://www.cdc.gov/hiv/pubs/hivcompendium/HIVcompendium.htm

Cohen, M. D., March, J. G., & Olsen, J. P. (1972). A garbage can model of organizational choice. *Administrative Science Quarterly, 17,* 1–15.

Crosby, R. A., Holtgrave, D. R., DiClemente, R. J., Wingood, G. M., & Gayle, J. A. (2003). Social capital as a predictor of adolescents' sexual risk behavior: A state-level exploratory analysis. *AIDS & Behavior, 7,* 245–252.

Crosby, R. A., & Holtgrave, D. R. (2006). The protective value of social capital against teen pregnancy: A state-level analysis. *Journal of Adolescent Health, 38* (5), 556–559.

Ferrari, M. D., Goadsby, P. J., Lipton, R. B., Dodick, D. W., Cutrer, F. M., McCrory, D., et al. (2005). The use of multiattribute decision models in evaluating triptan treatment options in migraine. *Journal of Neurology, 252,* 1026–1032.

Holtgrave, D. R. (Ed.) (1998). *Handbook of Economic Evaluation of HIV Prevention Programs.* New York: Plenum Publishing.

Holtgrave, D. R. (2004). The role of quantitative policy analysis in HIV prevention technology transfer. *Public Health Reports, 119,* 19–22.

Holtgrave, D. R., Pinkerton, S. D., Jones, T. S., Lurie, P., & Vlahov, D. (1998). Cost and cost-effectiveness of increasing access to sterile syringes and needles as an HIV prevention intervention in the U.S. *Journal of Acquired Immune Deficiency Syndromes, 18*(Suppl. 1), S133-S138.

Holtgrave, D. R., Thomas, C. W., Chen, H., Edlavitch, S., Pinkerton, S. D., & Fleming, P. (2000). HIV prevention community planning and communities of color: Do resources track the epidemic? *AIDS & Public Policy Journal, 15,* 75–81.

Holtgrave, D. R., & Crosby, R. A. (2003). Social capital, poverty and income inequality as predictors of gonorrhea, syphilis, chlamydia and AIDS case rates in the United States. *Sexually Transmitted Infections, 79,* 62–64.

Holtgrave, D. R., & Crosby, R. A. (2004). Social determinants of tuberculosis case rates in the United States. *American Journal of Preventive Medicine, 26,* 159–162.

Holtgrave, D. R., & Curran, J. W. (2006). What works, and what remains to be done in HIV prevention in the United States? *Annual Review of Public Health,* E-pub ahead of print.

Montaño, D. E., Kasprzyk, D., & Taplin, S. H. (1997). The theory of reasoned action and the theory of planned behavior. In K. Glanz, F. M. Lewis, and B. K. Rimer (Eds.), *Health Behavior and Health Education* (pp. 85–112). San Francisco: Jossey-Bass.

Office of Management and Budget (OMB). (2006). *Program assessment rating tool (PART)*. Retrieved April 14, 2006, from http://www.whitehouse.gov/omb/part/

Pick, S. (this volume) *Extension of TRA principles for health promotion programs with marginalized populations in Latin America.*

Pinkerton, S. D., Holtgrave, D. R., & Jemmott, J. B. (2000). Economic analysis of an HIV risk reduction intervention for male African American adolescents. *Journal of Acquired Immune Deficiency Syndromes, 25*, 164–172.

Pinkerton, S. D., Johnson-Masotti, A. P., Holtgrave, D. R., & Farnham, P. G. (2002). A review of the cost-effectiveness of interventions to prevent sexual transmission of HIV in the United States. *AIDS & Behavior, 6*, 15–31.

Rose, V. J., Gomez, C. A., & Valencia-Garcia, D. (2003). Do community planning groups (CPGs) influence HIV prevention policy? An analysis of California CPGs. *AIDS Education and Prevention, 15*, 172–183.

CHAPTER 19

A Reasoned Action Approach: Some Issues, Questions, and Clarifications

Martin Fishbein

University of Pennsylvania

The chapters in this volume have, each in their own way, raised some very important issues in relation to the reasoned action approach. Since the discussants have commented on each of the presentations, I will not try to do the same. Rather, I would like to address a number of issues that run through many of the chapters. It really is very rewarding to see that a reasoned action approach-represented by the Theories of Reasoned Action (Fishbein & Ajzen, 1975; Ajzen & Fishbein, 1980), Planned Behavior (Ajzen, 1985, 1991) and the Integrative Model (Fishbein, 2000)-continues to stimulate both proponents and critics to raise important questions about behavioral prediction and change. Indeed, although all the chapters in this volume are written by supporters of a reasoned action approach, several suggest additions or modifications to the theory. In this chapter I would like to address four of the themes that seem to run through a number of the chapters: the role of emotion; the prediction of complex and/or multiple behaviors; the role of perceived behavioral control as a moderator of intention's influence on behavior as well as of attitudinal and normative influences on intention; and finally, some concerns about the measurement of, and distinction between, attitudes, normative pressure, and perceived control.

RATIONALITY AND EMOTION

Almost from its inception, people have questioned the extent to which a reasoned action approach assumes rationality and ignores the role of emotion in the prediction and understanding of human behavior. Although Icek and I have addressed these issues in a number of articles (see e.g., Ajzen & Fishbein, 2005), we obviously haven't been as clear as we should have been. So let me again try to clarify our position. First, as we have repeatedly stated, there's a huge difference between *reasoned* and *rational*. All reasoned means is that people use whatever information is available to them in a reasonable fashion to arrive at a behavioral decision. According to the reasoned action approach, whether or not people will engage in a given behavior is ultimately based on the behavioral, normative, and control beliefs that they hold with respect to the behavior. This is true irrespective of whether these beliefs are veridical, biased, distorted or *irrational*. In this respect, a belief that "My performing behavior X will stop the voices in my head" is no different from a belief that "My performing behavior X will please my spouse." Both of these behavioral beliefs or outcome expectancies will contribute to the person's attitude toward performing the behavior. It is interesting to note that if it can be shown that a person's behavior is consistent with the latter belief, most people would consider the behavior to be rational, but if the behavior is consistent with the former belief, the behavior may appear to be quite irrational. What is rational or irrational is in the eye of the beholder. To put this somewhat differently, a reasoned action approach may help to explain what appear to be irrational as well as rational behaviors.

This however still does not address the more frequently asked question: Don't people behave *emotionally* as well as *rationally* (or cognitively)? The answer is "of course," but the real question is how do emotions affect behavior? Before addressing this question, it is worth considering the concept of affect as well as the distinction between affective states (i.e., moods and emotion) on one hand and affective evaluations (i.e., attitude) on the other.

Ever since Thurstone (1931; Thurstone & Chave, 1929) defined attitude as "the amount of affect for or against a psychological object," the term *affect* has been used in very different ways. For example, in their now classic chapter on the "cognitive, affective, and behavioral components of attitude," Rosenberg and Hovland (1960) used *affect* to refer to two different response classes. First, in a manner similar to Thurstone, affect referred to the overall feeling of favorableness or unfavorableness with respect to an attitude object. Second, they proposed that affect could also be assessed through "sympathetic nervous responses." However, in the very next chapter entitled, "An analysis of affective-cognitive consistency," Rosenberg (1960) essentially reverted to Thurstone's original use of the term. That is, in his demonstration that *attitudinal affect* could be predicted from a belief-based instrumentality-value index, the term *affect* referred to a measure of overall favorableness or unfavorableness. More specifically, the measure of attitudinal affect was obtained by giving subjects "an attitudinal questionnaire dealing with the issue of 'whether members of the Communist party should be allowed to address the public.' Each subject checked his first choice among five alternative statements" (Rosenberg, 1960, p. 18). Clearly, this measure of attitudinal affect is best viewed as a relatively direct measure of attitude. Consistent with this latter perspective, many social psychologists have employed the terms *affect and attitude* interchangeably (e.g., Chen & Bargh, 1999; Fishbein & Ajzen, 1975; Murphy & Zajonc, 1993).

With the introduction of the Semantic Differential as an attitude measurement instrument, the term affect was largely dropped and attitude quickly became identified with "the evaluative dimension of meaning." More specifically, after Osgood, Suci, & Tannenbaum (1957) demonstrated that an instrument comprised of bipolar evaluative scales could provide reliable and valid measures of attitude (i.e., the score on the evaluative dimension of meaning was highly correlated with the score on more traditional attitude measurement instruments such as Thurstone, Likert and Guttman scales), the Semantic Differential became the most widely used attitude measurement instrument. Based in part on Osgood, Suci, and Tannenbaum's (1957) tables of factor analytic results, bipolar evaluative adjective pairs such as good-bad, wise-foolish, pleasant-unpleasant, harmful-beneficial, enjoyable-unenjoyable were often used to assess attitude toward an object. On occasion, instead of, or in addition to, asking people to rate whether performing some behavior was good or bad, or pleasant or unpleasant, some investigators asked whether performing the behavior would make one *feel* good or bad, happy or sad, relaxed or tense. These latter measures were often viewed as measures of affective feelings or emotion. It can be argued, however, that rating some psychological object on any of these bipolar scales reflects an evaluative judgment. Consistent with this, factor analyses of sets of such evaluative and *emotion* scales often resulted in a single factor. But at least in certain behavioral domains, a two-factor structure emerged with items like wise-foolish, harmful-beneficial, and good-bad loading on one factor, and items like (makes me feel) pleasant-unpleasant and enjoyable-unenjoyable loading on the other. Although these two factors were often highly correlated, and although an internal consistency alpha coefficient based on all evaluative items (i.e., from both factors) was often as high as or higher than the alpha of either factor alone, a number of investigators took the two-factor solution as evidence for a distinction between cognitive (instrumental) and affective (experiential) aspects of attitude. It is important to note that this distinction is very different from Rosenberg and Hovland's (1960) distinction between cognitive and affective components of attitude. Both dimensions are a part of what Rosenberg and Hovland termed the affective component of attitude. Indeed, while a distinction between experiential and instrumental aspects of attitude may be intuitively appealing, it should be recognized that both dimensions are evaluative in nature, and that both aspects are a part of one's overall evaluation of (or attitude toward) a psychological object. Indeed, we (e.g., Ajzen & Fishbein, 2005) have argued that a good Semantic Differential measure of attitude should include both instrumental and experiential items. When only one aspect is assessed, the attitude measure is incomplete and will often be a poor predictor of intention and behavior.

Equally important, however, emphasizing the distinction between cognitive and affective *evaluations* confounds a truly significant distinction between attitude (evaluation) and affect. In contrast to some attitude researchers' use of the term *affect* to refer to an overall feeling of favorableness or unfavorableness toward an object (i.e., to attitude) or, more narrowly to only experiential evaluations, personality and clinical psychologists applied the term *affect* to considerations of mood, emotion, and arousal (see Giner-Sorolla, 1999; Schwarz & Clore, 1983, 1996). Rather than assessing evaluative judgments, these investigators assessed *affect* by means of physiological indicators, mood adjective check lists, or emotion inventories (see Giner-Sorolla, 1999; Petty & Cacioppo, 1983). Thus, like Rosenberg and Hovland's (1960) second indicator of attitudinal affect, the term was used to refer to a separate response system with a somatic component characterized by some degree of activation or deactivation (Crites, Fabrigar, & Petty, 1994; see Giner-Sorolla, 1999, for a discussion). When used in this way, affect includes generalized mood states without a well-defined object of reference (sadness versus happiness), as well as qualitatively different emotions (anger, fear, pride, dejection). I think it's safe to say that when people criticize a reasoned action approach for not taking emotion into account, they are referring to this definition of affect, not to an experiential evaluation. So what is the role of affective states—that is, moods and emotions—in a reasoned action approach?

From a reasoned action perspective, mood and emotions affect behavior in many ways. Perhaps the most common way is by influencing what we believe and how we value outcomes. When I'm in a good mood or when I'm feeling hopeful or excited, I may believe different things than when I'm in a bad mood or feeling scared, anxious, or depressed. There is considerable evidence that positive moods and emotions increase the perceived likelihood that good things will happen and decrease the perceived likelihood that bad things will happen (e.g., Forgas, Bower, & Krantz, 1984; Johnson & Tversky, 1983; Schaller & Cialdini, 1990). Similarly, if I'm scared, depressed or anxious, I may be more likely to believe that bad things will happen and good things will not. Moreover, evaluations of outcomes are also influenced by mood and emotion. Those in a good mood tend to increase their evaluations of positive outcomes and decrease their evaluations of negative outcomes. Similarly, those in a bad mood or who are anxious or frightened tend to view negative outcomes as more negative and positive outcomes as less positive. To put this somewhat differently, mood and emotion can have profound effects on behavioral beliefs and outcome evaluations and thus on attitudes, intentions and behavior.

In a similar fashion, mood and emotion may influence one's choice of relevant referents (e.g., I may think of different people when I'm happy than when I'm angry) as well as whether one perceives barriers or facilitators to action. So the question is not whether moods and emotions influence behavior, but rather whether moods and emotions have a direct influence on behavior, or, as suggested by the reasoned action approach, whether moods and emotions operate like other distal background variables by indirectly influencing intention and behavior through their impact on underlying behavioral, normative, or control beliefs.

Unfortunately, the problem is even more complex—as Ottati and Krumdick (this volume) point out, emotion comes in many guises. In addition to moods and emotions that are independent of any particular behavior (e.g., something at work made me angry; being with my family made me happy), moods and emotions may also be tied to the performance of the particular behavior one is trying to predict or understand (e.g., when we feel anxious about going to the dentist, fearful about flying, or proud about our decision to quit smoking). One question is whether these behavior-specific affective reactions influence intentions and behavior in a manner that is similar to, or different from, behavior-independent moods and emotions. On the one hand, it could be argued that once an emotion is aroused, irrespective of its source, it influences our beliefs and values. Thus behavior-specific and behavior-independent moods and emotions can perhaps be viewed as distal variables that influence intentions and behavior indirectly. Alternatively, it could be argued that behavior-specific affective reactions are best conceptualized as outcome expectancies; that is, as several investigators have pointed out (see e.g., Gorn, Ottati & Krumdick, and Cappella—all in this volume), people anticipate that certain emotional consequences will follow if they perform a certain behavior. Thus, for example, they may believe that quitting cigarettes would make them feel proud, that engaging in unprotected sexual intercourse would make them feel anxious or guilty, or that they would feel regret if they ate junk food or used drugs or alcohol (see Cappella, this volume; McMillan, Higgins & Conner, 2005; Richard, van der Pligt, & deVries 1995). Although one can conceptually distinguish between moods and emotions tied to a particular behavior and anticipated affective reactions, it seems to me that these are really very similar empirically. For example, feeling proud about my decision to quit smoking seems very similar to my belief that quitting will make me feel proud. Thus, in addition to viewing behavior-specific emotional reactions as distal variables, they may also be viewed as anticipated emotional consequences of performing the behavior. It is interesting to note that several investigators (e.g., McMillan et al., 2005; Richard et al., 1995) have argued for the inclusion of such anticipated emotions as an independent factor influencing intention.

According to Bandura (1997), anticipated emotions of this kind are considered self-evaluative outcome expectancies, which he distinguishes from physical and social outcome expectancies. From a reasoned action perspective, anticipated affective reactions (e.g., will make me feel guilty), like anticipated social (e.g., will please my friends) or physical (e.g., will prevent pregnancy) outcomes, are simply behavioral beliefs about the likely consequences of performing a behavior. Clearly, one could choose to classify behavioral beliefs in many ways: pros vs. cons; benefits vs. costs; short range vs. long range, personal vs. impersonal; etc. Essentially, however, each belief links the behavior to some outcome. To the extent that people anticipate positive outcomes (be they affective, physical, or social outcomes), their attitudes toward the behavior should become more favorable, and to the extent that they anticipate negative outcomes, their attitudes should become more unfavorable.

However, as several investigators have pointed out (see, e.g., Cappella, this volume; Gorn, this volume), elicitation of salient beliefs usually does not produce anticipated emotional reactions as likely consequences of a behavior. Although this type of outcome expectancy can be elicited by adding additional questions to an elicitation procedure, it is not clear that if this were done, the outcomes elicited would be among a person's chronically salient behavioral beliefs. Be that as it may, according to a reasoned action approach, these beliefs should be part of the cognitive base for attitude, and thus should not contribute to the prediction of behavior over and above the attitude construct. Nevertheless, at least some studies have found that such anticipated emotions (including anticipated regret) can explain additional variance in intentions and behavior not accounted for by direct measures of attitude. My guess is that when anticipated emotions account for variance over and above the direct measure of attitude, the direct measure of attitude used in the study is probably incomplete. More specifically, if the direct measure of attitude is based only upon instrumental items (e.g., wise-foolish, harmful-beneficial, good-bad), one would expect a set of experiential beliefs (i.e., beliefs linking performance of the behavior to anticipated emotional outcomes), to contribute to the prediction of behavior over and above the contribution of both a set of instrumental beliefs and the incomplete attitude measure. It is interesting to note that this is precisely what happened in the Cappella study in this volume. The hypothesis that anticipated emotions will contribute to behavioral prediction only when the attitude measure is incomplete should be empirically tested before accepting the notion that emotional outcome expectancies represent an additional, independent predictor of intentions and behavior.

To summarize, when one is considering performing a behavior, there is little difference between evaluations of the behavior (be they instrumental or experiential evaluations) and what have often been called emotional responses to the behavior.(i.e., ratings of the behavior on bipolar scales like "Makes me feel good-bad; happy-sad, frightened-relaxed"). As discussed previously, when such bipolar emotional ratings are included along with bipolar instrumental and experiential evaluations in the same factor analysis, one either finds them all loading on a single factor or, depending upon the behavior, on separate, experiential and instrumental factors. One does not arrive at a three-factor solution that distinguishes between experiential, instrumental, and emotional factors. Indeed, as long as we are considering behavior-specific judgments on bipolar evaluative or emotional scales, we are assessing attitude toward that behavior. This is very different from more general moods or emotions; that is, my feeling happy or sad, mellow or anxious, scared or hopeful can influence what I believe and the value I place on various outcomes, and, as indicated herein, mood and emotion thus play an important, but indirect, role in influencing my intentions and behaviors. Finally, whether one is dealing with outcome expectancies that concern physical outcomes, social outcomes, or emotional outcomes (feeling guilty, proud,), or those that concern anticipated regret, these are all behavioral beliefs that serve as the cognitive underpinning of attitude. Thus, I would argue that rather than ignoring emotion, a reasoned action approach allows one to determine exactly how emotions influence a given behavior, and I would encourage people who are interested in this issue to assess emotion in all of its aspects and to use the reasoned action approach to investigate whether the particular measure of emotion is a measure of attitude, a measure of outcome expectancies, or a distal variable that influences behavior directly or indirectly.

PREDICTING MULTIPLE BEHAVIORS

A second theme that runs through many of the chapters in this volume concerns the question of complex behaviors, or categories of behavior. For example, Bob Hornik (this volume) proposes a number of models to extend the theory to multiple behaviors, and Harry Triandis (this volume) wonders whether we need to be behavior specific if we are interested in a broader behavioral category. I'd like to address this issue it two ways—by considering the role of more traditional attitudes toward objects, and by distinguishing between prediction of intentions and prediction of behaviors.

First, as is now widely recognized, attitudes toward objects such as specific individuals, demographic groupings, and institutions are almost always very poor predictors of whether one will or will not engage in a specific behavior with respect to that object. What is often forgotten, however, is that these broad attitudes are very good predictors of patterns of behavior with respect to the object or institution. Thus, if prejudice indeed leads to discrimination and if I want to reduce the amount of discrimination that is taking place—without being concerned about any specific discriminatory behavior—it makes perfectly good sense to try to change people's prejudicial attitudes. The same is true with respect to attitudes toward engaging in a behavioral category. If all I want people to do is engage in some form of physical exercise, and if I don't care exactly what type of exercise they engage in, then it makes perfectly good sense for me to try to change their attitudes toward exercising . Similarly, if I want to increase the number of people who participate in politics, and if I really don't care how they participate (e.g., whether they make campaign contributions, volunteer to work for a candidate or an organization, vote, or attend community meetings), then changing their attitudes toward political participation makes good sense. But if I want to increase the number of people who walk 90 minutes a week, or who donate money to the Republican party, then it makes little sense to change attitudes toward exercising or political participation. Whether one wants to deal with broad dispositions or behavior-specific attitudes really depends upon what behavior or class of behaviors one is trying to predict, explain, or change.

It is important to recognize that a reasoned action approach is applicable to the prediction of any intention, be it an intention to perform a specific behavior, to engage in a class of behaviors, or to reach some goal. As long as one can clearly specify the intention to perform the behavior, to engage in the behavioral category, or to reach some goal, one can use a reasoned action approach to try to understand why some people do and others do not hold that intention. Thus for example, I can ask people if they intend to lose weight in the next 3 months and consistent with this I can assess their attitudes toward "My losing weight in the next 3 months"; their perception of the norms concerning "My losing weight in the next 3 months"; and their perceptions of control concerning "My losing weight in the next 3 months." Moreover, I can assess their beliefs that "My losing weight in the next 3 months" will lead to a number of salient outcomes, as well as their beliefs as to whether specific referent others think they should lose weight in the next 3 months and their beliefs that some of these referents (e.g., those that need to lose weight) will themselves lose or not lose weight in the next 3 months." Finally I can also ask them how likely it is that they will be in situations or experience internal or external conditions that will make it easy or difficult for them to "lose weight in the next 3 months." In the same fashion, I can try to understand the determinants of intentions to get an A on an exam, to get a particular job, or to diet, study, exercise, participate in politics, etc.

What I've tried to point out over the years is that while intentions to perform a specific behavior are usually very good predictors of whether or not that behavior will be performed, intentions to engage in behavioral categories and intentions to reach goals are often poor predictors of whether someone will engage in the behavioral category (at least as that category is defined by the investigator) or reach his or her goal. Thus, for example, intentions to lose weight are poor predictors of weight loss, and intentions to diet may or may not predict dieting behavior depending upon the extent to which the respondent and the investigator agree on the operational definition of dieting. In contrast, people's intention to eat or to not eat bread with dinner will probably be a very good predictor of whether they do or do not eat bread with their dinner. If the criterion to be predicted is goal attainment or engagement in a behavioral category, then it is incumbent upon the investigator to identify an intention that will in fact be significantly correlated with attainment of the goal in question or performance in the particular behavioral category. We never meant to imply that a reasoned action approach couldn't explain these types of intentions—only that the accuracy of predictions based on these intentions will vary depending upon the type of criterion being predicted.

Many years ago, I argued that while using a condom was a behavior for men, it was a goal for women, and thus I predicted that intentions to use a condom would be a good predictor of men's condom use behavior but a poor predictor of women's condom use behavior. Thus, I also argued that for women we should be measuring their intentions to "tell (or ask) their partner to use a condom." Interestingly, the data didn't support this hypothesis; indeed, women's intentions to "always use a condom for vaginal sex" were just as good predictors of condom use as were men's intentions to perform this behavior. The point I'm trying to make is this: If you have empirical evidence that intentions to achieve a goal will predict goal achievement, then by all means try to understand people's intentions to reach that goal. Similarly, if you know that intentions to engage in a behavioral category (e.g., to exercise or diet) accurately predict whether one will exercise or diet, then, again, by all means try to understand people's intentions to engage in these behaviors. But if intentions are not predictive of goal attainment or behavioral performance, then we need to identify specific behaviors that will increase the likelihood that the goal will be attained, or identify specific behaviors in the behavioral category that we are interested in. The relation between an intention and some dependent variable (be it a behavior, a behavioral category, or a goal) is an empirical question. As I mentioned previously, the evidence is quite strong that intentions to engage in a specific behavior are good predictors of whether or not one will engage in the behavior. The evidence is much weaker for intentions to engage in behavioral categories or to reach goals. And, at least in the case of goals, the problem is often that reaching the goal is not something that is completely under the actor's control. When we first introduced the reasoned action approach, we suggested that intentions would not be very good predictors of behaviors that were not under one's volitional control (Ajzen & Fishbein, 1980). Icek has tried to deal with these behaviors by introducing the concept of perceived behavioral control, arguing that taking control issues into account will help to predict behavioral performance and goal attainment. Let me use this as a way to move to the next broad issue, namely, the role of perceived control in predicting intentions, behavior, and other outcomes.

UNDERSTANDING THE ROLE OF PERCEIVED CONTROL

As Marco Yzer (this volume) has pointed out, according to a reasoned action approach, perceived behavioral control (PBC) should act as a moderator of both the intention-behavior relationship and the relationships of attitudes and norms with intention. Consider first the effect of PBC on intentions. According to the theory of reasoned action, if I have a favorable attitude toward performing some behavior and if I perceive social pressure to perform that behavior, then I should form an intention to perform that behavior. However, according to the theory of planned behavior, if I also believe that I don't have actual control over behavioral performance (i.e., if I believe that I don't have the necessary skills and abilities to perform the behavior, or if I believe that there are a number of environmental constraints that can prevent behavioral performance), it is considerably less likely that I will intend to perform the behavior. Thus, when I believe the behavior is under my control, intentions should be primarily determined by attitudes and perceived normative pressure. However, when I don't have PBC, the influence of attitudes and norms on intention should be greatly reduced (i.e., PBC should moderate the impact of attitudes and perceived norms on the intention).

In a similar fashion, the theory of reasoned action suggests that once I've formed an intention to engage in some behavior, the stronger the intention the more likely it is that I will, in fact, perform the behavior. However, as mentioned previously, if I don't have actual control over behavioral performance (i.e., if I don't have the necessary skills and abilities to perform the behavior or if there are a number of environmental constraints that can prevent behavioral performance), it is considerably less likely that, even if I have a positive intention to perform the behavior, I will be able to do so. Since we rarely have good measures of actual control (i.e., of skills and abilities or of environmental factors that can impede or facilitate behavioral performance), Icek, in his theory of planned behavior (Ajzen, 1985, 1991), suggested using PBC as a proxy for actual control, and he argued that the more veridical PBC was with actual control, the more it would act as a moderator of the intention-behavior relation. In addition, consistent with the work of Bandura, he also argued that the more I believe I can do something, the more persistent I may be in my attempts to carry out the behavior in question. In an analogous fashion, if I believe that performance of the behavior is not really up to me, an initial failure may lead to a rapid withdrawal. What Marco has elegantly pointed out is that in order to demonstrate the moderating effect of one variable on another (i.e., in order to find a statistically significant interaction), one needs to have a full range of responses on both variables. Clearly if everybody is at one side or the other of an intention, attitude, or perceived normative pressure scale, and if people are distributed across the PBC scale, then it will look like PBC is having a direct, rather than a moderating, effect on intention and behavior. Thus, finding a main effect of PBC and no interaction does not necessarily mean that PBC is not acting as a moderator. I leave it to those more statistically sophisticated than I am to figure out how best to determine whether PBC does, or does not, have a moderating effect on the prediction of intention and behavior.

MEASUREMENT OF ATTITUDE, PERCEIVED NORMS, AND PERCEIVED CONTROL

Given that we are discussing perceived control, let me address some of the issues that have arisen concerning this construct. Perhaps most problematic is the apparent attempt to distinguish between perceived control and self-efficacy. Factor analyses of items used to directly measure PBC have often arrived at a two-factor solution. More specifically, items such as "I can perform this behavior if I want to," "I have the necessary skills and abilities to perform this behavior," and "Performing this behavior is easy/difficult" typically load on one factor (which has often been labeled *self-efficacy*), while items such as "Performing this behavior is up to me/not up to me," "is under my control/not under my control" load on another (which is usually labeled *perceived control*). I'm amused by the fact that the first factor has often been labeled *self-efficacy* since Bandura (1997) has explicitly and repeatedly argued that the ease or difficulty of performing a behavior should not be confounded with perceived efficacy. Indeed, as Bandura has pointed out, being able to perform a behavior when it's easy has little to do with efficacy; it's only when you believe that you can perform difficult behaviors or a given behavior under difficult circumstances that you are truly efficacious. Thus using judgments of easy to imply efficacy and judgments of difficult to imply a lack of efficaciousness seems to totally change Bandura's meaning of the construct of self-efficacy. Perhaps more important, from a purely theoretical perspective, it is hard to conceptually distinguish between self-efficacy and perceived behavioral control. Icek acknowledged this conceptual similarity when he first introduced the PBC construct, and he has repeatedly pointed out that PBC is attempting to assess essentially the same latent construct as self-efficacy. Theoretically both PBC and self-efficacy are concerned with the belief that one is capable of (has the necessary skills and abilities for) performing the behavior in question. So how can we explain the two-factor solution and what should we call the two factors?

In order to answer this, it may be useful to digress for a moment and reconsider the attitude construct. As discussed herein, similar to factor analyses of control items, factor analyses of bipolar evaluative scales sometimes produce a two-factor solution. One factor, typically defined by items such as "good/bad," "wise/foolish," and "harmful/ beneficial" is often labeled "evaluative or instrumental" while the other, typically defined by items such as "pleasant/unpleasant" and "enjoyable/unenjoyable" is often labeled "affective or experiential." Interestingly, even when this two-factor structure emerges, combining items from both factors in a single scale typically results in a very good unidimensional scale, with internal consistency, alpha = .80. Thus, we have argued that there is a single attitude construct, and that one should always include both experiential and instrumental items to capture the full meaning of this construct.

I would argue that the same is true for perceived control. Just as combining experiential and instrumental items results in an internally consistent measure of attitude, combining items from the two control factors typically results in an internally consistent measure of perceived control (alpha is usually greater than or equal to .75). Unlike the attitude construct however, the meaning of the two aspects of control (i.e., the two factors) is not immediately obvious. In fact, in addition to those who have labeled one factor self-efficacy and the other perceived behavioral control, at least some investigators have argued that these factors represent internal and external control. Unfortunately, observing the items that load on the two factors does not support either of these sets of labels. Instead, the two factors seem to represent what can best be described as judgments of capability and controllability.

Thus, just as attitude is comprised of both instrumental and experiential evaluations, one could argue that perceived control is comprised of both perceptions of capability and perceptions of controllability. That is, for people to perceive that they have complete control over behavioral performance, they must not only believe that they have the necessary skills and abilities required for behavioral performance (capability), but they must also believe that performance of the behavior is up to them, that is, is under their control (controllability). Thus, I would argue that, similar to attitude, it becomes incumbent on investigators to make sure that their measure of perceived control takes both of these aspects into account.

There is however, an alternative explanation which is more methodological than theoretical. Specifically, items loading on the capability factor are typically assessed in a direct *unipolar* fashion (e.g., I can perform this behavior, I have the skills and abilities to perform this behavior), while items loading on the controllability factor are typically assessed in a *bipolar* fashion (e.g., *whether or not* I do this is up to me, *whether or not* I do this is under my control). This methodological difference, rather than any substantive differences, could produce the two-factor structure. But whether the two-factor solution is substantive or methodological in nature, it seems necessary to assess both of these aspects of control in order to fully represent the control construct.

THE NORMATIVE COMPONENT

Turning to perceived norms, I must say I've been somewhat surprised by the fact that none of the chapters in this volume address the role of descriptive norms. Indeed, there is a growing body of literature that suggests that our initial conception of subjective norm did not fully capture normative influence. We had originally defined the subjective norm as one's perception of whether one's important others thought one should or should not engage in the behavior. But in addition to knowing what others think one should (or should not) do, normative pressure can also be a result of one's perception of others' behavior. That is, if most "people like me" or if "most of the people who are important to me" are performing a behavior, I will also feel social pressure to engage in that behavior. This distinction between my beliefs about what others think I should do (which is now referred to as an injunctive norm) and what I believe others are doing (a descriptive norm) is to some extent analogous to the distinction between experiential and instrumental indicators of attitude, and the capability and controllability indicators of perceived control. It seems quite clear that in order to fully capture perceived normative pressure, one must assess both injunctive and descriptive norms.

I find it interesting that the constructs of attitude, subjective norm and perceived behavioral control have, in some ways, become more complex over the years. I suppose that the big question is whether, as we have done with attitude, we should combine the two control and the two normative aspects to create single measures of perceived control and perceived normative pressure, if we should look at the two aspects of each construct as lower order components of a higher order factor, or if we should maintain the distinction between the two aspects of each construct and wind up with six rather than with three predictors. There is some empirical evidence to suggest that we should be dealing with three higher-order constructs (see e.g., Hagger & Chatzisarantis, 2005) and I would argue that from a practical perspective, as well as for the sake of parsimony, we should develop instruments that provide the best single measures of attitudes, perceived normative pressure, and perceived control. Once we've established that one or more of these constructs are important determinants of a given behavior, we can then determine the relative importance of each aspect of that construct.

It should be clear from this discussion that despite being around for over 40 years, the reasoned action approach is still in a developmental stage. There are many unanswered questions that need to be addressed if we are truly going to be able to understand, predict, and change important behaviors. For example, I'm not quite sure how to deal with Susan Pick's concern (this volume) that, at least in some marginalized communities, people cannot form or express intentions without first being empowered. I must admit that although I know it is sometimes difficult to translate the concept of intention into other languages, I have always assumed that it would be possible to develop items to tap the intention construct, and I would find it surprising if someone couldn't tell me whether they will or will not perform a given behavior or if their performance of a behavior is likely or unlikely. One of the nice things about the reasoned action approach is that it has been applied in numerous developing and developed countries, and the four main constructs (i.e., attitudes, norms, perceived control, and intention) seem to be applicable in all cultures. But there can, of course, be exceptions and thus Susan raises an interesting empirical question.

And like Jim Jaccard (Jaccard & Blanton, this volume), I wonder what the Implicit Attitudes Test (IAT) is really measuring. I'm pretty convinced it has little if anything to do with one's implicit or explicit feelings of favorableness or unfavorableness toward some object (i.e., an attitude), but at the same time I wonder if there are *implicit attitudes* that are different from *explicit* ones. More important, if they do exist, can they contribute to our understanding of whether one does or does not perform some specific behavior. Clearly, as Jim pointed out, as long as assessments of implicit attitudes focus on attitudes toward objects, rather than on attitudes toward the performance of a behavior, it is very unlikely that they will contribute to our ability to predict and understand socially relevant behaviors.

CONCLUSION

Clearly, although there are some limitations and unanswered questions surrounding a reasoned action approach, I still am excited by the fact that this approach continues to provide important insights into socially relevant behaviors (see e.g., the applications of the theory in this volume). I am truly gratified by the extent to which a reasoned action approach has led to the development of interventions to increase safer and decrease riskier behavior.

Let me conclude these comments by thanking Icek Ajzen, Dolores Albarracín, and Bob Hornik for putting together this volume and the symposium that led to it. I cannot tell you how nice it is to be recognized by one's colleagues and students. I am deeply honored by the number of students and colleagues who attended and participated in the symposium. I also want to thank Michael Deli Carpini, the dean of the Annenberg School for Communication, and Kathleen Hall-Jamieson, the director of the Annenberg Public Policy Center, for making the symposium possible. Without their support, and that of the National Cancer Institute, this volume would not have happened. But it really wouldn't have happened without the truly generous support of Ambassadors Walter and Lee Annenberg, who created a school and an environment that fosters and supports events like this. I also want to thank Debra Willliams and Mirka Cortes for their incredible logistical support, and Kyle Cassidy for the amazing art work on the invitations and the poster.

Finally, I want to thank all of the contributors to this volume who represent the many different stages in my career. I was at Illinois from 1961 to 1997 and in that time I had some remarkable PhDs—five of whom have contributed to this book: From early to late (at least at Illinois) they are Icek Ajzen, Jim Jaccard, Victor Ottatti, David Trafimow and Dolores Albarracín. I could not ask for a better legacy. I've also been blessed with some extraordinary colleagues both at Illinois and at Penn and I want to thank Harry Triandis, Joseph Cappella, Robert Hornik, and John and Loretta Jemmott for their support and friendship over the years. Early in my career, I spent two sabbaticals at the London School of Economics and Political Science (LSE) and it gives me a great deal of pleasure to see contributions from students from each of those years (Gerry Gorn, 1967–68 and Susan Pick, 1974–75). I've also worked with some great post-doctoral students and my first post-doc (Susan Middlestadt) as well as one of my most recent (Marco Yzer) have also contributed to this volume. And last, but certainly not least, there are my colleagues who I've had the pleasure of working with in the area of HIV/STD prevention. Some of these I had actually known from their earlier lives—as students at Illinois (Dan Montano, Danka Kaspryzk, David Holtgrave), but most I've met as a result of the time I spent at the CDC, as a consultant to NIMH, or as a member of the AIDS Impact international board (Rich Wolitski, Kees Reitmeijer, Seth Kalichman, and Lorraine Sherr).

As a final note, I should make it clear that this volume does not mark my retirement. I am still fascinated by the problems associated with predicting, understanding, and changing socially relevant behaviors, and I hope to be able to pursue these interests for many more years. And for better or worse, I'm happy to report that Icek and I are currently working on a new book that will not only address many of the questions and issues surrounding our reasoned action approach, but will also consider some of the new directions in attitude theory and research .

ACKNOWLEDGMENTS

Preparation of this chapter was supported by a grant from the National Cancer Institute P50 CA095856.

REFERENCES

Ajzen, I. (1985). From intention to actions: A theory of planned behavior. In J. Kuhl & J. Beckman (Eds.), *Action-control: From cognition to behavior* (pp. 11–39). Heidelberg, Germany: Springer.

Ajzen, I. (1991). The theory of planned behavior. *Organizational Behavior and Human Decision Processes, 50,* 170–211.

Ajzen, I. & Fishbein, M. (1980). *Understanding attitudes and predicting social behavior.* Englewood Cliffs, NJ: Prentice Hall.

Ajzen, I. & Fishbein, M. (2005). The influence of attitudes on behavior. In D. Albarracín, B. T. Johnson, & M. P. Zanna (Eds.), *The handbook of attitudes* (pp. 173–221). Mahwah, NJ: Lawrence Erlbaum Associates.

Bandura, A. (1997). *Self-efficacy: The exercise of control.* New York: Freeman.

Chen, M. & Bargh, J. A. (1999). Consequences of automatic evaluation: Immediate behavioral predispositions to approach or avoid the stimulus. *Personality and Social Psychology Bulletin, 25,* 215–224.

Crites, S. L., Fabrigar, L. R. & Petty, R. E. (1994). Measuring the affective and cognitive properties of attitudes: Conceptual and methodological issues. *Personality and Social Psychology Bulletin, 20,* 619–634.

Fishbein, M. & Ajzen, I. (1975). *Belief, attitude, intention and behavior: An introduction to theory and research.* Reading, MA: Addison-Wesley.

Fishbein, M. (2000) The role of theory in HIV prevention. *AIDS Care, 12,* 273–278

Forgas, J. P., Bower, G. H. & Krantz, S. E. (1984). The influence of mood on perceptions of social interactions. *Journal of Experimental Social Psychology, 20,* 497–513.

Giner-Sorolla, R. (1999). Affect in attitude: Immediate and deliberative perspectives. In S. Chaiken & Y. Trope (Eds.), *Dual process theories in social psychology* (pp. 441–461). New York: Guilford.

Hagger, M. S., & Chatzisarantis, N. L. D. (2005). First- and higher-order models of attitudes, normative influence, and perceived behavioural control in the theory of planned behaviour. *British Journal of Social Psychology, 44,* 513–535

Johnson, E. J., & Tversky, A. (1983). Affect, generalization, and the perception of risk. *Journal of Personality and Social Psychology, 45,* 20–31.

McMillan, B., Higgins, A. R. & Conner, M. (2005). Using an extended theory of planned behavior to understand smoking amongst schoolchildren. *Addiction Research and Theory, 13,* 293–306.

Murphy, S. & Zajonc, R. B. (1993). Affect, cognition, and awareness: Affective priming with optimal and suboptimal stimulus exposures. *Journal of Personality and Social Psychology, 64(5),* 723–739.

Osgood, C. E., Suci, G. J.& Tannenbaum, P. H. (1957). *The measurement of meaning.* Champaign, IL: University of Illinois Press.

Petty, R. E. & Cacioppo, J. T. (1983). The role of bodily responses in attitude measurement and change. In J. T. Cacioppo & R. T. Petty (Eds.), *Social Psychology: A Sourcebook* (pp. 51–101). New York: Guilford.

Richard, R., van der Pligt, J, & deVries, N. (1995). Anticipated affective reactions and prevention of AIDS. *British Journal of Social Psychology, 34,* 9–21.

Rosenberg, M. J. (1960). An analysis of affective-cognitive consistency. In M. J. Rosenberg, C. I. Hovland, W. J. McGuire, R. P. Abelson, & J. W. Brehm (Eds.), *Attitude organization and change* (pp 15–64). New Haven: Yale University Press.

Rosenberg, M. J. & Hovland, C. I. (1960). Cognitive, affective and behavioral components of attitude. In M. J. Rosenberg, C. I. Hovland, W. J. McGuire, R. P. Ableson & J. W. Brehm (Eds.), *Attitude organization and change* (pp. 1–14). New Haven: Yale University Press.

Schaller, M. & Cialdini, R. B., (1990). Happiness, sadness, and helping: A motivational integration. In E. T. Higgins & R. M. Sorrentino (Eds.), *Handbook of Motivation and Cognition: Foundations of Social Behavior* (Vol. 2, pp. 265–296). New York: Guilford.

Schwarz, N. & Clore, G. L. (1983). Mood, misattribution, and judgments of well-being: Informative and directive functions of affective states. *Journal of Personality and Social Psychology. 45,* 513–523

Schwarz, N. & Clore, G.L. (1996). Feelings and phenomenal experiences. In E. T. Higgins & A. W. Kruglanski (Eds.), *Social psychology: Handbook of basic principles* (pp. 433–465). New York: Guilford Press.

Thurstone, L. L. (1931). The measurement of social attitudes. *Journal of Abnormal and Social Psychology, 26,* 249–269.

Thurstone, L. L. & Chave, E. J. (1929). *The measurement of attitude: A psychophysical method and some experiments with a scale for measuring attitude toward the church.* Chicago: University of Chicago Press.

Index